DYSTONIA – THE MANY FACETS

Edited by **Raymond L. Rosales**

Dystonia – The Many Facets
Edited by Raymond L. Rosales

Published by InTech
Janeza Trdine 9, 51000 Rijeka, Croatia

Publishing Process Manager Martina Durovic

Technical Editor Teodora Smiljanic

Cover Designer InTech Design Team

Additional hard copies can be obtained from orders@intechopen.com

Dystonia – The Many Facets, Edited by Raymond L. Rosales
p. cm.
ISBN 978-953-51-0329-5

For EU product safety concerns:
IN TECH d.o.o., Prolaz Marije Krucifikse Kozulić 3, 51000 Rijeka, Croatia,
info@intechopen.com or visit our website at intechopen.com.

Meet the editor

Raymond L. Rosales is a Full Professor in the Department of Neurology and Psychiatry of the University of Santo Toma s (UST) and Hospital, Metro Manila, Philippines. At the Metropolitan Medica I Center, a Iso in Ma nila, he is a chief of Neurology, head of the Center for Neurodiagnostic and Thera peutic Services, and chair of the hospital's Trials Institutional Review Board. He is likewise a staff member of the Movement Disorders and Clinical Neurophysiology Clinics of St. Luke's Medical Center, Quezon City. He obtained his BS and MD degrees from the UST, and a PhD in Neuroscience from the Kagoshima University Graduate School of Medicine, Japan. His PhD dissertation was on the botulinum toxin effects in the extrafusal and intrafusal muscles of animal models. He completed a Fellowship in Electrophysiology of Neuromuscular and Movement disorders at Kagoshima University Department of Neurology and Geriatrics, followed by an Exchange Scientist Programme in the same institution through the Japan Society for the Promotion of Science and the Philippine Dept. of Science and Technology. He undertook a Clinician's programme at the Dystonia Clinic of Columbia University, New York, USA. He was a Iso a Visiting Professor in the Movement Disorder Clinics of the University of Florida, Brain McKnight Institute and the Cleveland Clinic Center for Neurological Restoration.

Contents

Preface

Dystonia has many facets, and among those, this book commences with the increasingly associated genes identified, including a construct on how biology interacts with the dystonia genesis. The clinical phenomenology of dystonia as approached in the book is interesting because, not only were the cervical, oromandibular/lingual/laryngeal, task-specific and secondary dystonias dealt with individually, but that the associated features such as parkinsonism, tremors and spasticity were also separately presented. Advances in dystonia management followed, and they ranged from dopaminergic therapy, chemodenervation, surgical approaches and rehabilitation, effectively complementing the approach in dystonia at the clinics. A timely critical pathophysiologic review, including muscle spindle involvement in dystonia, is highlighted at the book's end. Clearly, dystonia, once thought to be a psychiatric disorder, will even become a greater topic in the generations to come as new genes, therapy and pathophysiologic precepts evolve. This book relates these facets for future comprehensive coverage, as developments abound.

Meanwhile, my support staff (Drs. Arlene Ng, Mary Mildred De Los Santos and Criscely Go, as well as PT Michelle Tanglao) from the movement disorders and neuromuscular divisions of the CNS-Metropolitan Medical Center are acknowledged for their invaluable assistance in providing editorial, literature search and review work, to have this book come into fruition.

Raymond L. Rosales, MD, PhD
Department of Neurology and Psychiatry
University of Santo Tomas Hospital, Manila,
Philippines

1

Dystonia and Genetics

Shih-Fen Chen[1] and Yu-Chih Shen[2,3]
[1]*Department of Life Science and Graduate Institute of Biotechnology, Dong-Hwa University*
[2]*Department of Psychiatry, Tzu-Chi General Hospital*
[3]*School of Medicine and Department of Human Development, Tzu-Chi University*
Taiwan

1. Introduction

In recent years, the identification of several new dystonia genes has provided important insights into the nature of this clinically and genetically heterogeneous disorder. Currently, about twenty different forms of monogenic dystonia are distinguished genetically and have been designated DYT 1–13; DYT 14, which has been redefined as DYT 5; and DYT 15–21 (Ozelius et al., 2011; Wider et al., 2008). Among these DYTs, ten genes have been identified using linkage analysis in families: DYT 1, 3, 5/14, 6, 8, 11, 12, 16, and 18 (See Table 1 and Figure 1) (Ozelius et al., 2011).

A DYT is designated based on phenotype or chromosomal location. Therefore, it represents a clinically heterogeneous group of disorders that include primary dystonia, where dystonia is the only phenotype (DYT 1, 2, 4, 6, 7, 13, 17, and 21); dystonia plus syndromes, where other phenotypes in addition to dystonia, such as parkinsonism or myoclonus, are seen (DYT 3, 5/14, 11, 12, 15, and 16); and paroxysmal forms of dystonia/dyskinesia (DYT 8, 9, 10, 18, 19, and 20) (Table 1) (Ozelius et al., 2011).

2. Primary dystonia

The clinical phenotype of primary dystonia is broad, ranging from early-onset generalized to late onset focal. Early-onset dystonia is rare, often starts in a limb, tends to generalize, and frequently has a monogenic origin. Late-onset dystonia is relatively common, rarely involves the lower extremities, has a tendency to remain focal, and appears to be sporadic in most cases (Schmidt & Klein, 2010). Six of the primary dystonia are associated with an early-onset generalized phenotype (DYT 1, 2, 4, 6, 13, and 17), whereas two of them are characterized by a late-onset focal phenotype (DYT 7 and 21) (Ozelius et al., 2011). Genes have been identified for DYT 1 and 6 (See Table 1).

2.1 Early-onset primary dystonia

2.1.1 DYT1

DYT1 dystonia is the most common and severe form of hereditary dystonia, with an estimated frequency of 1/9000 in the Ashkenazi Jewish and 1/160000 in the non-Jewish population. The onset age of affected members ranges from 6 to 42 years, and the severity of the disease varies considerably. In very early-onset cases, symptoms typically begin in a lower limb and progress up the body over the following years. In contrast, later-onset cases are usually limited to upper-body parts, correlating with a somatotopic gradient in the basal ganglia (Bressman et al., 2000).

Dystonia type	Designation	Mode of inheritance	Gene locus	Protein (Gene)
Primary dystonia				
Early-onset primary dystonia	DYT1	Autosomal dominant	9q34	TorsinA (TOR1A)
	DYT2	Autosomal recessive	Unknown	Unknown
	DYT4	Autosomal dominant	Unknown	Unknown
	DYT6	Autosomal dominant	8p21-22	Thanatos-Associated Protein 1 (THAP1)
	DYT13	Autosomal dominant	1p36	Unknown
	DYT17	Autosomal recessive	20p11-q13	Unknown
Late-onset primary dystonia	DYT7	Autosomal dominant	18p	Unknown
	DYT21	Autosomal dominant	2q14-21	Unknown
Dystonia plus syndrome				
Dystonia plus parkinsonism	DYT3	X-chromosomal recessive	Xq13	Gene transcription factor (TAF1)
	DYT5/14	Autosomal dominant	14q22	GTP cyclohydrolase I (GCH1)
		Autosomal recessive	11p15	Tyrosine hydroxylase (TH)
	DYT12	Autosomal dominant	19q12-13	Na^+/K^+ATPaseα3 subunit (ATP1A3)
	DYT16	Autosomal recessive	2q31	Stress-response protein (PRKRA)
Dystonia plus myoclonus	DYT11	Autosomal dominant	7q21	ε-sarcoglycan (SCGE)
	DYT15	Autosomal dominant	18p11	Unknown
Paroxysmal dystonia/dyskinesia				
Non-kinesigenic form	DYT8	Autosomal dominant	2q33-36	Myofibrillogenesis regulator 1 (MR1)
	DYT20	Autosomal dominant	2q31	Unknown
Kinesigenic form	DYT10	Autosomal dominant	16p11-q12	Unknown
	DYT19	Autosomal dominant	16q13-22	Unknown
Exercise-induced forms	DYT9	Autosomal dominant	1p21-13	Unknown
	DYT18	Autosomal dominant	1p35-31	Glucose transporter (SLC2A1)

Table 1. Twenty forms of monogenic dystonia are distinguished genetically and have been designated DYT 1–13; DYT 14, which is redefined as DYT 5; and DYT 15–21

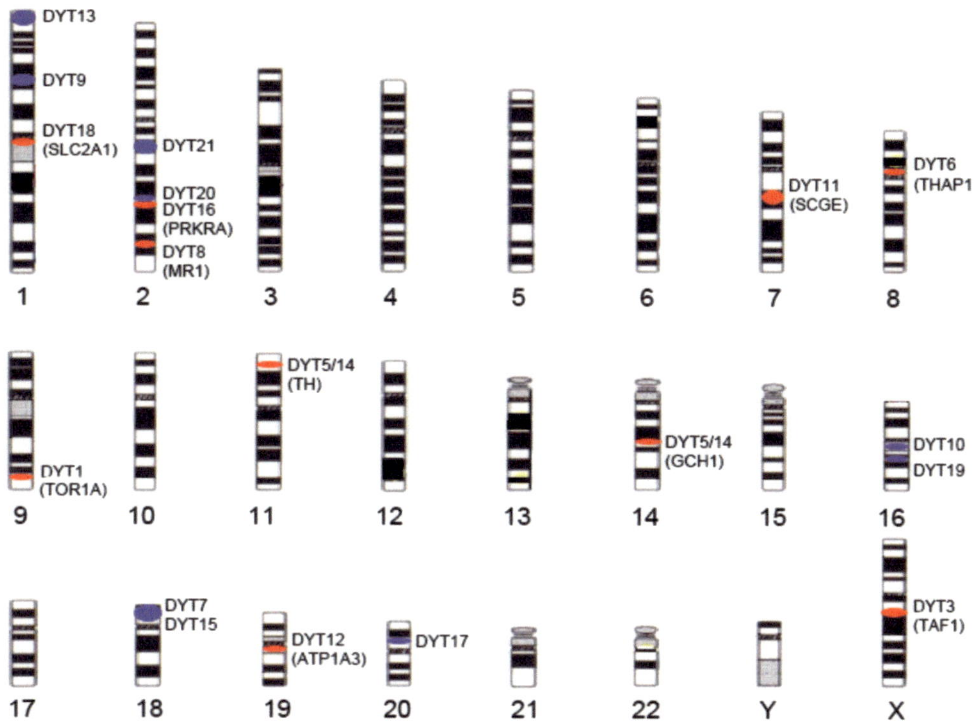

Fig. 1. Ideogram showing major chromosomal regions implicated by linkage studies of dystonia. Red circles indicate areas for which DYT genes have been found. Blue circles indicate areas for which there is suggestive evidence of linkage to different DYT loci.

DYT1 dystonia is inherited in an autosomal dominant pattern with 30% penetrance (Bressman et al., 2000). Regardless of ethnic background, most cases are caused by a three base pair (GAG) deletion in the coding region of the TOR1A gene on chromosome 9q34, leading to the loss of a glutamic acid in the carboxy terminal region of the encoded protein TorsinA (Ozelius et al., 1997). The Asparagine to Histidine substitution at position 216 moderates the effects of the DYT1 GAG deletion. Haplotype analysis demonstrates Asp216 in cis is required for the disease to be penetrant (Risch et al., 2007).

TorsinA is a member of the AAA family (ATPases Associated with diverse cellular Activities), which has many different functions, including cytoskeletal dynamics, protein processing and degradation, vesicle recycling, and intracellular trafficking (Neuwald et al., 1999). TorsinA is predominantly located within the lumen of the endoplasmatic reticulum. The mutant form relocates to the nuclear envelope, where it alters connections between the inner and outer nuclear membranes, suggesting DYT1 dystonia may be one of a group of diseases associated with defects in nuclear membrane structure and function (Goodchild & Dauer, 2004; Naismith et al., 2004). In addition, loss of TorsinA activity would lead to a dysfunction of protein processing through the secretary pathway and defective degradation of mutant proteins in the cell (Hewett et al., 2007). Furthermore, TorsinA is expressed prominently in the substantia nigra, and its staining pattern is granular and present in the neuronal processes, suggesting that DYT1 dystonia may be associated with a dysfunction of dopamine transmission (Konakova et al., 2001; Shashidharan et al., 2005).

2.1.2 DYT2

DYT2 dystonia is clinically similar to DYT1 dystonia, but it is inherited in an autosomal recessive manner (Schmidt & Klein, 2010). Nevertheless, some experts posit that DYT2 dystonia is unlikely for recessive inheritance but is consistent with dominant inheritance with low penetrance (Zlotogora, 2004). Until now, no gene locus has been identified.

2.1.3 DYT4

DYT4 dystonia has been described in a large Australian family containing members of at least five generations distributed in an autosomal dominant pedigree pattern. Onset age ranges from 13 to 37 years. Dystonia first involves speech, then torticollis, and later develops dysphonia. Some patients have been identified with Wilson disease (Ahmad et al., 1993). Until now, no gene locus has been identified. Linkage studies exclude location of the responsible locus on 9q (see DYT1) (Ahmad et al., 1993). Investigation for linkage using markers flanking the Wilson disease locus likewise also yields negative results (Ahmad et al., 1993).

2.1.4 DYT6

DYT6 dystonia is characterized by early involvement of craniofacial muscles with secondary generalization often involving the arms and is characterized by laryngeal dystonia that causes speech difficulties. The mean age at onset is 16 years, with more than half of the patients developing symptoms before age 16 years. It is inherited in an autosomal dominant pattern with 60% penetrance (Djarmati et al., 2009).

DYT6 dystonia is caused by mutations in the THAP1 gene, which encodes the Thanatos-Associated Protein 1 on chromosome 8p21-22 (Schmidt & Klein, 2010). The protein belongs to the family of sequence-specific DNA-binding cellular factors that functions as a nuclear proapoptotic protein and regulates endothelial cell proliferation (Kaiser et al., 2010). THAP1 interacts with prostate apoptosis response 4 protein (Par-4) (Roussigne et al., 2003), an effector of cell death linked to neurodegenerative diseases, including Parkinson's disease (Duan et al., 1999). Additionally, THAP1 has been shown to bind to the TorsinA promoter and repress its expression. DNA binding is disrupted and expression decreased by pathogenic THAP1 mutations (Kaiser et al., 2010). These data link the molecular pathways underlying DYT1 and DYT6 dystonia and highlight transcriptional dysregulation as a cause of primary dystonia (Gavarini et al., 2010).

2.1.5 DYT13

DYT13 dystonia is reported in a large non-Jewish Italian family with autosomal dominant idiopathic torsion dystonia spanning three generations. Eight members have definite torsion dystonia characterized by average onset at 15 years of age, symptoms beginning in the cervical or craniocervical region or in the upper limbs, and slow progression to other body regions (more than 18 years). Two treated patients are unresponsive to dopaminergic medication (Bentivoglio et al., 1997). Linkage analysis on this family identifies a locus within a 22-cM interval on chromosome 1p36 (Valente et al., 2001).

2.1.6 DYT17

DYT17 dystonia is reported in a large, consanguineous Lebanese family, in which three sisters have primary focal torsion dystonia beginning with torticollis at ages 17, 19, and 14 years, respectively. Two years after onset, the symptoms spread, causing segmental dystonia for two patients and generalized dystonia for the third. At the time of examination, when the sisters were in their thirties, all had severe dysphonia and dysarthria (Chouery et al., 2008). DYT17 dystonia is inherited in an autosomal recessive manner. The responsible gene locus is linked to a 20.5-Mb interval on chromosome 20p11-q13 (Chouery et al., 2008).

2.2 Late-onset primary dystonia

2.2.1 DYT7

DYT7 dystonia was first described in a German family. Family members are primarily affected with cervical dystonia beginning in mid-adulthood (mean age of onset: 43). The dystonic symptoms remain focal in all cases of over 9 years of disease duration (Leube et al., 1996). The mode of inheritance is autosomal dominant with reduced penetrance. The family shows linkage to chromosome 18p (Leube et al., 1996). Following the above study, eighteen nuclear adult-onset focal dystonia families from central Europe were studied by genotyping with 18p microsatellites. In three families, the affected relatives do not share an 18p haplotype, suggesting locus heterogeneity in this disorder (Leube et al., 1997).

2.2.2 DYT21

DYT21 dystonia was first described in a family from northern Sweden. The phenotype in this family is characterized by later onset (mean: 27 years; range, 13-50 years) and mainly multifocal dystonia, with onset in the cranial/cervical muscles in most and the hands in about 25% (Norgren et al., 2011). The disease is inherited in an autosomal dominant manner with a penetrance that may be as high as 90%. The DYT21 locus in this family is mapped to chromosome 2q14-21 (Norgren et al., 2011).

3. Dystonia plus syndrome

Dystonia associated with but not secondary to other movement disorders, such as parkinsonism or myoclonus, are classified as dystonia plus syndrome (Schmidt & Klein, 2010). Within the dystonia plus classification there are four forms that include parkinsonism as part of their phenotype (DYT 3, 5/14, 12, and 16), and two that have myoclonus in addition to dystonia (DYT 11 and 15). Genes have been identified for all these forms except DYT 15 (Ozelius et al., 2011).

3.1 Dystonia plus parkinsonism

3.1.1 DYT3

DYT3 dystonia was first identified in an island of the Philippines (Lee et al., 1976). First manifestations are noted in the head and neck in 39%, in the lower limbs in 33%, in the upper limbs in 24%, and in the trunk in 9%. At least one "parkinsonian symptom" (bradykinesia, rigidity, loss of postural reflexes, and resting tremor) is found in 36% of the cases. The mean age of onset is 34.8 years, which is similar to that in the adult-onset autosomal dominant form. Nevertheless, DYT3 dystonia tends to generalize in most patients within 7 years of onset (Kupke et al., 1990b; Lee et al., 2011).

DYT3 dystonia is inherited in an X-linked recessive pattern (Kupke et al., 1990a). It is caused by an SVA (short interspersed nuclear element, variable number of tandem repeats, and Alu composite) retrotransposon insertion in intron 32 of the TAF1 gene (TATA box binding protein associated factor) on Xq13, which encodes the largest component of the TFIID complex (Makino et al., 2007; Pasco et al., 2011). The insertion is 2,627 bp in length. SVA retrotransposon insertions are thought to be active in the human genome and are thought to alter the expression level of adjacent genes that cause diseases. The insertion has a high GC content (approximately 70%) and a large number of CpG sites (more than 150) in its nucleotide sequence, so it is frequently hypermethylated in its insertion site (Hancks & Kazazian, 2010). In DYT3 dystonia, the decreased expression of the neuron-specific TA14-391 isoform, and probably other TAF1 isoforms, results in transcriptional dysregulation of many neuronal genes, including that which encodes the dopamine receptor (Makino et al., 2007; Pasco et al., 2011).

3.1.2 DYT5/14

The symptom presentation of DYT5 dystonia ranges from spasticity in early childhood to dystonia in mid-childhood, and finally becomes parkinsonism in later life. It is characterized by a dramatic response to L-dopa therapy and by diurnal fluctuation in the severity of symptoms (Ozelius et al., 2011).

DYT5 dystonia is inherited in either an autosomal dominant or recessive manner. The autosomal dominant form is mostly caused by mutations in the gene encoding GTP cyclohydrolase I (GCH1) on chromosome 14q22 (Ichinose et al., 1994). GCH1 is rate-limiting in the conversion of GTP to tetrahydrobiopterin (BH4), the cofactor for tyrosine hydroxylase (TH), which is the rate-limiting enzyme for dopamine synthesis (Gesierich et al., 2003). An autosomal recessive form of DYT5 dystonia that is associated with infantile parkinsonism is caused by mutations in the TH gene on chromosome 11p15 (Gorke & Bartholome, 1990). Other forms of DYT5 dystonia result from a deficiency of other enzymes in the biosynthetic pathway for biopterins, such as sepiapterin reductase (Asmus & Gasser, 2010). All of these defects diminish the activity of TH, which explains the molecular basis for the efficacy of L-dopa treatment, as this drug bypasses the enzymatic defect (Breakefield et al., 2008). The diurnal variation of symptoms, which typically are worse during the course of the day and improve overnight with sleep, is thought to derive from use-dependent depletion of BH4 in dopamine-producing neurons (Breakefield et al., 2008).

A dopa-responsive dystonia in the family reported by Grotzsch et al. was originally thought to be at a locus on chromosome 14, separate from the DYT5 locus, and was designated DYT14 (Grotzsch et al., 2002). Wider et al. restudied the same family and determined that the disorder is indeed DYT5 caused by mutation in the GCH1 gene (Wider et al., 2008).

3.1.3 DYT12

DYT12 dystonia is characterized by abrupt onset of dystonia with parkinsonism over a few minutes to 30 days, a clear rostrocaudal (face, arm, leg) gradient of involvement, and prominent bulbar findings, and it is triggered by stress. Onset age is usually in late adolescence or early adulthood (range 15 to 45 years). Treatment with dopaminergic medications is usually not effective (Brashear et al., 2007).

DYT12 dystonia is inherited in an autosomal dominant pattern with reduced penetrance. It is caused by heterozygous mutations in the ATP1A3 gene encoding the α3 subunit of the Na^+/K^+ATPase on chromosome 19q12-13 (de Carvalho Aguiar et al., 2004). Na^+/K^+ATPase maintains an electrochemical gradient across the plasma membrane. It consists of α, β, and γ subunits, with the human α3 subunit only expressed in the brain and heart, indicating a specialized role in excitable tissues (Hilgenberg et al., 2006). DYT12 dystonia could result from reduced function of this ion transporter and could appear to exacerbate the physiologic response to stress, as in stress-induced channelopathies (Cannon, 2006).

3.1.4 DYT16

DYT16 dystonia is characterized by early-onset (2-18 years) gait abnormalities and leg pain, followed by dysphagia, spasmodic dysphonia generalized dystonia, torticollis, upper limb dystonia, and opisthotonic posturing. Orofacial dystonia and facial grimacing are prominent features. Possible parkinsonian signs are reported in a minority of patients, are limited to bradykinesia in the presence of severe generalized dystonia, and are not responsive to dopaminergic medication (Camargos et al., 2008).

DYT16 dystonia is inherited in an autosomal recessive pattern. It is caused by mutations in the PRKRA gene on chromosome 2q31, which encodes the protein kinase, interferon-inducible double-stranded RNA-dependent activator (Camargos et al., 2008; Seibler et al., 2008). The function of the protein remains largely unknown.

3.2 Dystonia plus myoclonus

3.2.1 DYT11

DYT11 dystonia is characterized by myoclonic jerks affecting mostly proximal muscles, occurring at rest and increasing with activity or changes in posture. Onset age is in childhood or adolescence. Symptoms often respond to alcohol, and patients may have psychiatric abnormalities (Saunders-Pullman et al., 2002).

DYT11 dystonia is inherited in an autosomal dominant pattern. It is caused by loss-of-function mutations in the SGCE gene encoding ε-sarcoglycan on chromosome 7q21. Maternal imprinting of SGCE results in reduced penetrance of the disorder when the mutation is inherited from the mother (Zimprich et al., 2001). ε-sarcoglycan is highly expressed during brain development and is highly expressed in dopaminergic neurons, as well as in other neuronal subtypes (Chan et al., 2005). The mutant proteins are unable to reach the cell surface and are retained intracellular and degraded (Esapa et al., 2007). The exact pathophysiology is thought to be similar to the sarcoglycans that are mutated in limb girdle muscular dystrophies (Chen et al., 2006). More studies are needed to determine whether ε-sarcoglycan participates in the formation of dystrophin-glycoprotein complexes in the brain like it does in muscles.

3.2.2 DYT15

DYT15 dystonia is reported in a large Canadian family, in which twelve members over four generations have alcohol-responsive myoclonic dystonia characterized by jerky movements of the upper limbs, hands, and axial muscles. Four members also have dystonia of the upper limbs, and one has dystonia of the leg (Grimes et al., 2001). Mutation in the SGCE gene is excluded (DYT11), and linkage of the disorder to a 17-cM region on chromosome 18p11 is seen. Two unaffected obligate carriers and all affected members carried the same haplotype. Five other unaffected members also carried at least part of the haplotype, suggesting reduced penetrance of the disorder in this family (Grimes et al., 2001).

4. Paroxysmal dystonia/dyskinesia

This is a heterogeneous group of disorders characterized by sudden transient attacks of involuntary movements. They are subdivided into non-kinesigenic (DYT 8 and 20), kinesigenic (DYT 10 and 19), and exercise-induced forms (DYT 9 and 18). The genes for DYT 8 and 18 have been identified (Ozelius et al., 2011).

4.1 Non-kinesigenic form

4.1.1 DYT8

DYT8 dystonia is characterized by attacks of uncontrollable dystonic choreoathetosis and onset in infancy or childhood. The attacks last only a few minutes, occur a few times a day, and are not accompanied by unconsciousness. Alcohol, coffee, hunger, fatigue, and tobacco are precipitating factors. Between attacks, affected individuals are phenotypically normal (Ozelius et al., 2011).

DYT8 dystonia is inherited in an autosomal dominant pattern with incomplete penetrance. It is caused by mutations in the gene for the myofibrillogenesis regulator-1 (MR1) on chromosome 2q33-36, which lead to valine-to-alanine substitutions at positions 7 and 9 and also are predicted to disrupt α-helix structures of MR1 proteins (Rainier et al., 2004). MR1 long isoform (MR1L) is likely to have similar enzymatic activity to hydroxyl-acyl glutathione hydrolase (HAGH), which functions in a pathway to detoxify methylglyoxal, a compound present in coffee and alcoholic beverages and produced as a byproduct of oxidative stress (Lee et al., 2004). Thus, in this form of dystonia, toxins and stress could combine with abnormal MR-1 activity to exacerbate neuronal toxicity. Recently, a mutation in the N-terminal mitochondrial targeting sequence (MTS) of the MR1 gene has been reported in a three-generation family (Ghezzi et al., 2009). Their results differ from the above findings with regard to localization of the MR1L and suggest a novel disease mechanism based on a deleterious action of the MTS.

4.1.2 DYT20

DYT20 dystonia was reported in a Canadian family of European descent, in which 10 members spanning 4 generations have PNKD. This disorder is characterized by episodic dystonia primarily affecting the hands and feet symmetrically. Age at onset ranged from childhood to age 50 years. Episodes last 2 to 5 minutes (up to 10 minutes in 1 patient) and occur daily or several times per month. Alcohol, caffeine, and excitement are not obvious triggers (Spacey et al., 2006).

DYT20 dystonia is inherited in an autosomal dominant manner. The gene locus is linked to chromosome 2q31, which is distinct from the DYT8 locus on chromosome 2q33-36 (Spacey et al., 2006).

4.2 Kinesigenic form

4.2.1 DYT10

DYT10 dystonia is characterized by recurrent and brief attacks of involuntary movement precipitated by sudden unexpected movements. Onset age is in childhood or adolescence. It differs from the DYT8 dystonia by later onset in many cases; by briefer duration of attacks (seconds to minutes), which usually occur daily; and by good response to anticonvulsants. About 40% of patients have afebrile, general convulsions in infancy (Bennett et al., 2000).

Both autosomal dominant and autosomal recessive inheritance of this disorder is proposed. The cases interpreted as autosomal recessive may have been instances of reduced penetrance in an affected parent or new mutation. The gene locus maps to chromosome 16p11-q12 (Tomita et al., 1999). DYT10 dystonia shares some clinical features with benign familial infantile convulsions (BFIC2) and with infantile convulsions and paroxysmal choreoathetosis (ICCA). The three disorders overlap across a pericentromeric region of chromosome 16, suggesting that they may be allelic disorders (Caraballo et al., 2001).

4.2.2 DYT19

DYT 19 dystonia is reported in a large Indian clan in which thirteen individuals have received a definite diagnosis. The onset age ranges from 7 to 13 years. It is characterized by brief attacks of up to 2 minutes consisting of dystonic or choreic movements precipitated by sudden movements, with a frequency of 1 to 20 episodes per day. None of the affected patients have a history of benign infantile convulsions. Some of them, however, have sporadic episodes of generalized tonic-clonic seizures in their teenage years that spontaneously resolve (Valente et al., 2000).

DYT19 dystonia is inherited in an autosomal dominant manner with incomplete penetrance (75%). The gene locus is linked to chromosome 16q13-22, which is distinct from the DYT10 locus (16p11-q12) (Valente et al., 2000).

4.3 Exercise-induced form

4.3.1 DYT9

DYT9 dystonia is characterized by paroxysmal choreoathetosis, ataxia, and spasticity. Onset age ranges from 2 to 15 years, with most patients presenting clear symptoms before attending school. The episodes last approximately 20 minutes and occur at frequencies ranging from twice a day to twice a year. The involuntary movements and dystonia are similar to those in DYT8 dystonia. In both disorders, episodes can be induced by alcohol, fatigue, and emotional stress; nevertheless, in DYT9 dystonia, physical exercise can precipitate the episodes (Auburger et al., 1996).

Inheritance is clearly autosomal dominant. By linkage analysis, the gene for this disorder probably lies in a 2-cM region on chromosome 1p21-13, where a cluster of potassium channel genes is located. Until now, the precise gene locus has not been identified (Auburger et al., 1996).

4.3.2 DYT18

DYT18 dystonia is characterized primarily by onset in childhood of paroxysmal exercise-induced dyskinesia. The dyskinesia involves transient abnormal involuntary movements, such as dystonia and choreoathetosis, induced by exercise or exertion, and affecting the exercised limbs. Some patients may also have epilepsy, most commonly childhood absence epilepsy, with an average onset of about 2 to 3 years. Mild mental retardation may also occur (Margari et al., 2000).

DYT18 dystonia is inherited in an autosomal dominant manner. It is caused by heterozygous mutations in the SLC2A1 gene, which encodes the GLUT1 transporter, on chromosome 1p35-31 (Schneider et al., 2009; Weber et al., 2008). A defect in the GLUT1 glucose transporter causing decreased glucose concentration in the central nervous system is part of a spectrum of neurologic phenotypes resulting from GLUT1 deficiency. A ketogenic diet often results in marked clinical improvement of the motor and seizure symptoms (Kamm et al., 2007; Pascual et al., 2004)

5. Conclusion

Currently, the dystonias represent a clinically and genetically heterogeneous set of movement disorders. Although the identified dystonia genes are diverse and the underlying mechanisms of how they cause dystonia remain wanting, their identification has led basic research to understand the pathophysiology of dystonia. For example, DYT6 THAP1 has been shown to bind to the DYT 1 TorsinA promoter and repress its expression (Kaiser et al., 2010), suggesting that common pathways may be involved in dystonia, and novel treatments targeting these common pathways may be effective for the treatment of different forms of dystonia. Next, better understanding of the underlying mechanisms of these dystonia genes and their interactions would allow researchers to compare and reclassify the dystonia subtypes that would help direct therapies and define endophenotypes. Finally, new genetic technologies, including SNP based genome-wide association study, microarray comparative genomic hybridization study, next-generation exomic and whole-genome sequencing, should accelerate gene discovery for dystonias that should further elucidate the underlying pathways.

6. References

Ahmad, F.; Davis, M. B.; Waddy, H. M.; Oley, C. A.; Marsden, C. D. & Harding, A. E. (1993). Evidence for locus heterogeneity in autosomal dominant torsion dystonia. *Genomics*, Vol. 15, No. 1, pp. 9-12, ISSN 0888-7543

Asmus, F. & Gasser, T. (2010). Dystonia-plus syndromes. *European Journal of Neurology*, Vol. 17, Suppl 1, pp. 37-45, ISSN 1468-1331

Auburger, G.; Ratzlaff, T.; Lunkes, A.; Nelles, H. W.; Leube, B.; Binkofski, F.; Kugel, H.; Heindel, W.; Seitz, R.; Benecke, R.; Witte, O. W. & Voit, T. (1996). A gene for autosomal dominant paroxysmal choreoathetosis/spasticity (CSE) maps to the vicinity of a potassium channel gene cluster on chromosome 1p, probably within 2 cM between D1S443 and D1S197. *Genomics*, Vol. 31, No. 1, pp. 90-94, ISSN 0888-7543

Bennett, L. B.; Roach, E. S. & Bowcock, A. M. (2000). A locus for paroxysmal kinesigenic dyskinesia maps to human chromosome 16. *Neurology*, Vol. 54, No. 1, pp. 125-130, ISSN 0028-3878

Bentivoglio, A. R.; Del Grosso, N.; Albanese, A.; Cassetta, E.; Tonali, P. & Frontali, M. (1997). Non-DYT1 dystonia in a large Italian family. *Journal of Neurology, Neurosurgery, and Psychiatry*, Vol. 62, No. 4, pp. 357-360, ISSN 0022-3050

Brashear, A.; Dobyns, W. B.; de Carvalho Aguiar, P.; Borg, M.; Frijns, C. J.; Gollamudi, S.; Green, A.; Guimaraes, J.; Haake, B. C.; Klein, C.; Linazasoro, G.; Munchau, A.; Raymond, D.; Riley, D.; Saunders-Pullman, R.; Tijssen, M. A.; Webb, D.; Zaremba, J.; Bressman, S. B. & Ozelius, L. J. (2007). The phenotypic spectrum of rapid-onset dystonia-parkinsonism (RDP) and mutations in the ATP1A3 gene. *Brain*, Vol. 130, No. Pt 3, pp. 828-835, ISSN 1460-2156

Breakefield, X. O.; Blood, A. J.; Li, Y.; Hallett, M.; Hanson, P. I. & Standaert, D. G. (2008). The pathophysiological basis of dystonias. *Nature Reviews Neuroscience*, Vol. 9, No. 3, pp. 222-234, ISSN 1471-0048

Bressman, S. B.; Sabatti, C.; Raymond, D.; de Leon, D.; Klein, C.; Kramer, P. L.; Brin, M. F.; Fahn, S.; Breakefield, X.; Ozelius, L. J. & Risch, N. J. (2000). The DYT1 phenotype and guidelines for diagnostic testing. *Neurology*, Vol. 54, No. 9, pp. 1746-1752, ISSN 0028-3878

Camargos, S.; Scholz, S.; Simon-Sanchez, J.; Paisan-Ruiz, C.; Lewis, P.; Hernandez, D.; Ding, J.; Gibbs, J. R.; Cookson, M. R.; Bras, J.; Guerreiro, R.; Oliveira, C. R.; Lees, A.; Hardy, J.; Cardoso, F. & Singleton, A. B. (2008). DYT16, a novel young-onset dystonia-parkinsonism disorder: identification of a segregating mutation in the stress-response protein PRKRA. *Lancet Neurology*, Vol. 7, No. 3, pp. 207-215, ISSN 1474-4422

Cannon, S. C. (2006). Pathomechanisms in channelopathies of skeletal muscle and brain. *Annual Review of Neuroscience*, Vol. 29, pp. 387-415, ISSN 0147-006X

Caraballo, R.; Pavek, S.; Lemainque, A.; Gastaldi, M.; Echenne, B.; Motte, J.; Genton, P.; Cersosimo, R.; Humbertclaude, V.; Fejerman, N.; Monaco, A. P.; Lathrop, M. G.; Rochette, J. & Szepetowski, P. (2001). Linkage of benign familial infantile convulsions to chromosome 16p12-q12 suggests allelism to the infantile convulsions and choreoathetosis syndrome. *American Journal of Human Genetics*, Vol. 68, No. 3, pp. 788-794, ISSN 0002-9297

Chan, P.; Gonzalez-Maeso, J.; Ruf, F.; Bishop, D. F.; Hof, P. R. & Sealfon, S. C. (2005). Epsilon-sarcoglycan immunoreactivity and mRNA expression in mouse brain. *The Journal of Comparative Neurology*, Vol. 482, No. 1, pp. 50-73, ISSN 0021-9967

Chen, J.; Shi, W.; Zhang, Y.; Sokol, R.; Cai, H.; Lun, M.; Moore, B. F.; Farber, M. J.; Stepanchick, J. S.; Bonnemann, C. G. & Chan, Y. M. (2006). Identification of functional domains in sarcoglycans essential for their interaction and plasma membrane targeting. *Experimental Cell Research*, Vol. 312, No. 9, pp. 1610-1625, ISSN 0014-4827

Chouery, E.; Kfoury, J.; Delague, V.; Jalkh, N.; Bejjani, P.; Serre, J. L. & Megarbane, A. (2008). A novel locus for autosomal recessive primary torsion dystonia (DYT17) maps to 20p11.22-q13.12. *Neurogenetics*, Vol. 9, No. 4, pp. 287-293, ISSN 1364-6753

de Carvalho Aguiar, P.; Sweadner, K. J.; Penniston, J. T.; Zaremba, J.; Liu, L.; Caton, M.; Linazasoro, G.; Borg, M.; Tijssen, M. A.; Bressman, S. B.; Dobyns, W. B.; Brashear, A. & Ozelius, L. J. (2004). Mutations in the Na^+/K^+ ATPase alpha3 gene ATP1A3 are associated with rapid-onset dystonia parkinsonism. *Neuron*, Vol. 43, No. 2, pp. 169-175, ISSN 0896-6273

Djarmati, A.; Schneider, S. A.; Lohmann, K.; Winkler, S.; Pawlack, H.; Hagenah, J.; Bruggemann, N.; Zittel, S.; Fuchs, T.; Rakovic, A.; Schmidt, A.; Jabusch, H. C.; Wilcox, R.; Kostic, V. S.; Siebner, H.; Altenmuller, E.; Munchau, A.; Ozelius, L. J. & Klein, C. (2009). Mutations in THAP1 (DYT6) and generalised dystonia with prominent spasmodic dysphonia: a genetic screening study. *Lancet Neurology*, Vol. 8, No. 5, pp. 447-452, ISSN 1474-4422

Duan, W.; Zhang, Z.; Gash, D. M. & Mattson, M. P. (1999). Participation of prostate apoptosis response-4 in degeneration of dopaminergic neurons in models of Parkinson's disease. *Annals of Neurology*, Vol. 46, No. 4, pp. 587-597, ISSN 0364-5134

Esapa, C. T.; Waite, A.; Locke, M.; Benson, M. A.; Kraus, M.; McIlhinney, R. A.; Sillitoe, R. V.; Beesley, P. W. & Blake, D. J. (2007). SGCE missense mutations that cause myoclonus-dystonia syndrome impair epsilon-sarcoglycan trafficking to the plasma membrane: modulation by ubiquitination and torsinA. *Human Molecular Genetics*, Vol. 16, No. 3, pp. 327-342, ISSN 0964-6906

Gavarini, S.; Cayrol, C.; Fuchs, T.; Lyons, N.; Ehrlich, M. E.; Girard, J. P. & Ozelius, L. J. (2010). Direct interaction between causative genes of DYT1 and DYT6 primary dystonia. *Annals of Neurology*, Vol. 68, No. 4, pp. 549-553, ISSN 1531-8249

Gesierich, A.; Niroomand, F. & Tiefenbacher, C. P. (2003). Role of human GTP cyclohydrolase I and its regulatory protein in tetrahydrobiopterin metabolism. *Basic Research in Cardiology*, Vol. 98, No. 2, pp. 69-75, ISSN 0300-8428

Ghezzi, D.; Viscomi, C.; Ferlini, A.; Gualandi, F.; Mereghetti, P.; DeGrandis, D. & Zeviani, M. (2009). Paroxysmal non-kinesigenic dyskinesia is caused by mutations of the MR-1 mitochondrial targeting sequence. *Human Molecular Genetics*, Vol. 18, No. 6, pp. 1058-1064, ISSN 1460-2083

Goodchild, R. E. & Dauer, W. T. (2004). Mislocalization to the nuclear envelope: an effect of the dystonia-causing torsinA mutation, *Proceedings of the National Academy of Sciences of the United States of America*, Vol. 101, No. 3, pp. 847-852, ISSN 0027-8424

Gorke, W. & Bartholome, K. (1990). Biochemical and neurophysiological investigations in two forms of Segawa's disease. *Neuropediatrics*, Vol. 21, No. 1, pp. 3-8, ISSN 0174-304X

Grimes, D. A.; Bulman, D.; George-Hyslop, P. S. & Lang, A. E. (2001). Inherited myoclonus-dystonia: evidence supporting genetic heterogeneity. *Movement Disorders*, Vol. 16, No. 1, pp. 106-110, ISSN 0885-3185

Grotzsch, H.; Pizzolato, G. P.; Ghika, J.; Schorderet, D.; Vingerhoets, F. J.; Landis, T. & Burkhard, P. R. (2002). Neuropathology of a case of dopa-responsive dystonia associated with a new genetic locus, DYT14. *Neurology*, Vol. 58, No. 12, pp. 1839-1842, ISSN 0028-3878

Hancks, D. C. & Kazazian, H. H. Jr. (2010). SVA retrotransposons: Evolution and genetic instability. *Seminars in Cancer Biology*, Vol. 20, No. 4, pp. 234-245, ISSN 1096-3650

Hewett, J. W.; Tannous, B.; Niland, B. P.; Nery, F. C.; Zeng, J.; Li, Y. & Breakefield, X. O. (2007). Mutant torsinA interferes with protein processing through the secretory pathway in DYT1 dystonia cells, *Proceedings of the National Academy of Sciences of the United States of America*, Vol. 104, No. 17, pp. 7271-7276, ISSN 0027-8424

Hilgenberg, L. G.; Su, H.; Gu, H.; O'Dowd, D. K. & Smith, M. A. (2006). Alpha3Na^+/K^+-ATPase is a neuronal receptor for agrin. *Cell*, Vol. 125, No. 2, pp. 359-369, ISSN 0092-8674

Ichinose, H.; Ohye, T.; Takahashi, E.; Seki, N.; Hori, T.; Segawa, M.; Nomura, Y.; Endo, K.; Tanaka, H.; Tsuji, S. (1994). Hereditary progressive dystonia with marked diurnal fluctuation caused by mutations in the GTP cyclohydrolase I gene. *Nature Genetics*, Vol. 8, No. 3, pp. 236-242, ISSN 1061-4036

Kaiser, F. J.; Osmanoric, A.; Rakovic, A.; Erogullari, A.; Uflacker, N.; Braunholz, D.; Lohnau, T.; Orolicki, S.; Albrecht, M.; Gillessen-Kaesbach, G.; Klein, C. & Lohmann, K. (2010). The dystonia gene DYT1 is repressed by the transcription factor THAP1 (DYT6). *Annals of Neurology*, Vol. 68, No. 4, pp. 554-559, ISSN 1531-8249

Kamm, C.; Mayer, P.; Sharma, M.; Niemann, G. & Gasser, T. (2007). New family with paroxysmal exercise-induced dystonia and epilepsy. *Movement Disorders*, Vol. 22, No. 6, pp. 873-877, ISSN 0885-3185

Konakova, M.; Huynh, D. P.; Yong, W. & Pulst, S. M. (2001). Cellular distribution of torsin A and torsin B in normal human brain. *Archives of Neurology*, Vol. 58, No. 6, pp. 921-927, ISSN 0003-9942

Kupke, K. G.; Lee, L. V. & Muller, U. (1990a). Assignment of the X-linked torsion dystonia gene to Xq21 by linkage analysis. *Neurology*, Vol. 40, No. 9, pp. 1438-1442, ISSN 0028-3878

Kupke, K. G.; Lee, L. V.; Viterbo, G. H.; Arancillo, J.; Donlon, T. & Muller, U. (1990b). X-linked recessive torsion dystonia in the Philippines. *American Journal of Medical Genetics*, Vol. 36, No. 2, pp. 237-242, ISSN 0148-7299

Lee, H. Y.; Xu, Y.; Huang, Y.; Ahn, A. H.; Auburger, G. W.; Pandolfo, M.; Kwiecinski, H.; Grimes, D. A.; Lang, A. E.; Nielsen, J. E.; Averyanov, Y.; Servidei, S.; Friedman, A.; Van Bogaert, P.; Abramowicz, M. J.; Bruno, M. K.; Sorensen, B. F.; Tang, L.; Fu, Y. H. & Ptacek, L. J. (2004). The gene for paroxysmal non-kinesigenic dyskinesia encodes an enzyme in a stress response pathway. *Human Molecular Genetics*, Vol. 13, No. 24, pp. 3161-3170, ISSN 0964-6906

Lee, L. V.; Pascasio, F. M.; Fuentes, F. D. & Viterbo, G. H. (1976). Torsion dystonia in Panay, Philippines. *Advances in Neurology*, Vol. 14, pp. 137-151, ISSN 0091-3952

Lee, L. V.; Rivera, C.; Teleg, R. A.; Dantes, M. B.; Pasco, P. M.; Jamora, R. D.; Arancillo, J.; Villareal-Jordan, R. F.; Rosales, R. L.; Demaisip, C.; Maranon, E.; Peralta, O.; Borres, R.; Tolentino, C.; Monding, M. J. & Sarcia, S. (2011). The unique phenomenology of sex-linked dystonia parkinsonism (XDP, DYT3, "Lubag"). *International Journal of Neuroscience*, Vol. 121, Suppl 1, pp. 3-11, ISSN 1563-5279.

Leube, B.; Hendgen, T.; Kessler, K. R.; Knapp, M.; Benecke, R. & Auburger, G. (1997). Evidence for DYT7 being a common cause of cervical dystonia (torticollis) in Central Europe. *American Journal of Medical Genetics*, Vol. 74, No. 5, pp. 529-532, ISSN 0148-7299

Leube, B.; Rudnicki, D.; Ratzlaff, T.; Kessler, K. R.; Benecke, R. & Auburger, G. (1996). Idiopathic torsion dystonia: assignment of a gene to chromosome 18p in a German family with adult onset, autosomal dominant inheritance and purely focal distribution. *Human Molecular Genetics*, Vol. 5, No. 10, pp. 1673-1677, ISSN 0964-6906

Makino, S.; Kaji, R.; Ando, S.; Tomizawa, M.; Yasuno, K.; Goto, S.; Matsumoto, S.; Tabuena, M. D.; Maranon, E.; Dantes, M.; Lee, L. V.; Ogasawara, K.; Tooyama, I.; Akatsu, H.; Nishimura, M. & Tamiya, G. (2007). Reduced neuron-specific expression of the TAF1 gene is associated with X-linked dystonia-parkinsonism. *American Journal of Human Genetics*, Vol. 80, No. 3, pp. 393-406, ISSN 0002-9297

Margari, L.; Perniola, T.; Illiceto, G.; Ferrannini, E.; De Iaco, M. G.; Presicci, A.; Santostasi, R. & Ventura, P. (2000). Familial paroxysmal exercise-induced dyskinesia and benign epilepsy: a clinical and neurophysiological study of an uncommon disorder. *Neurological Sciences*, Vol. 21, No. 3, pp. 165-172, ISSN 1590-1874

Naismith, T. V.; Heuser, J. E.; Breakefield, X. O. & Hanson, P. I. (2004). TorsinA in the nuclear envelope, *Proceedings of the National Academy of Sciences of the United States of America*, Vol. 101, No. 20, pp. 7612-7617, ISSN 0027-8424

Neuwald, A. F.; Aravind, L.; Spouge, J. L. & Koonin, E. V. (1999). AAA+: A class of chaperone-like ATPases associated with the assembly, operation, and disassembly of protein complexes. *Genome Research*, Vol. 9, No. 1, pp. 27-43, ISSN 1088-9051

Norgren, N.; Mattson, E.; Forsgren, L. & Holmberg, M. (2011). A high-penetrance form of late-onset torsion dystonia maps to a novel locus (DYT21) on chromosome 2q14.3-q21.3. *Neurogenetics*, Vol. 12, No. 2, pp. 137-143, ISSN 1364-6753

Ozelius, L. J.; Hewett, J. W.; Page, C. E.; Bressman, S. B.; Kramer, P. L.; Shalish, C.; de Leon, D.; Brin, M. F.; Raymond, D.; Corey, D. P.; Fahn, S.; Risch, N. J.; Buckler, A. J.; Gusella, J. F. & Breakefield, X. O. (1997). The early-onset torsion dystonia gene (DYT1) encodes an ATP-binding protein. *Nature Genetics*, Vol. 17, No. 1, pp. 40-48, ISSN 1061-4036

Ozelius, L. J.; Lubarr, N. & Bressman, S. B. (2011). Milestones in dystonia. *Movement Disorders*, Vol. 26, No. 6, pp. 1106-1126, ISSN 1531-8257

Pasco, P. M.; Ison, C. V.; Munoz, E. L.; Magpusao, N. S.; Cheng, A. E.; Tan, K. T.; Lo, R. W.; Teleg, R. A.; Dantes, M. B.; Borres, R.; Maranon, E.; Demaisip, C.; Reyes, M. V. & Lee, L. V. (2011). Understanding XDP through imaging, pathology, and genetics. International Journal of Neuroscience, Vol. 121, Suppl 1, pp. 12-17, ISSN 1563-5279

Pascual, J. M.; Wang, D.; Lecumberri, B.; Yang, H.; Mao, X.; Yang, R. & De Vivo, D. C. (2004). GLUT1 deficiency and other glucose transporter diseases. *European Journal of Endocrinology*, Vol. 150, No. 5, pp. 627-633, ISSN 0804-4643

Rainier, S.; Thomas, D.; Tokarz, D.; Ming, L.; Bui, M.; Plein, E.; Zhao, X.; Lemons, R.; Albin, R.; Delaney, C.; Alvarado, D. & Fink, J. K. (2004). Myofibrillogenesis regulator 1 gene mutations cause paroxysmal dystonic choreoathetosis. *Archives of Neurology*, Vol. 61, No. 7, pp. 1025-1029, ISSN 0003-9942

Risch, N. J.; Bressman, S. B.; Senthil, G. & Ozelius, L. J. (2007). Intragenic Cis and Trans modification of genetic susceptibility in DYT1 torsion dystonia. *American Journal of Human Genetics*, Vol. 80, No. 6, pp. 1188-1193, ISSN 0002-9297

Roussigne, M.; Cayrol, C.; Clouaire, T.; Amalric, F. & Girard, J. P. (2003). THAP1 is a nuclear proapoptotic factor that links prostate-apoptosis-response-4 (Par-4) to PML nuclear bodies. *Oncogene*, Vol. 22, No. 16, pp. 2432-2442, ISSN 0950-9232

Saunders-Pullman, R.; Ozelius, L. & Bressman, S. B. (2002). Inherited myoclonus- dystonia. *Advances in Neurology*, Vol. 89, pp. 185-191, ISSN 0091-3952

Schmidt, A. & Klein, C. (2010). The role of genes in causing dystonia. *European Journal of Neurology*, Vol. 17 Suppl 1, pp. 65-70, ISSN 1468-1331

Schneider, S. A.; Paisan-Ruiz, C.; Garcia-Gorostiaga, I.; Quinn, N. P.; Weber, Y. G.; Lerche, H.; Hardy, J. & Bhatia, K. P. (2009). GLUT1 gene mutations cause sporadic paroxysmal exercise-induced dyskinesias. *Movement Disorders*, Vol. 24, No. 11, pp. 1684-1688, ISSN 1531-8257

Seibler, P.; Djarmati, A.; Langpap, B.; Hagenah, J.; Schmidt, A.; Bruggemann, N.; Siebner, H.; Jabusch, H. C.; Altenmuller, E.; Munchau, A.; Lohmann, K. & Klein, C. (2008). A heterozygous frameshift mutation in PRKRA (DYT16) associated with generalised dystonia in a German patient. *Lancet Neurology*, Vol. 7, No. 5, pp. 380-381, ISSN 1474-4422

Shashidharan, P.; Sandu, D.; Potla, U.; Armata, I. A.; Walker, R. H.; McNaught, K. S.; Weisz, D.; Sreenath, T.; Brin, M. F. & Olanow, C. W. (2005). Transgenic mouse model of early-onset DYT1 dystonia. *Human Molecular Genetics*, Vol. 14, No. 1, pp. 125-133, ISSN 0964-6906

Spacey, S. D.; Adams, P. J.; Lam, P. C.; Materek, L. A.; Stoessl, A. J.; Snutch, T. P. & Hsiung, G. Y. (2006). Genetic heterogeneity in paroxysmal nonkinesigenic dyskinesia. *Neurology*, Vol. 66, No. 10, pp. 1588-1590, ISSN 1526-632X

Tomita, H.; Nagamitsu, S.; Wakui, K.; Fukushima, Y.; Yamada, K.; Sadamatsu, M.; Masui, A.; Konishi, T.; Matsuishi, T.; Aihara, M.; Shimizu, K.; Hashimoto, K.; Mineta, M.; Matsushima, M.; Tsujita, T.; Saito, M.; Tanaka, H.; Tsuji, S.; Takagi, T.; Nakamura, Y.; Nanko, S.; Kato, N.; Nakane, Y. & Niikawa, N. (1999). Paroxysmal kinesigenic choreoathetosis locus maps to chromosome 16p11.2-q12.1. *American Journal of Human Genetics*, Vol. 65, No. 6, pp. 1688-1697, ISSN 0002-9297

Valente, E. M.; Bentivoglio, A. R.; Cassetta, E.; Dixon, P. H.; Davis, M. B.; Ferraris, A.; Ialongo, T.; Frontali, M.; Wood, N. W. & Albanese, A. (2001). DYT13, a novel primary torsion dystonia locus, maps to chromosome 1p36.13--36.32 in an Italian family with cranial-cervical or upper limb onset. *Annals of Neurology*, Vol. 49, No. 3, pp. 362-366, ISSN 0364-5134

Valente, E. M.; Spacey, S. D.; Wali, G. M.; Bhatia, K. P.; Dixon, P. H.; Wood, N. W. & Davis, M. B. (2000). A second paroxysmal kinesigenic choreoathetosis locus (EKD2) mapping on 16q13-q22.1 indicates a family of genes which give rise to paroxysmal disorders on human chromosome 16. *Brain*, Vol. 123 (Pt 10), pp. 2040-2045, ISSN 0006-8950

Weber, Y. G.; Storch, A.; Wuttke, T. V.; Brockmann, K.; Kempfle, J.; Maljevic, S.; Margari, L.; Kamm, C.; Schneider, S. A.; Huber, S. M.; Pekrun, A.; Roebling, R.; Seebohm, G.; Koka, S.; Lang, C.; Kraft, E.; Blazevic, D.; Salvo-Vargas, A.; Fauler, M.; Mottaghy, F. M.; Munchau, A.; Edwards, M. J.; Presicci, A.; Margari, F.; Gasser, T.; Lang, F.; Bhatia, K. P.; Lehmann-Horn, F. & Lerche, H. (2008). GLUT1 mutations are a cause of paroxysmal exertion-induced dyskinesias and induce hemolytic anemia by a cation leak. *The Journal of Clinical Investigation*, Vol. 118, No. 6, pp. 2157-2168, ISSN 0021-9738

Wider, C.; Melquist, S.; Hauf, M.; Solida, A.; Cobb, S. A.; Kachergus, J. M.; Gass, J.; Coon, K. D.; Baker, M.; Cannon, A.; Stephan, D. A.; Schorderet, D. F.; Ghika, J.; Burkhard, P. R.; Kapatos, G.; Hutton, M.; Farrer, M. J.; Wszolek, Z. K. & Vingerhoets, F. J. (2008). Study of a Swiss dopa-responsive dystonia family with a deletion in GCH1: redefining DYT14 as DYT5. *Neurology*, Vol. 70, No. 16 Pt 2, pp. 1377-1383, ISSN 1526-632X

Zimprich, A.; Grabowski, M.; Asmus, F.; Naumann, M.; Berg, D.; Bertram, M.; Scheidtmann, K.; Kern, P.; Winkelmann, J.; Muller-Myhsok, B.; Riedel, L.; Bauer, M.; Muller, T.; Castro, M.; Meitinger, T.; Strom, T. M. & Gasser, T. (2001). Mutations in the gene encoding epsilon-sarcoglycan cause myoclonus- dystonia syndrome. *Nature Genetics*, Vol. 29, No. 1, pp. 66-69, ISSN 1061-4036

Zlotogora, J. (2004). Autosomal recessive, DYT2-like primary torsion dystonia: a new family. *Neurology*, Vol. 63, No. 7, pp. 1340, ISSN 1526-632X

2

Dystonias of the Neck: Clinico-Radiologic Correlations

Gerhard Reichel
Department of Movement Disorders, Paracelsus Clinic, Zwickau, Germany

1. Introduction

Idiopathic cervical dystonias (CD), the most prevalent form of defined dystonias in adults, are characterized by involuntary, abnormal movements of the head, and/or by the involuntary adoption of various head postures. With the exception of a few patients, the course of the condition is not progressive[1,2].

Since the clinical description of the four basic dystonic head/neck movements in 1953 by Hassler[3] there have been no publications concerning the further differentiation of these forms of CD. Also, it has not been attempted to define muscles affected by dystonia with the help of imaging procedures. A new book called "Imaging of Movement Disorders" does not contain a single image of dystonic muscles in its eleven chapters[4].

Since botulinum toxin has become available for the symptomatic treatment of CD, an exact differentiation between dystonic and non-dystonic muscles is very important.

Botulinum toxin is an established treatment for CD[5] and has gained widespread acceptance since its first use in 1985[6], based on a large body of evidence[7,8]. Response rates of approximately 80% have been achieved in patients with CD in open and double-blind studies[9-11]. Furthermore, treatment is generally well tolerated even following long-term administration[12, 13] and the risk of adverse events may also be minimized using well-defined injection procedures.

Nevertheless, unsatisfactory treatment outcomes have been observed in patients with CD[14]. These may generally be attributed to incorrect muscles selected for treatment administration and suboptimal dosing and distribution to the affected muscles. Moreover, in some cases, poor treatment outcomes may reflect failure to treat all the affected muscles or the influence of toxins on healthy muscles. Although imaging[15], electromyography[16] and modifications of injection technique[17] have all been used to improve treatment outcomes, the influence of these methods on treatment outcome requires further clarification[17].

In patients with CD, dystonic nodding movements, rotatory movements and lateral flexion can originate from the head joints and from the cervical spine. The combination of nodding movements of the upper head joint with rotatory movements of the lower head joint can result in movements in all three spatial planes. Dystonic movement disorders occur in the majority of patients in two planes (50%), less commonly in one plane (approximately 35%) and, rarely, in three planes (11%)[18].

The localization of dystonic movements is dependent on the origin and insertion of the muscles involved in dystonia. As not all potentially affected muscles are dystonic in each form of CD, clinical decisions must be based on findings from the clinical examination, including palpation, electromyographic analysis and, in cases of ambiguity, imaging (computed tomography [CT] and magnetic resonance imaging [MRI]). Although dystonic head postures are traditionally classified according to four different movement planes (rotation, lateral flexion, forward/backward flexion and sagittal shift), our clinical experience suggests that this system of classification is not sufficient for the accurate identification of muscles that should be targeted for botulinum toxin treatment. Thus, we conducted a large, non-intervention study using clinical examination, CT and MRI, with the overall aim of elucidating a more precise method of differentiating forms of head and neck postures in patients with CD. Initial results of the MRI analyses have been published previously[19].

2. Methodology

2.1 Setting and study population

Patients treated in our specialist movement disorders clinic with documented primary CD – established by clinical examination, electromyography, MRI of the neurocranium, laboratory tests and data relating to the patient's medical history - were eligible for inclusion. Patients were enrolled from 2007 to 2009. This sample represents all the patients in our clinic in this time period, with the exception of pregnant patients (n=1) or those who refused to participate (n=1). Written informed consent was given by all included patients and the study was approved by the local ethics committee.

2.2 Study assessments

Characterization of the different forms of the abnormal head (-caput) and neck (-collis) postures in patients with CD was conducted by clinical evaluation and radiological examination. For complicated or unclear cases, CT and/or MRI was also used.

Radiological examinations involved: 1) CT scanning of the soft tissues of the neck as single layers at the section level of cervical vertebrae 3 and 7; and 2) MRI of the cervical spine and the soft parts of the neck (with T1- and T2-weighting in 2 mm slices), and the deep neck muscles (examined at an angle with T1 weighting). During the examination, patients were requested to assume a relaxed head or neck posture. For patients with lateral flexion, electronic 'straightening' of the tomograph was performed to enable muscles to be visualized at the same height on both sides of the image (Figure 1). For evaluation of MRI data, images from 50 patients who did not suffer from CD (prior condition documented as mild trauma or suspected radicular disorder) were used as retrospective controls.

2.3 Statistical analyses

Following CT and MRI, the relationships of the skull to the cervical spine and of the cervical spine to the thoracic spine were analyzed. CT images were also used to obtain measurements and shapes of muscles in the neck region, as clinically appropriate. Results of analyses for CT and MRI data for patients with CD are presented descriptively as percentages.

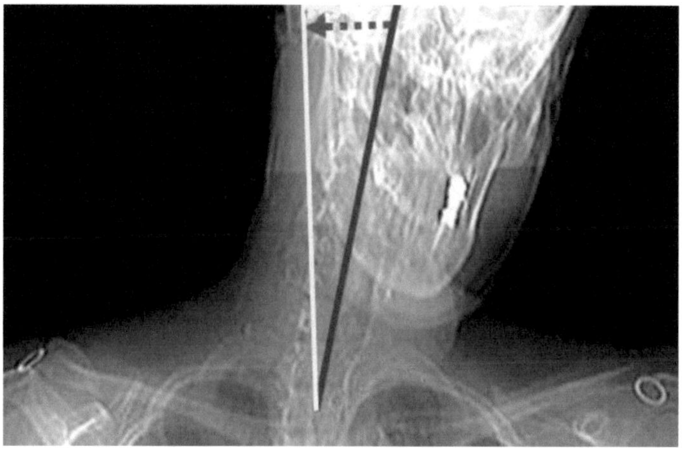

Fig. 1. 'Straightening' by computer tomography in the case of lateral flexion.

3. Results

Overall, 95 patients (55 female, 40 male) with established primary CD were included in the study. The patient population had a mean age of 48.5 years, with a mean age at disease onset of 41.6 years.

The incidences of abnormal head posture, categorized according to the traditional classification of four different movement planes (rotation, lateral flexion, forward/backward flexion and sagittal shift), are presented in Table 1. The most frequent form of CD presented as lateral flexion and rotation (34%). The incidence of pure backward flexion was rare (5%), and there were no cases of pure forward flexion.

Abnormal head posture	**n (%)**
Lateral flexion alone	13 (14)
Rotation alone	10 (11)
Lateral flexion + rotation	32 (34)
Lateral flexion + lateral shift	2 (2)
Lateral flexion + backward flexion	9 (10)
Lateral flexion + forward flexion	2 (2)
Lateral flexion + forward flexion + lateral shift	2 (2)
Lateral flexion + rotation + forward flexion	12 (13)
Lateral flexion + rotation + forward flexion + lateral shift	1 (1)
Backward flexion alone	5 (5)
Rotation + forward flexion	2 (2)
Forward sagittal shift	4 (4)
Backward sagittal shift	1 (1)

Table 1. Incidence of differing abnormal head postures in patients with cervical dystonia (N=95)

The majority of patients (78%; n=73) experienced lateral flexion followed by rotation (61%; n=57), forward flexion (20%; n=19), backward flexion (15%; n=14), and, less frequently, lateral shift (9%; n=8) and sagittal shift (5%; n=5).

The four types of abnormal head posture were characterized further using clinical findings and MRI and CT imaging, and are summarized in Tables 2 and 3.

	-Caput	**-Collis**	**Both**	**Total (n [%])***
Lateral flexion	14 (19.2)	16 (21.9)	43 (58.9)	73 (44.8)
Rotation	11 (19.3)	10 (17.5)	36 (63.2)	57 (35.0)
Forward flexion	3 (15.8)	5 (26.3)	11 (57.9)	19 (11.7)
Backward flexion	3 (21.4)	2 (14.3)	9 (64.3)	14 (8.6)
Total (n [%])	**31 (19)**	**33 (20)**	**99 (61)**	**163 (100)**

*Patients were included more than once in any subgroup.

Table 2. Patient subgroups by flexion or rotation type (latero/antero/retro/torticaput or -collis; n [%])

Clinical manifestation	Dystonic muscles acting on the skull or head joints	Dystonic Muscles acting on C2–7
Lateral flexion	Laterocaput	Laterocollis
Rotation	Torticaput	Torticollis
Forward flexion	Anterocaput	Anterocollis
Backward flexion	Retrocaput	Retrocollis
Combination of laterocollis and contralateral laterocaput	Lateral shift	
Combination of anterocollis and retrocaput	Forward sagittal shift	
Combination of anterocaput and retrocollis	Backward sagittal shift	

Table 3. Proposed subdivisions of cervical dystonia forms

3.1 Flexion

Clinical examination alone was sufficient to determine the variant of lateral flexion that was present in the majority of patients (Figure 2a and b). In a few cases, imaging was used to confirm the clinical decision (Figure 2c).

Clinical and imaging observations revealed that 19% of patients had lateral flexion that was located in the head joints, whereas flexion in the cervical spine or between the cervical spine and the thoracic spine was present in 22% of patients (Table 2). Most (59%) patients exhibited simultaneous lateral flexion of the head and of the cervical spine (Table 2).

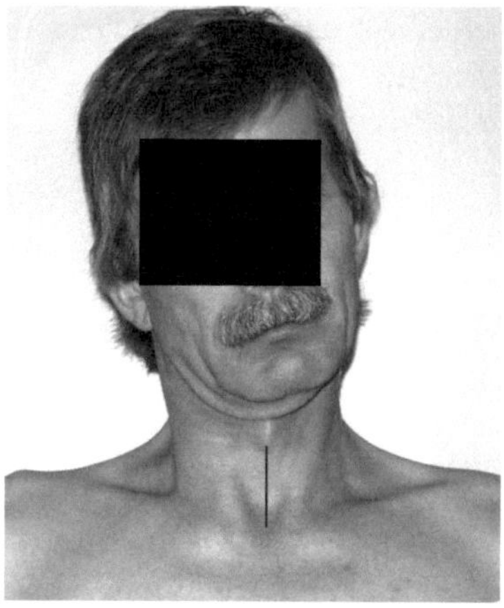

a.

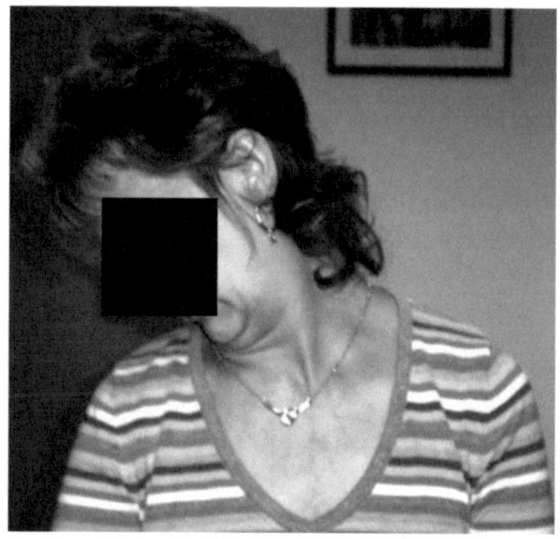

b.

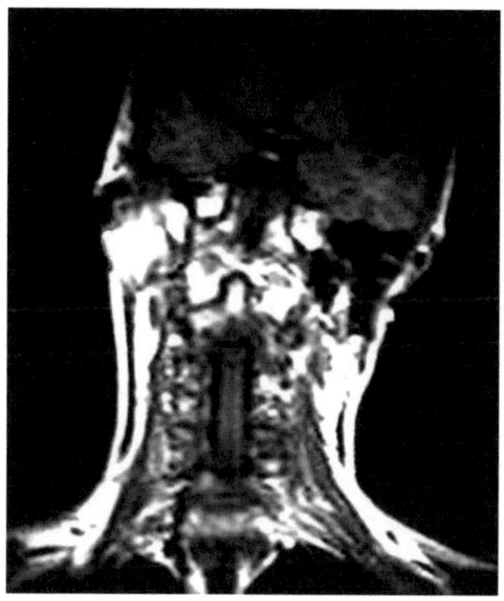

c.

Fig. 2. a.–c. Lateral flexion: a) Laterocaput; b) Laterocollis; c) Computer tomograph-reconstruction in the case of laterocaput.

As observed for lateral flexion, clinical impression was accurate in the majority of patients with backward and forward flexion (Figure 3). The incidence of backward and forward flexion was similar to observations for lateral flexion, with approximately 16 (forward) and 21 (backward) % of cases caused by flexion in the head joints and 14 (forward) and 26 (backward) % by flexion of the cervical spine. Both forms of these posture disorders were present in 58 (forward) and 64 (backward) % of the patients (Table 2).

3.2 Rotation

In analyses of head rotation, clinical differentiation between rotation in the head joints and the cervical spine region was frequently inaccurate (Figures 4 and 5). Guidance was provided by the position of the readily palpable incisura jugularis sterni with respect to the incisura thyreoidea superior (for example, in the case of rotation in the head joints, the notches are positioned directly above each other; Figure 4d).

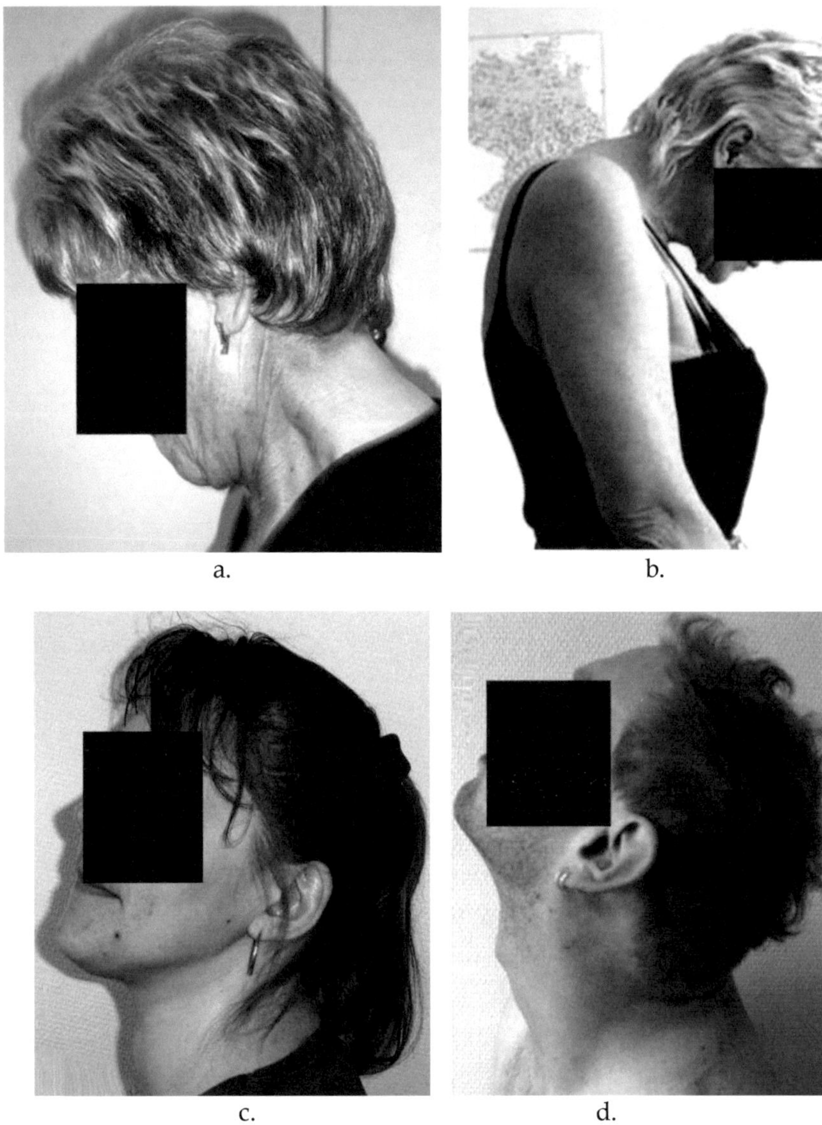

Fig. 3. a.–d. Patients with forward and backward flexion forms of cervical dystonia: a) Forward flexion, anterocaput; b) Forward flexion, anterocollis; c) Backward flexion, retrocaput; d) Backward flexion, retrocollis.

Results using CT-slices to compare the position of the vertebrae in both planes (C3 and C7) allowed more reliable differentiation between torticollis and torticaput. In the case of torticaput, rotation was observed only in the lower head joint (articulatio atlantoaxialis).

Thus, in the C3 image, only the skull (easy to recognize by the lower jaw) is positioned in the rotated direction, whereas cervical vertebrae 3 and 7 are not rotated towards each other (Figure 4b and c). By contrast, the upper cervical vertebrae are rotated towards the lower cervical vertebrae in the presence of torticollis, and the third cervical vertebra points in the direction of the lower jaw (Figure 5b and c). Correspondingly, CT images demonstrated differences between the diameters of the muscles on each side, and therefore the muscles affected by dystonia.

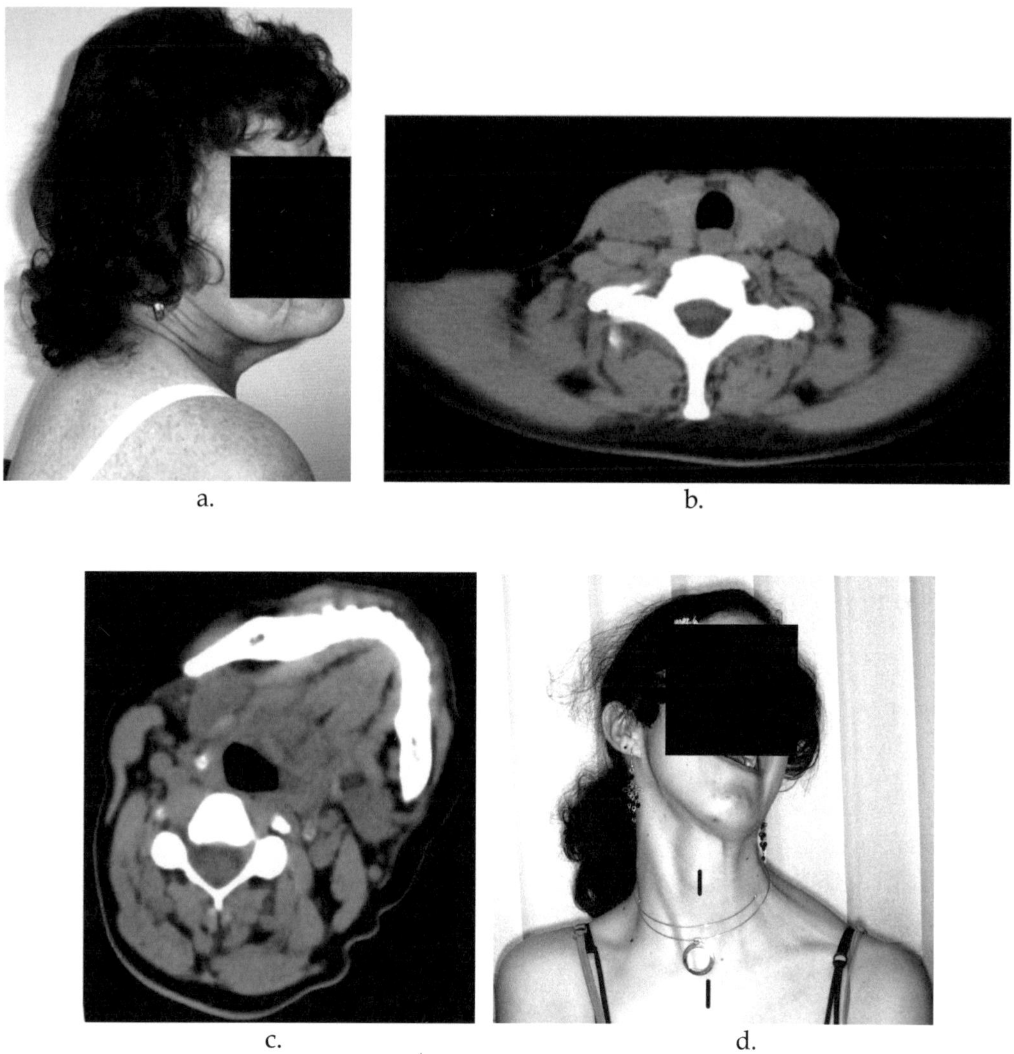

Fig. 4. a.-d. Clinical and imaging evaluations of torticaput: a) Patient with torticaput; b) Computer tomograph at section C7; c) Computer tomograph at C3 (the cervical vertebra is not rotated towards C7 but towards the skull); d) Torticaput (laterocaput and retrocaput, the larynx is positioned above the sternum).

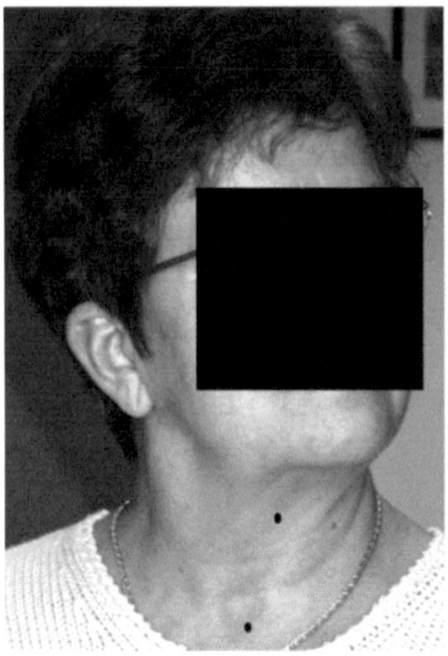

a.

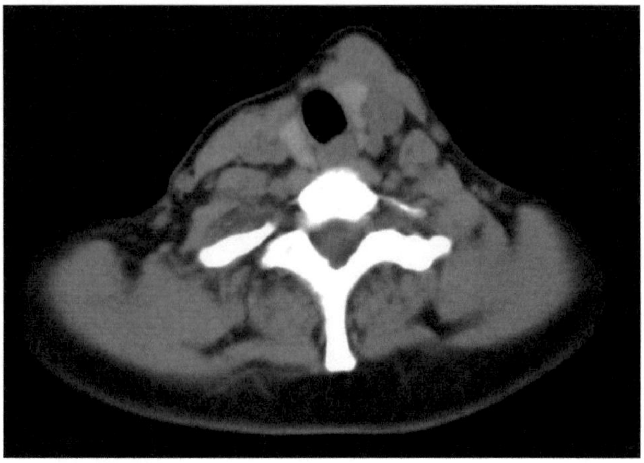

b.

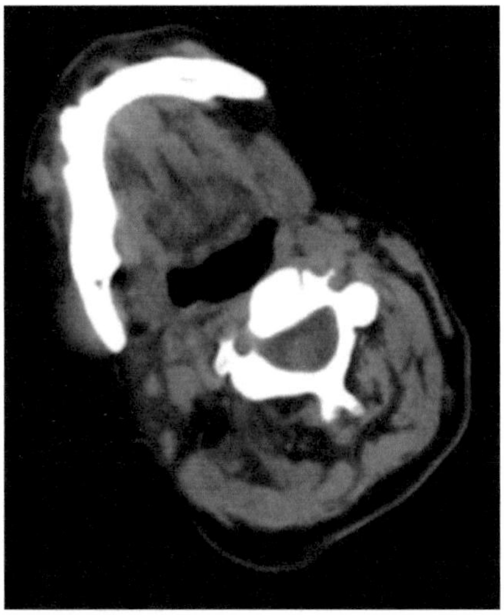

c.

Fig. 5. a.–c. Clinical and imaging evaluations of torticollis: a) Patient with torticollis (the larynx is not positioned above the sternum); b) Computer tomograph at section C7; c) Computer tomograph at C3 (the cervical vetebra is rotated towards C7 but not towards the skull).

3.3 Shift

Lateral shift was evident as a combination of lateral flexion of the cervical spine with flexion in the head joints to the opposite side (Figure 6a), whereas sagittal shift presented as a combination of forward flexion of the cervical spine with backward flexion in the head joints (Figure 6b). In contrast, backward shift developed from a combination of retrocollis and anterocaput (Figure 6c).

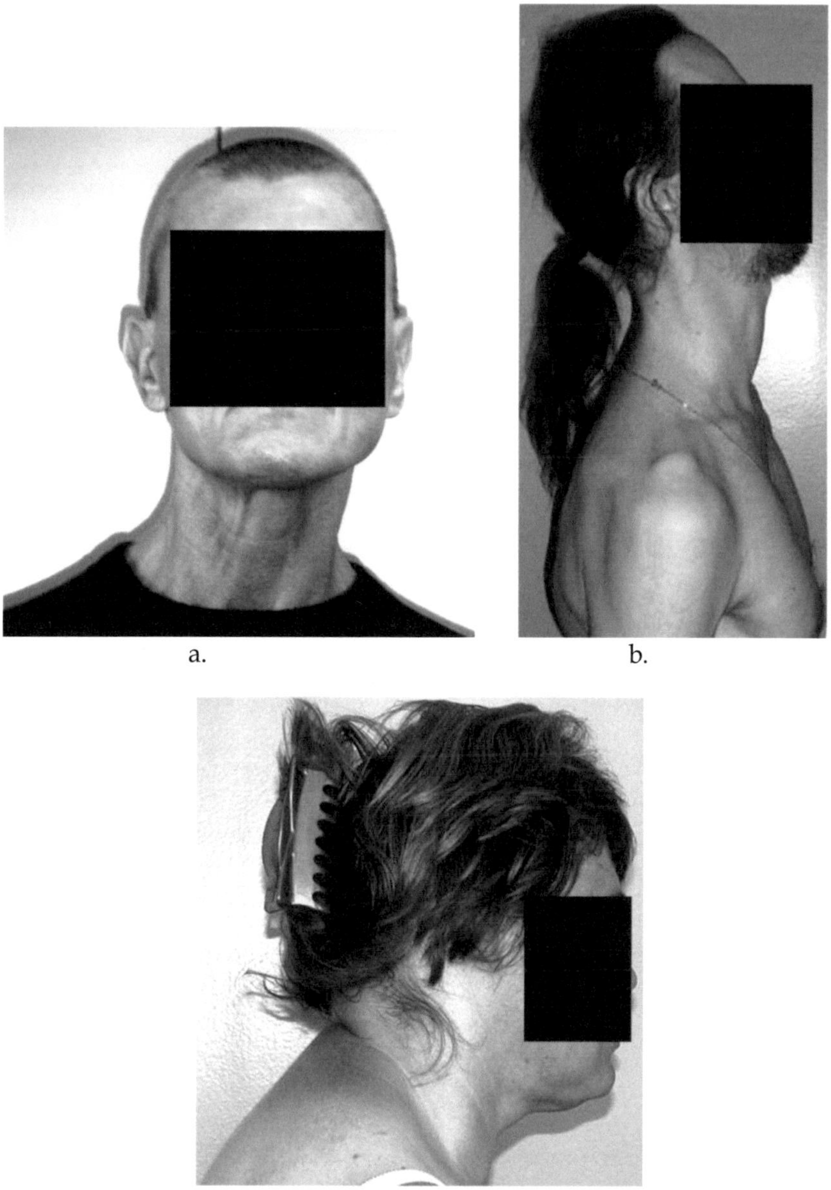

a. b.

c.

Fig. 6. a.–c. Patients with cervical dystonia characterized by lateral or sagittal shift: a) Lateral shift; b) Backward sagittal shift; c) Forward sagittal shift.

3.4 Muscle size

Measurement of maximum muscle diameters using MRI[15] revealed that, in addition to the large neck muscles, musculus obliquus capitis inferior was the only small muscle that was asymmetrical in the majority of patients (73%; Figure 7a). This muscle, when dystonic, induced rotation and backward flexion in the head joints. Therefore, separate analysis of this muscle is advised given the difficulty of localized treatment with botulinum toxin. For reasons of safety, treatment should only be performed if administration is monitored by CT (Figure 7b).

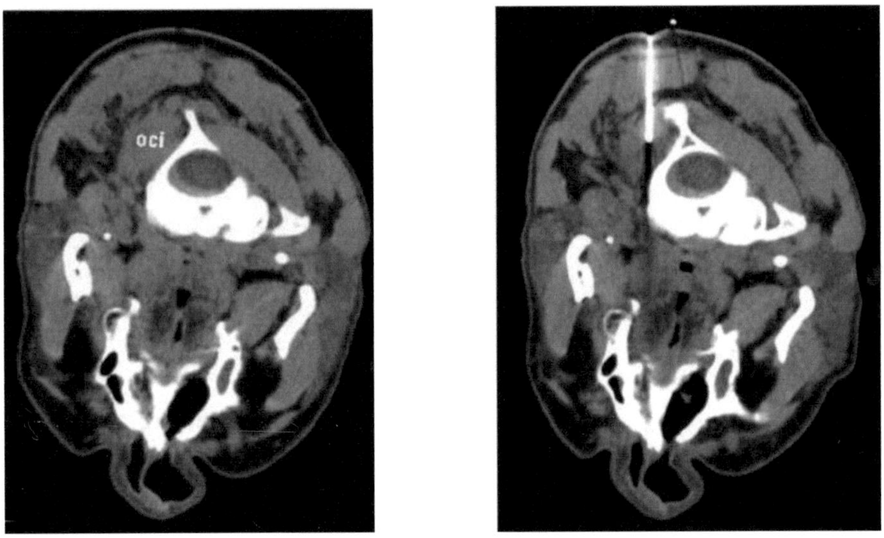

a. b.

Fig. 7. a.-b. Computertomographic evaluations of dystonic small neck muscle: a) Hypertrophy of the musculus obliquus capitis inferior (oci); b) Botulinum toxin therapy of the musculus obliquus capitis inferior monitored by CT.

4. Botulinum toxin targeting in CD based on clinic-radiologic correlates

This was a large study that was conducted to elucidate the characteristics of abnormal head and neck postures among patients with CD in order to maximize treatment outcomes with botulinum toxin. In contrast to the previously accepted classification of CD (four basic forms), our clinical and imaging findings support the differentiation of the disorder into 10 variations of posture and/or movement (Figure 8), which allows better delineation of the muscles involved in the particular form of CD (Table 4).

Analyses of the prevalence of the characterized forms of CD in our study population revealed that, in the case of lateral flexion and rotation, the abnormal movement and/or posture involved only the head joints (latero- and/or torticaput) in approximately 20% of patients and only the region of the cervical spine (latero- and/or torticollis) in approximately a further 20% of patients. The remaining patients, approximately 60%, had both disorders, albeit with varying degrees of involvement of -caput and -collis. Thus, the incidence of these three forms represented a ratio of 1:1:3. A similar ratio of incidence was observed for forward and backward flexion forms involving the head joints (antero- and/or retrocaput) or the cervical spine (antero- and/or retrocollis) or both in our study population.

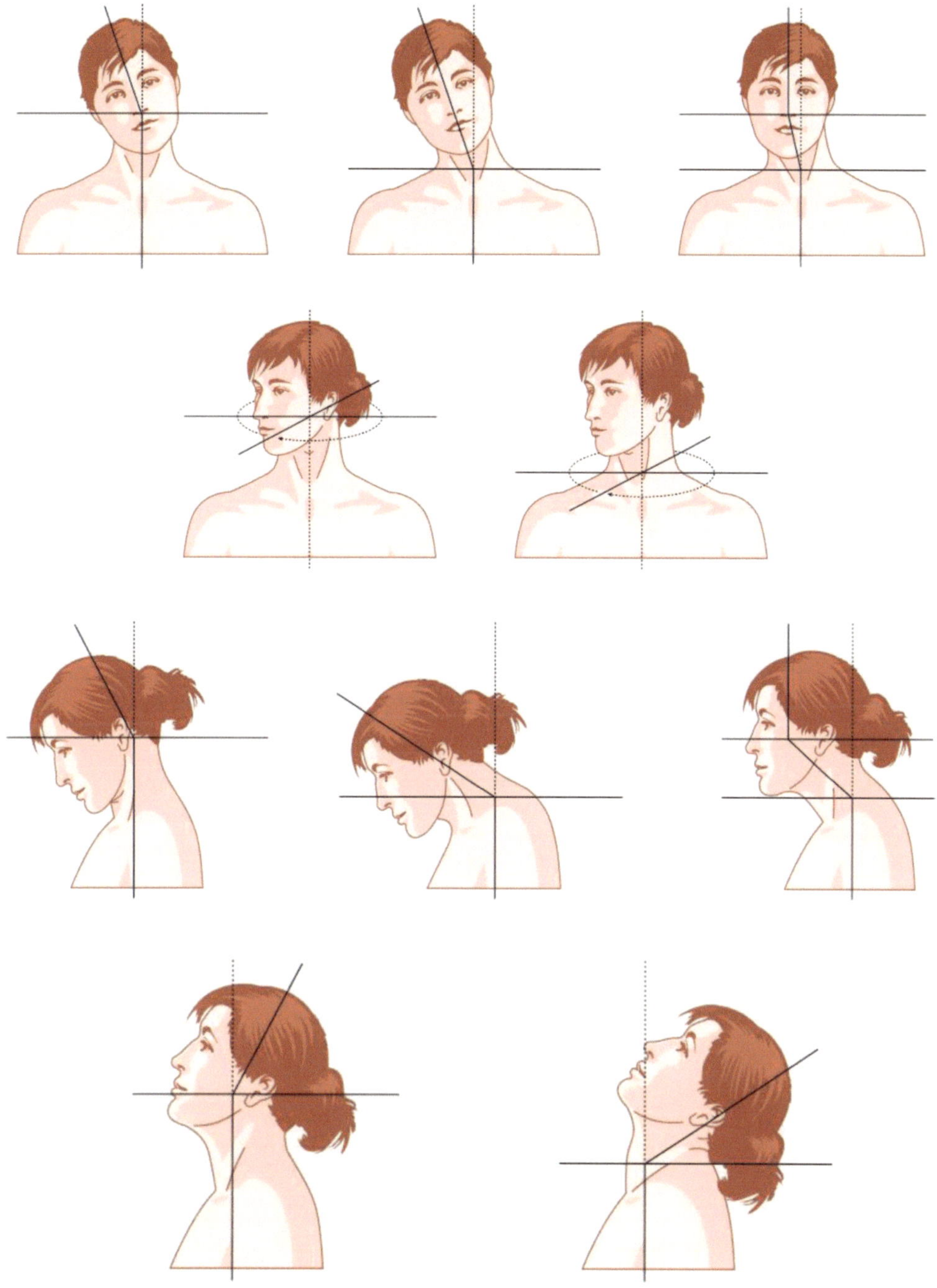

Fig. 8. Schematic representation of all forms of cervical dystonia: From the left: upper row - laterocaput, laterocollis, lateral shift; second row - torticaput, torticollis; third row - anterocaput, anterocollis, forward sagittal shift; bottom row - retrocaput, retrocollis.

Form	**Muscle**	**Origin**	**Insertion**
Laterocollis	Levator scapulae	Proc. transv. CV 1-4	Angulus superior scapulae
	Scalenus anterior	Proc. transv. CV 4-6	Rib 1
	Scalenus medius	Proc. transv. CV 2-7	Rib 1
	Semispinalis cervicis	Proc. transv. upper TV	Proc. spin. lower 4 CV
	Longissimus cervicis	Proc. transv. 6 upper TV	Proc. transv. CV 2-5
Laterocaput	Sternocleidomastoideus	Sternum, clavicula	Proc. mastoideus + linea nuchae superior
	Splenius capitis	Proc. spinosus CV 4-7	Proc. mastoideus
	Splenius cervicis	Proc. spinosus TV 4-6	Proc. transv. CV 1 + 2
	Trapezius pars descendens	Linea nuchae	Lateral third of clavicula
	Semispinalis capitis	Proc. transv. CV 4-7	Linea nuchae
	Longissimus capitis	Proc. transv. CV 5-7 and TV 1-4	Proc. mastoideus
	Levator scapulae	Proc. transv. CV 1-4	Angulus superior scap
Torticollis	Longissimus cervicis	Proc. transv. 6 upper TV	Proc. transv. CV 2-5
	Semispinalis cervicis	Proc. transv. upper TV	Proc. spin. lower 4 CV
Torticaput	**Sternocleidomastoideus**	Sternum, clavicula	Proc. mast. + linea nuchae superior
	Trapezius pars descendens	Linea nuchae	Lateral third of clavicula
	Semispinalis capitis	Proc. transv. CV 4-7	Linea nuchae
	Splenius capitis	Proc. spinosus CV 4-7	Proc. mastoideus
	Splenius cervicis	Proc. spinosus TV 4-6	Proc. transv. CV 1 + 2
	Longissimus capitis	Proc. transv. TV 5-7 and TV 1-4	Proc. mastoideus
	Obliquus capitis inferior	Proc. spinosus axis	Proc. transv. atlantis
Anterocollis bilateral	Scalenus anterior	Proc. transv. CV 4-6	Rib 1
	Scalenus medius	Proc. transv. CV 2-7	Rib 1
	Levator scapulae	Proc. transv. CV 1-4	Angulus superior scapulae
	Longus colli	Proc. transv. CV 2-7	Rib 1
Anterocaput bilateral	**Longus capitis**	Proc. CV 3-6	Pars basilaris ossis occipitalis

Form	Muscle	Origin	Insertion
Retrocollis bilateral	Longissimus cervicis	Proc. transv. 6 upper TV	Proc. transv. CV 2-5
	Semispinalis cervicis	Proc. transv. upper BW	Proc. spin. lower 4 CV
Retrocaput bilateral	**Sternocleidomastoideus**	Sternum, clavicula	Proc. mast. + linea nuchae superior
	Trapezius pars descendens	Linea nuchae	Lateral third of clavicula
	Semispinalis capitis	Proc. transv. CV 4-7	Linea nuchae
	Splenius capitis	Proc. spinosus CV 4-7	Proc. mastoideus
	Splenius cervicis	Proc. spinosus TV 4-6	Proc. transv. CV 1 + 2
	Obliquus capitis inferior	Proc. spinosus axis	Proc. transv. atlantis

Table 4. Muscles involved in the different head posture variants (bold: most frequently affected; from MRI measurements[15]).

Treatment strategies for the individual abnormal dystonic postures will differ according to the function of the muscles in the neck region. For example, in the event of lateral bending, dystonia of the muscles originating from, or inserted in, the head or the first cervical vertebra causes abnormal head posture only when normal alignment of the cervical spine is present (Figure 2). With the involvement of muscles that originate from, or are inserted in, the cervical spine, 'genuine' laterocollis occurs if the relationship of the head to the cervical spine is normal. If both muscle groups are dystonic in the same direction, both muscle groups must be treated. However, dosage must be evaluated for both groups, and final dose is dependent on which of the two groups is most affected. If both muscle groups are affected in opposite directions (i.e. laterocollis and laterocaput), this presents clinically as lateral shift (Figure 6). In this study, sagittal backward shift, a rare presentation, was shown to be a complex cervical dystonia with involvement of the muscles for retrocollis and anterocaput. In contrast, forward sagittal shift, in most cases, was solely caused by bilateral dystonia of the musculus sternocleidomastoidei. Contrary to many earlier reports, bilateral tonus of the musculus sternocleidomastoidei does not cause anterocaput; the head is turned backwards in the sagittal plane and the upper cervical spine is pulled downwards, representing a forward shift (Figure 6c). This was first described in 1895[20], and has been confirmed more recently[21].

The results of this study are intended to provide a more precise differentiation of the variants of CD and thus to maximize the effectiveness of treatment with botulinum toxin. For purposes of treatment, it is necessary to decide which of the muscle groups are primarily dystonic; it is often sufficient to treat only severely affected muscles[22].

It is important to treat the most involved dystonic muscles, but it is just as important not to treat muscles that are not affected; a healthy muscle injected accidentally causes a significant change in the pattern of movement and posture and thus renders it difficult to select strategies for further treatment. If an injection plan is prepared on the basis of the clinical examination and consequently optimum treatment results are achieved (i.e. no complaints for several weeks), further diagnostic procedures are not required. If treatment results are inadequate, imaging procedures should also be used to modify the injection plan.

5. Recommendations for the differentiation and treatment of CD with botulinum toxin and conclusion

Based on our classification of CD, we propose the following recommendations for the treatment of CD with botulinum toxin:

1. To confirm *lateral bending,* it is usually possible to differentiate clinically between laterocollis and laterocaput. In addition, an analysis of the position of the incisura jugularis sterni towards the incisura thyreoidea superior (Figure 4d) is helpful. Should the diagnosis remain unclear, a simple anterior-posterior X-ray is normally sufficient to resolve the problem. In the event of a combination of laterocaput and laterocollis, the relationship of the angles between the thoracic spine and the cervical spine and/or between the cervical spine and the skull is adequate to determine the distribution of botulinum toxin dose between the two different muscle groups.
2. *Lateral shift* inevitably occurs when laterocollis occurs on one side and laterocaput on the other side. Thus, muscles attached to the cervical spine on the side of the shift, and the muscles attached to the skull on the opposing side, require treatment.
3. In the case of *rotation,* reliable clinical differentiation between torticollis and torticaput is difficult. The position of the larynx may be helpful. In the case of torticaput, it tends to remain in the middle, whereas in the presentation of torticollis it tends to be turned to the side. To confirm this form of CD, CT sections at planes C3 and C7 should always be obtained. By comparing the position of the vertebra in both planes, torticollis and torticaput can be reliably differentiated. Additionally, measurements of muscle diameters and shapes on both sides can be extracted from the CT images at C3 and C7, enabling capture of almost all of the muscles involved in CD.
4. An analysis of *forward* flexion (i.e. differentiation between anterocollis and anterocaput) can be performed by lateral examination of the angles between the cervical spine and the thoracic spine and/or between the cervical spine and the base of the skull. This also applies to the analysis of *backward* movement (the differentiation between retrocollis and retrocaput).
5. A *forward sagittal* shift (a combination of anterocollis and retrocaput) is generally caused by bilateral dystonic activity of the musculus sternocleidomastoidei. Conversely, a *backward sagittal shift* is a combination of anterocaput and retrocollis.

In considering our findings, a potential methodological limitation of note was that this study constituted neither a prospective nor a controlled design. However, by recruiting patients without using strict inclusion and exclusion criteria (with the exception of pregnancy and lack of consent), the observed results can be considered to be more representative of the real-life treatment population.

Botulinum toxin administration to the affected muscles is the treatment of choice for primary CD. In order to differentiate between the dystonia affecting muscles inserted in, or originating from, the cervical spine and/or muscles inserted in, or originating from, the skull, supplementation of the clinical examination with CT or MRI is advised. Given the involvement of different muscle groups, it is essential to differentiate between -collis and -caput forms of CD. We have proposed a classification system of 10 basic subtypes of abnormal dystonic positions and postures that we envisage will aid the selection of optimal treatment strategies with botulinum toxin.

6. Acknowledgments

Grateful thanks to Andrea Stenner, MD, Director of the Neurological Specialist Department of the MVZ[1] of the Paracelsus clinik, Zwickau, and Anke Jahn, MD, Member of staff of the Radiological group practice at the Paracelsus clinic, Zwickau, for their expert support and kind help. Thank you also to David Caird, PhD, Ipsen Pharma GmbH, Ettlingen, for help in preparation of the manuscript. Editorial assistance for the preparation of this manuscript was provided by Ogilvy Healthworld Medical Education; funding was provided by Ipsen Pharma GmbH .

7. References

[1] Stacy M, ed. Handbook of dystonia. 2007, Informa: New York.
[2] Jankovic J. Treatment of cervical dystonia. In: Dystonia. M Brin, C Comella, and J Jankovic (eds). Lippincott Williams & Wilkins: Philadelphia, 2004. pp. 159-166.
[3] Hassler R. Torticollis spasticus. In: Begmann G, Frey W, Schwiegk H, editors. Handbuch der Inneren Medizin. Part 3 Neurologie, vol. 5. Berlin: Springer; 1953. p. 774–9.
[4] Yousry T, A. Leews. Imaging of Movement Disorders. An Issue of Neuroimaging Clinics of North America. 2010 Saunders W B Co
[5] Simpson DM, Blitzer A, Brashear A, Comella C, Dubinsky R, Hallett M, et al. Assessment: Botulinum neurotoxin for the treatment of movement disorders (an evidence-based review): Report of the therapeutics and technology assessment subcommittee of the american academy of neurology. Neurology 2008;70(19):1699-706.
[6] Tsui JK, Eisen A, Mak E, Carruthers J, Scott A, Calne DB. A pilot study on the use of botulinum toxin in spasmodic torticollis. Can J Neurol Sci 1985;12(4):314-6.
[7] Costa J, Espirito-Santo C, Borges A, Ferreira JJ, Coelho M, Moore P, et al. Botulinum toxin type a therapy for cervical dystonia. Cochrane Database Syst Rev 2005(1):CD003633.
[8] Swope D, Barbano R. Treatment recommendations and practical applications of botulinum toxin treatment of cervical dystonia. Neurol Clin 2008;26 Suppl 1:54-65.
[9] Jost WH. [clinical use of botulinum toxin]. Nervenarzt 2008;79 Suppl 1:9-14.
[10] Vogt T, Lussi F, Paul A, Urban P. [Long-term therapy of focal dystonia and facial hemispasm with botulinum toxin a]. Nervenarzt 2008;79(8):912-7.
[11] Jankovic J, Schwartz K. Botulinum toxin injections for cervical dystonia. Neurology 1990;40(2):277-80.
[12] Truong D, Brodsky M, Lew M, Brashear A, Jankovic J, Molho E, et al. Long-term efficacy and safety of botulinum toxin type a (Dysport) in cervical dystonia. Parkinsonism Relat Disord 2010;16(5):316-23.
[13] Mohammadi B, Buhr N, Bigalke H, Krampfl K, Dengler R, Kollewe K. A long-term follow-up of botulinum toxin a in cervical dystonia. Neurol Res 2009;31(5):463-6.
[14] Comella CL. The treatment of cervical dystonia with botulinum toxins. J Neural Transm 2008;115(4):579-83.
[15] Reichel G. Therapy guide spasticity - dystonia. 2nd revised & expanded ed: Uni-Med Verlag Bremen 2011.

[1] Medizinisches Versorgungszentrum – AHCC (ambulatory health care center)

[16] Lee LH, Chang WN, Chang CS. The finding and evaluation of emg-guided botox injection in cervical dystonia. Acta Neurol Taiwan 2004;13(2):71-6.
[17] Jost W. Pictorial atlas of botulinum toxin injection: Dosage, localization, application. Berlin: Quintessence Pub Co, 2008.
[18] Camargo CH, Teive HA, Becker N, Baran MH, Scola RH, Werneck LC. Cervical dystonia: Clinical and therapeutic features in 85 patients. Arq Neuropsiquiatr 2008;66(1):15-21.
[19] Reichel G, Stenner A, Jahn A. Zur Phänomenologie der zervikalen Dystonien [the phenomenology of cervical dystonia]. Fortschr Neurol Psychiatr 2009;77(5):272-7.
[20] Mikulicz J. Über die Exstirpation des Kopfnickers beim muskulären Schiefhals, nebst Bemerkungen zur Pathologie dieses Leidens. Centralblatt für Chirurgie 1895;22:1-10.
[21] Platzer W. Color atlas of human anatomy 1. Locomotor system. Vol 1. New York: Thieme Stuttgart, 2003.
[22] Hefter H. [Aspects of the complexity of cervical dystonia]. Nervenarzt 2008;79 Suppl 1:15-8.

3

Dystonia of the Oromandibular, Lingual and Laryngeal Areas

Karla Odell and Uttam K. Sinha
University of Southern California, Keck School of Medicine
USA

1. Introduction

Head and neck dystonias, like in other types of dystonias, are defined clinically by the presence of involuntary sustained, forceful muscle contractions leading to characteristic rhythmic movements and abnormal postures.[1,2] Cranio-cervical manifestations of dystonia can have a significant effect on a person's quality of life by impacting the ability for speech, swallowing and social interaction. Oromandibular, lingual, laryngeal and cervical dystonias can occur as part of a generalized neurodegenerative disorder or can be a focal primary dystonia.[3, 4] Focal primary dystonias of the head and neck can be task specific where the dystonic action is triggered by speaking. In some cases, the dystonic action can be overcome with a "geste antagoniste" or sensory trick. Tactile or sensory stimulation in the region of the affected muscle group causes relaxation of the dystonic muscles.[5] Understanding the particular muscle involved in the dystonia and that muscle's normal function is important to diagnose and treat cranio-cervical dystonias.

The mainstay of treatment for focal dystonia of the head and neck is Botulinum toxin (BoNT) injection.[6] Since its introduction in 1980 to treat childhood strabismus, BoNT has become the treatment of choice in a number of conditions characterized by focal involuntary muscle over activity. Patients suffering from head and neck dystonias require repeated injections to treat symptoms.[8] This present chapter focuses on BoNT treatment protocols for oromandibular, lingual and laryngeal dystonia. BoNT for cervical dystonia is discussed in related chapters.

2. Oromandibular dystonia

Oromandibular dystonia (OMD) is a disorder where repetitive or sustained spams of the masticatory muscles result in involuntary jaw opening, closing or a combination. [12] This disorder can produce painful muscle contractions resulting in abnormal positions of the mouth, jaw or tongue affecting speech and swallow function. OMD can be idiopathic, either focal or as part of generalized dystonia, or secondary to medications, trauma, metabolic disorders or other neurologic movement disorders.[13-15] Focal oromandibular dystonia is rare.[3] In the focal idiopathic form, disease onset typically occurs between 30-70 years of age and occurs twice as frequently in women.[13,16] Initially, dystonic episodes may be triggered by specific tasks such as eating, speaking or swallowing. Later less specific motor tasks induce the symptoms and in advanced stages dystonic movements can occur at rest.[17,18] The majority of cases are idiopathic though can occur with phenothiazine use or head injury.[19] A 12 year follow up study on a patient with OMD, highlighted the influence of hormonal factors on OMD as more severe symptoms occur during stress or menses.[12] Although the exact pathogenesis is unknown, neurotransmitter abnormalities which result in disturbed firing pattern of the basal ganglia are likely involved in the abnormal muscle contraction.[20]

Oromandibular dystonia can be classified as jaw opening or jaw closing dystonia. Knowing the muscles of mastication, their actions and attachments is important to understanding the symptoms and treatment of OMD. The muscles of mastication are innervated by the trigeminal nerve and include the temporalis, masseter and medial and lateral pterygoids. The temporalis muscle originates in the temporalis fossa of the temporal bone and inserts on the cornoid process and anterior surface the mandible ramus and functions to elevate and retract the mandible. The masseter originates at the zygomatic arch and attaches to the angle and ramus of the mandible and functions to elevate the mandible. The medial pterygoid originates from the medial surface of the lateral pterygoid plate and the tuberosity of maxilla and attaches to the medial surface of the mandible angle and ramus. It functions to elevate and protract the mandible. The lateral pterygoid muscle has a superior and inferior head. The superior head originates at the greater wing of sphenoid and attaches to the capsule and articular disk of temporomandibular joint. The inferior head originates at lateral surface of lateral pterygoid plate superior head and attaches to the neck of mandible. The lateral pterygoid elevates and protrudes the mandible.[21]

Jaw opening dystonia is caused by sustained contraction of the lateral pterygoid muscle resulting in the inability to close the mouth. Prolonged jaw opening results in difficulty with mastication, swallowing and causes drooling. Patients have difficulty articulating and have unintelligible speech.[22]The dystonic movements can impact chewing and swallowing so much the significant weight loss can occur.[23] Often idiopathic jaw opening dystonia may be misdiagnosed as dental problems, bruxism or temporo-mandibular joint disorders.[12,24]

Jaw closing dystonias can occur alone or in association with jaw opening dystonias as general OMD dysfunction.[14] Involuntary contraction of the masseter muscle results in sustained trismus and jaw clenching. Jaw closing dystonias have been described in musicians who play wind instruments and develop task specific dystonia in response to attempting to play their instrument.[25]

Assessment of patients with OMD requires exclusion of brain injury or other secondary causes. MRI is performed to evaluate for stroke or mass involving the basal ganglia. Basic laboratory tests are also performed. A blood ceruloplasmin level and slit lamp exam to rule out Wilson's disease should be performed.[26] Also a thorough evaluation of the temporomandibular joint should be performed to evaluate for other disorders. A non-reducing TMJ disk displacement disorder can mimic jaw clenching (closing) dystonia.[3]

Therapeutic options for OMD include systemic medications, BoNT injections, speech therapy and the use of oral sensory devices. Both jaw opening and jaw closing OMD can be treated with oral anti dystonic therapies such as tetrabenazine, diazepam and carbamazepine. Anticholinergic drugs reduce muscle spasm by centrally inhibiting the parasympathic system. Benzodiazepine decreases monosynaptic and polysynaptic reflexes by increasing presynaptic GABA inhibition a similar action to Baclofen. Anticonvulsants such as carbamazepine reduce severe muscle spasm by decreasing polysynaptic response. Carbidopa/levodopa in low dose may help dopa-responsive dystonia.[26] Effectiveness of medical therapy for OMD is variable in the literature but only approximately 17% of patients with OMD responded reported significant benefit from medical therapy.[14]

For focal dystonias, BoNT has been shown to be superior to medical therapy. For jaw opening dystonias the target muscle is the lateral pterygoid muscle.[27] The technique is an intraoral injection performed by following the ramus of the mandible to locate the lateral ptyergoid and injecting approximately 45 units on each side.[28] For jaw closing dystonia, BoNT is injected into the masseter muscle. Palpation of the muscle at the angle of the mandible is performed and 20 units of BoNT are injected into each site. The use of BoNT injections have been shown to improve the quality of life and have a significant perceived benefit from patients.[29] In a study comparing jaw opening and jaw closing dystonias, jaw opening dystonias have been shown to respond better to BoNT therapy.[14] Jaw deviation dystonia may likewise occur and BoNT injections are done at the temporalis muscle (best approached injecting anterior fibers of muscle) ipsilateral to the jaw deviation and at the lateral pterygoid muscle in the contralateral side.[27] Side effects of BoNT injection for OMD include jaw weakness, loss of smile, jaw tremor, dysphagia and nasal regurgitation, but side effects are decreased with dose adjustment and accurate injection.[3,30]

"Geste antagoniste" or oral sensory feedback devices can be used in the treatment of OMD and as an adjunct to BoNT therapy. The use of an oral sensory device has been shown to decrease the frequency and dose of BoNT required to treat OMD.[24] For jaw opening dystonia, the device is a custom molded retainer that fits the mandibular teeth. Over the molars there is an extra prominence that, when the patient bites down, stimulates the lateral pterygoid muscle to overcome the dystonic action and results in relaxation of the muscle. [24] For jaw closing dystonia, a prostodontist device that fits over the teeth prevents complete jaw closing. This device helps to inhibit masseter muscle firing to overcome jaw closing dystonia.[25]

OMD can dramatically affect communication and swallowing function and it is therefore important to address the social, emotional and nutritional impact of the disorder. A multidisplinary approach with combining medical treatment with speech therapy and a nutritionist are important in address the needs of patients with OMD.

3. Lingual dystonia

Lingual dystonia affects the intrinsic muscles of the tongue resulting in repetitive tongue protrusion or tongue contraction.[31,32] Dystonic movements of the tongue are a well-recognized feature of tardive dystonia which develops secondary to first generation anti-psychotic medication.[33] Primary or idiopathic lingual dystonia is a very rare disabling cranial dystonia that impacts speaking, chewing and swallowing. The movements vary from repetitive to sustained tongue tip protrusion or contraction which can be action induced with speaking, eating and whistling.[34-36] In severe cases it is associated with tongue biting and has even caused life threatening airway obstruction.[37] Speech can be unintelligible and lingual dystonia can impact swallowing significantly resulting weight loss.[38]

While idiopathic lingual dystonia does occur, it is very rare and therefore it is important to evaluate for secondary causes. In addition to medications, lingual dystonia has been reported to occur secondary to head injury, electrical injury, varicella infection or part of a neurodegenerative disease. [39-42]Action induced lingual dystonia can be a striking and early finding in chorea-acanthocytosis. It is also a characteristic of pantothenate kinase associated neurodegeneration (PKAN), Lesch-Nyhan syndrome and Wilsons disease.[38] In one of the largest series of lingual dystonia cases, Esper et al reported the 41% of cases were secondary to medications, 18% heredodegenerative and post encephalitic, 12% generalized dystonia and 29% focal primary lingual dystonia.[34]

Evaluation of a patient with lingual dystonia requires a complete history especially a detailed drug history. History of trauma, infections and the association of symptoms with a specific action or the improvement of symptoms with a sensory trick are important to elucidate. A full neurologic evaluation is required, as lingual dystonia associated with neurodegenerative diseases often presents with other neurologic symptoms. Laboratory tests including creatinine kinase and ceruloplasmin level and brain imaging should be performed.[40]

While BoNT injections have been the mainstay of treatment for other primary focal dystonias, in lingual dystonia BoNT has been approached with caution. There is limited experience and have been reports of severe dysphagia and dysarthria after injection. Blitzer et al cautioned against using BoNT injections in patients with focal lingual dystonia as results are often disappointing and half of his patients developed significant dysphagia and aspiration pneumonia.[43] Esper et al recently published one of the largest series of patients with lingual dystonia and the use of BoNT. Their results found it to be a safe and effective treatment with a 55% of the patients sustaining a marked improvement and 97.8% of BoNT sessions without any significant adverse effects.[34] They used a submandibular approach to inject the genioglossus muscles. The patient is positioned supine with the head tilted back. The placement of the needle is approximately two fingerbreadths back from the midline body of the mandible and 1-2cm lateral. The needle is placed with EMG guidance through the digastric muscle into the genioglossus muscle approximately 2cm deep. The position is confirmed with EMG when the patient protrudes the tongue. The BoNT is injected into a single location. They recommend starting with 5 units in each genioglossus muscle with an increased by 2.5 units in each successive treatment until the patients achieves a reasonable response.[34]

Oral medications for the treatment of lingual dystonia are similar to the medical treatment of other focal dystonias. Medical management includes tetrabenazine, anticholinergics, benzodiazepines and levodopa with variable success reported in the literature.[31,32,35,36,40] Sensory tricks such as chewing bubble gum or sucking on a fruit seed may give patients relief from their symptoms or as an adjuvant to pharmacologic therapy.[36] Deep brain stimulation performed in patients with generalized dystonia, has been shown to improve tongue protrusion dystonia. Therefore deep brain stimulation should be considered in severe or medically refractive cases of lingual dystonia.[38]

4. Laryngeal dystonias

Laryngeal dystonia, also referred to as spasmodic dysphonia is a focal, action-induced dystonia that affects the laryngeal muscles. Involuntary muscle contraction of the vocal folds produces vocal strain, breathiness and phonatory breaks.[44] Laryngeal dystonia can be classified as adductor type, abductor type, mixed type or adductor laryngeal breathing dystonia.[1] The adductor type accounts for 80% of laryngeal dystonia and results from spasms of vocal fold adductor muscles resulting in inappropriate closing of the vocal folds with speech.[45] With the adductor type extreme effort is exerted to achieve fluent speech and the patient's voice quality is harsh and strained with voice breaks. The abductor type is rarer, with uncontrolled spasms of the vocal fold abductors resulting in speech with sustained breathiness and breathy voice breaks, sometimes to the point of aphonia. Mixed laryngeal dystonia has characteristics of the adductor and abductor types. Adductor laryngeal breathing dystonia is characterized by persistent inspiratory stridor and usually a normal voice with a paroxysmal cough. In all types of laryngeal dystonia, the dystonic muscles contractions are task specific usually affecting speech while sparing other laryngeal tasks such as breathing, singing, swallowing or coughing.[1] Laryngeal dystonia can also be associated with other dystonias such as blepharospasm, cervical dystonia or writer's cramp.[46]

Initially thought to be psychogenic in origin, the current thinking is laryngeal dystonia is a central neurologic processing disorder.[1] There have been several studies that demonstrate differences on neuroimaging and postmortem tissues in the basal ganglia and brainstem in patients with laryngeal dystonia compared to controls. [47,48] However these neuroimaging studies can be difficult to interpret and the knowledge regarding the pathologic mechanism are limited. [47]

Understanding the anatomy of the larynx and the function of intrinsic muscles of the larynx can elucidate the symptoms and treatment for different types of dystonia. There are six intrinsic muscles of the larynx and all are innervated by the recurrent laryngeal nerve, except the cricothyroid muscle which is innervated by the external branch of the superior laryngeal nerve.[21] The vocal fold adductors are the lateral cricoarytenoid, throarytenoid, cricothyroid and interarytenoid muscles. The thyroarytenoids are broad, thin muscles that lies parallel with and lateral to the vocal fold. It arises in front from the lower half of the angle of the thyroid cartilage, and from the middle cricothyroid ligament. Its fibers pass backward and laterally, to be inserted into the base and anterior surface of the arytenoid cartilage. In addition to adduction, the thyroarytenoid increases vocal fold tension and is the muscle target for BoNT injection in adductor laryngeal dystonia. The only abductor of the vocal folds is the posterior cricoarytenoid muscles. They are paired muscles that extend from the posterior cricoid cartilage to the arytenoid cartilages in the larynx, and abduct the vocal folds by rotating the arytenoid cartilages laterally.[21] This is the muscle targeted for BoNT injection in abductor laryngeal dystonia.

Diagnosis of laryngeal dystonia requires multidisplinary evaluation by an otolaryngologist, speech therapist and neurologist. A history of progressive symptoms with onset after a stressful life event, association with other dystonias or family history of dystonia supports the diagnosis of laryngeal dystonia. Similar to other focal dystonias, sensory tricks such as humming are effective in reducing the dystonic movement. As mentioned previously, other functions of the vocal folds such as laughing, coughing, or crying are not affected in laryngeal dystonia and unlike other functional voice disorders laryngeal dystonia does not improve with speech therapy alone.[1] Neurological evaluation includes evaluating for other neurodegenerative diseases such as Wilsons or Parkinson's disease which can cause secondary laryngeal dystonia. Flexible laryngoscopy and strobe exam are essential to diagnosis, to evaluate for other causes of voice problems and access the severity of the dystonia. During laryngoscopy, glottic function is observed for disruptions, spasms, breathy breaks and tremor while the patient speaks sentence segments.[49] Laryngeal EMG is useful to diagnosis laryngeal dystonia though no specific findings are pathognomonic for this form of dystonia. Adductor laryngeal dystonia may show abnormally high activity in the thyroartenoid and cricothyroid muscles. Posterior cricoarytenoid and thyroaryentoid will have abnormally high activity in abductor laryngeal dystonia. Large polyphasic motor unit potentials with phonation and irregular tremor can also be seen. [50]

The mainstay of treatment for laryngeal dystonia is BoNT injection. Oral medications, speech therapy, surgery and deep brain stimulation are used as adjuvants or in patients non responsive to BoNT injection. Pharmacotherapies for laryngeal dystonia are similar to other types of dystonias and include anticholinergics, benzodiazepines, or baclofen.[51] Long term relief of symptoms with systemic agents is limited in laryngeal dystonia.[52]

The first BoNT toxin injection for the treatment of laryngeal dystonia was given by Biltzer in 1984 and since then BoNT injection has become the main treatment modality. [53]For adductor laryngeal dystonia, injection of one or both of the thyroarytenoid muscles is performed. Using EMG, a needle is passed through the cricothyroid membrane in the midline and is angled superior lateral in the direction of the thyroarytenoid muscles. Confirmation is made with EMG by asking the patient to phonate. Injection of 0.625-4units of botox is performed per muscle depending on the individual. For new patients, an initial dose of 1-2.5 units per thyroarytenoid muscle has been proposed as a starting dose.[54] If the patient does not tolerate bilateral injections, the injections can be staggered several weeks apart. Blitzer et al showed BoNT injections for laryngeal dystonia had an average onset of action to be 2.4 days with peak effect of 9 days. Patients received an average of 15 weeks of benefit and achieved a voice quality 92% of normal.[54] For abductor laryngeal dystonia, BoNT is injected into the posterior cricoarytenoid muscles. Since the posterior cricoarytenoid muscle is the only abductor of the vocal folds, over injection of botulism can result in the inability to abduct the vocal folds during inspiration causing stridor and dyspnea. Therefore, unilateral injection of the posterior cricoarytenoid muscle that appears to have the greatest spasm on laryngoscopy is performed.[54] The technique for posterior cricoarytenoid muscle injection involves rotating the patient's larynx away from side of injection and passing the needle just posterior to the posterior edge of the thyroid cartilage at the level of the cricoid. The needle is advanced to the posterior plate of the cricoid and correct position is confirmed with EMG by asking the patient to sniff. A dose of 3.75 units is initially used. If injection of one side only is not sufficient, a repeat dose of the same side or a conservative contralateral injection can be performed a later time. Concurrent bilateral injections are avoided because of airway compromise. If stridor or significant narrowing of the glottis occurs no further injections are performed.[55] The dose requirements vary between patients and are not specific to the age or gender of the patient.[56]

Complications of BoNT injections include transient breathy hypophonia, hoarseness, swallowing difficulties and pain. More serious complications include more severe dysphagia or airway compromise.[49,54,55,57] While BoNT is effective in treating the symptoms of laryngeal dystonia, it requires multiple physician visits for repeat injections and the decline in voice quality before the next injection has an impact on the patient's quality of life.[58]

Various surgical procedures have been developed to provide a long term benefit for patients with adductor laryngeal dystonia. Procedures include a recurrent laryngeal nerve section, thyroarytenoid myectomy, expansion laryngoplasty and selective laryngeal denervation-reinnervation.[57] First described by Dedo in the 1970s unilateral recurrent laryngeal nerve section was an initial surgical treatment for laryngeal dystonia.[59] However, with high long term failure rates and poorer voice outcomes this technique has fallen out of favor. Berke et al described a selective denervation of the adductor branches of the recurrent laryngeal nerve bilaterally with immediate reinnevervation using the ansa cervicalis but long term data on this procedure is limited.[60] In general, surgical treatment is reserved for patients who do not respond to BoNT treatment.

Speech and physical therapy are important adjuvants to the treatment of laryngeal dystonia. Where speech therapy has its greatest value is in teaching patients who do not go through injection therapy or are in-between injections to manage the symptoms of the disorder with proper compensatory strategies. These include relaxation techniques, use of diaphragmatic breathing and easy onset tone production, reduced number of words per utterance, with the goals of reducing both excessive adduction and increased subglottal pressure. Sometimes, slight pitch elevation for automatic responses and use of vegetative gestures also help as 'starters' of clearer vocalizations.[61] Physical therapy includes myofascial release, integrated manual therapies and laryngeal manipulation.

5. Conclusions

Focal dystonia of the oromandibular, lingual and laryngeal areas are particularly debilitating because they affect the basic human functions of breathing, eating and communicating. While BoNT is effective for the treatment of these forms of dystonia, it is only a temporary treatment and has side effects. Surgery and deep brain stimulation offer the potential for longer lasting symptom relief but there is still much work to be done to perfect techniques. Research is focused on better understanding of the underlying brain pathophysiology causing the focal dystonia and to develop targeted treatments.

6. References

[1] Grillone GA, Chan T. Larygeal dystonia. Otolaryngologic Clinics of North America 2006;39(1):87-100.

[2] Colosimo C, Suppa A, Fabbrini G, Bologna M, Berardelli A. Craniocervical dystonia: clinical and pathophysiological features. European Journal of Neurology 2010;17(1):15-21.

[3] Lee KH. Oromandibular dystonia. Oral Surg Oral Med Oral Pathol Oral Radiol Endod 2007;104(4):491-496

[4] Tintner R, Jankovic J. Botulism Toxin type A in the management of oromandibular dystonia and bruxism. Scientific and Theraputic aspects of Botulism Toxin. Phildelphia, PA: Lippincott Williams and Wilkins; 2002 p 1-12.

[5] Filipovic SR, Jahanshahi M, Viswanathan R, Heywood P, Rodger D, Bhatia KP. Clinical Features of the geste antagoniste in cervical dystonia. Adv Neurol. 2004;94:191-201

[6] Albanese A, Asmus F, Bhatia KP, Elia AE, Elibol B, Filippini G, Gasser T, Krauss JK, Nardocci N, Newton A, Valls-Sole J. EFNS guidelines on diagnosis and treatment of primary dystonias. European Journal of Neurology 2011;18:5-18.

[7] Braun T, Gurkov R, Hempel JM, Berghaus A, Krause E. Patient benefit from treatment with botulinum neurotoxin A for functional indications in otorhinolaryngology. Eur Arch Otorhinolaryngol 2010;267:1963-1967
[8] Michelotti A, Silva R, Paduano S, Cimino R, Farella M. Oromandibular dystonia and hormonal factors: twelve years follow-up of a case report. J Oral Rehabil. 2009 Dec;36(12):916-21
[9] Balasubramaniam R, Rasmussen J, Carlson LW, Van Sickels JE, Okeson JP. Oromandibular dystonia revisited: a review and a unique case. J Oral Maxillofac Surg 2008;66:379-386.
[10] Singer C, Papapetropoulos S. A comparison of jaw-closing and jaw opening idiopathic oromandibular dystonia. Parkinsonism and Related Disorders 2006;12:115-118.
[11] Heise GJ, Mullen MP. Oromandibular dystonia treated with botulinum toxin: report of case. J Oral Maxillofac Surg 1995;53:332-335
[12] Epidemiologic Study of Dystonia in Europe (ESDE) Collaborative Group. Sex related influences on the frequency and age of onset of primary dystonia. Neurology.1999;53:1871-1873.
[13] Moore P, Naumann M. Handbook of botulism toxin treatment. Oxford: Blackwell Science Ltd; 2003
[14] Stacy MA. Handbook of dystonia. London: Informa Health Care; 2006
[15] Ngeow JYY, Prakash KM, Chowbay B, Quek ST, Choo S. Capecitabine-induced oromandibular dystonia: a case report and literature review. Acta Oncol. 2008;47(6):1161-5.
[16] Berardelli A, Rothwell JC, Hallett M, Thompson PD, Manfredi M, Marsden CD. The pathophysiology of primary dystonia. Brain 1998; 121:1195-1212.
[17] Moore KL, Dalley AF, Agur AMR Clinically Oriented Anatomy. Lippincott Williams and Wilkins. 6th Edition ; Feb 2009.
[18] Merz RI, Deakin J, Hawthorne MR. Oromandibular dystonia questionnaire (OMDQ-25): a valid and reliable instrument for measuring health-related quality of life. Clin Otolaryngol 2010;35:390-396.
[19] Papapetropoulos S, Singer C. Eating dysfunction associated with oromandibular dystonia: clinical characteristics and treatment considerations Head & Face Medicine 2006, 2:47.
[20] Verma SP, Sinha UK. Use of an oral sensory feedback device in the management of jaw-opening dystonia. Otolaryngology - Head and Neck Surgery 2009;141:142-143
[21] Frucht S, Fahn S, Ford B. A geste antagoniste device to treat jaw-closing dystonia. Movement Disorders 1999;14(5):883-885.
[22] Balasubramaniam R, Ram S. Orofacial Movement Disorders. Oral Maxillofacial Surg Clin N Am 20 (2008) 273–285.
[23] Moller E, Bakke M, Dalager T, Werdelin LM. Oromandibular dystonia involving the lateral pterygoid muscles: four cases with different complexity. Movement Disorders 2007;22(6):785-790.
[24] Mendes A, Upton LG. Management of dystonia of the lateral pterygoid muscle with botulinum toxin A. British Journal of Oral Maxillofacial Surg 2009;47:481-483.
[25] Bhattacharyya N, Tarsy D. Impact on quality of life of botulinum toxin treatments for spasmodic dysphonia and oromandibular dystonia. Arch Otorhinolaryngol Hean and Neck Sugery 2001;127:389-392.

[26] Adler CH, Factor SA, Brin M, Sethi KD. Secondary nonresponsiveness to botulinum toxin type A in patients with oromandibular dystonia. Movement Disorders 2002;17(1):158-161.
[27] Rosales RL, Ng AR, Delos Santos MM, Fernandez HH. The Broadening Application of Chemodenervation in X-Linked Dystonia-Parkinsonism (Part II): An Open-Label Experience With Botulinum Toxin-A (Dysport_R) Injections for Oromandibular, Lingual, and Truncal Dystonias. International Journal of Neuroscience, 121, 44–56, 2011.
[28] Baik SB, Park JH, Kim JY. Primary lingual dystonia induced speaking. Movement Disorders 2004;19:1251-1252.
[29] Papapetropoulos S, Singer C. Primary focal lingual dystonia. Movement Disorders 2006;21(3):429-430.
[30] Hennings JMH, Krause E, Botzel K, Wetter TC. Successful treatment of tardive lingual dystonia with botulinum toxin: Case report and review of the literature. Progress in Neuro-Psychopharmacology & Biological Psychiatry 2008;32:1167-1171.
[31] Esper CD, Freeman A, Factor SA. Lingual protrusion dystonia: Frequency, etiology and botulinum toxin therapy. Parkinsonism and Related Disorders 2010;16:438-441.
[32] Ishii K, Tamaoka A, Shoji S. A case of primary focal lingual dystonia induced by speaking. Eur J Neurol 2001;8:507.
[33] Tan EK, Chan LL. Sensory tricks and treatment in primary lingual dystonia. Movement Disorders 2005;3:388.
[34] Jacobsen R. Out-of-Hospital Lingual Dystonia Resulting in Airway Obstruction Prehosp Emerg Care. 2011 Oct-Dec;15(4):537-40.
[35] Schneider SA, Aggarwal A, Bhatt M, Dupont E, Tisch S, Limousin P, Lee P, Quinn N, Bhatia KP. Severe tongue protrusion dystonia Neurology 2006;2:940-943.
[36] Bader B, Walker, RH, Vogel M, Prosiegel M, McIntosh J, Danek A. Tongue protrusion and feeding dystonia: A hallmark of chorea-acanthocytosis. Movement Disorders 2010;25:127-129.
[37] Felicio AC, Godeiro-Junion C, Moriyama TS, Laureano MR, Felix EPV, Borges V, Silva SMA, Ferraz HB. Speech-induced lingual dystonia. Arq Neuropsiquiatr 2010;68(4):653-655.
[38] Ondo W. Lingual dystonia following electrical injury. Movement Disorder 1997;12:253.
[39] Gollomp SM, Fahn S. Transient dystonia as a complication of varicella. J Neurology Neurosurgery Psychiatry 1987;50:1228-1229.
[40] Blitzer A, Brin MF, Fahn S. Botulinum toxin injections for lingual dystonia. Laryngoscope 1991;101:799.
[41] Bailey B, Johnson JT. Head and Neck Surgery Otolaryngology. Lippincott Williams and Wilkins. 4th Edition 2006:876-877.
[42] Blitzer A, Brin MF, Stewart C. Botulism toxin management of spasmodic dysphonia: a 12-year experience in more than 900 patients. Laryngoscope 1998; 108:1435-1441
[43] Brin MF, Fahn S, Blitzer A. Movement Disorders of the larynx. Neurological disorders of the larynx .Thieme Medical Publishers; 1992:240-248
[44] Ludlow CL. Treatment for spasmodic dysphonia: limitations of current approaches. Curr Opin Otolaryngol Head Neck Surg 2009;17(3):160-165.
[45] Simoyan K, Ludlow CL, Vortmeyer AO. Brainstem pathology in spasmodic dysphonia. Laryngoscope 2010;120:121-124

[46] Gibbs SR, Blitzer A. Botulinum toxin for the treatment of spasmodic dysphonia. Otolaryngologic Clinics of North America 2000;33(4):879-894.
[47] Blitzer A, Lovelace RE, Brin MF. Electromyographic findings in focal laryngeal dystonia. Ann Otol Rhinol Laryngol. 1985;94:591-594
[48] Blitzer A, Brin M. Spasmodic dysphonia: evaluation and management. The larynx: a multidisciplinary approach 2nd Edition. Salem: Mosby Year Book Inc, 1996:187-198
[49] Watts C, Nye C, Whurr R. Botulinum for treating spasmodic dysphonia (laryngeal dystonia): a systematic Cochrane review. Clin Rehabil 2006;20:112-122.
[50] Blitzer A, Brin M, Fahn S, Lovlace RE. The use of Botulism toxin in the treatment of focal laryngeal dystonia. Laryngoscope 1988;98:193.
[51] Blitzer A. Spasmodic dysphonia and botulinum toxin: experience from the largest treatment series. European Journal of Neurology 2010;17(1):28-30.
[52] Ludlow CL. Spasmodic dysphonia: a laryngeal control disorder specific to speech. The Journal of Neuoscience 2011;31(3):793-797.
[53] Vasconcelos S, Birkent H, Sardesai MG, Merati AL, Hillel AD. Influence of age and gender on dose and effectiveness of botulinum toxin for laryngeal dystonia. Laryngoscope 2009;119:2004-2007.
[54] Merati AL, Heman-Ackah YD, Abaza M, Altman KW, Sulica L, Belamowicz S. Otolaryngology - Head and Neck Surgery 2005;133:654-665.
[55] Paniello RC, Barlow J, Serna JS. Longitudinal follow-up of adductor spasmodic dysphonia patients after botulism toxin injection: quality of life results. Laryngoscope 2008; 118:564-568.
[56] Dedo HH. Recurrent laryngeal nerve section for spasmodic dysphonia. Ann Otol Rhinol Laryngol 1976;85:451-459
[57] Tassorelli C, Mancini F, Balloni L. Botulism Toxin and Neuromotor Rehabilation. An integrated approach to idiopathic cervical dystonia. Movement Disorders 2006;21:2240-2243
[58] Ramdharry G. Case Report: physiotherapy cuts the dose of botulism toxin. Physiotherapy Research International 2006;11:117-122.

4

Dystonia Arising from Occupations: The Clinical Phenomenology and Therapy

Criscely L. Go[1,2] and Raymond L. Rosales[1,3,*]
[1]*Center for Neurodiagnostic and Therapeutic Services (CNS), Metropolitan Medical Center, Manila,*
[2]*University of Florida Center for Movement Disorders and Neurorestoration Gainesville, Florida,*
[3]*Dept. of Neurology and Psychiatry, University of Santo Tomas and Hospital, Manila,*
[1,3]*Philippines*
[2]*USA*

1. Introduction

Dystonia is generally referred to belong to the generic terms, *muscle spasm* and *muscle stiffness*. *Muscle spasms* would be any involuntary abnormal muscle contraction, regardless of whether it is painful or not, that cannot be usually terminated by voluntary relaxation. *Muscle stiffness* is an involuntary muscle shortening that usually lasts for seconds to minutes, but may be sustained. Sustained muscle contraction may lead to posturing and even pain as seen in tetany, dystonia, spasticity, and contracture. Whereas *tetany* is brisk, short-lived, and associated with paresthesiae, *dystonia* is a slow, more sustained co-contraction of the agonist and antagonist muscles, that may characteristically be task-specific and abolished by "sensory tricks."(1)

Limb Dystonia is a movement disorder characterized by excessive and overflow muscle contraction leading to abnormal limb postures (i.e. flexion, extension, twisting, abducting and adducting) and impaired movement. Limb dystonia may be focal (limited to a single body area), segmental (affecting at least two adjacent muscle groups), or a component of hemidystonia and generalized dystonia. It has been described in writers, typists, golfers, musicians, and many other occupations, and is often associated with markedly disabling loss of function.

Focal hand dystonia was first recognized by its characteristic impairment of specific tasks. It has a tendency to cluster in those with particular occupations so that it was once thought of as psychogenic in origin. The task specific focal hand dystonia arising from occupations (i.e. occupational cramp) include variants like writer's cramp, musician's cramp and sports' cramp (e.g. golfer's cramp). Embouchure's dystonia, mainly affecting the lips, jaw and tongue, is included in this category. In task specific dystonia, primary sensory modalities are

* Corresponding Author

intact, although impaired spatial or temporal discrimination may be identified if specifically sought(2). The neurological examination is essentially normal except for the dystonic movements. Actions eliciting the dystonia may be performed slowly and irregularly but there is no ataxia. This chapter aims to highlight the phenomenology, pathophysiology, clinical course and management of occupationally-related dystonias. Not only are these forms of dystonias characteristically mistaken to have psychogenic origins, but also that these disorders impinge on the profession and quality of life of the affected individuals. We cap this chapter with a peculiar illustrative case if only to emphasize the precepts of the phenomenology and management strategy of this kind of a dystonia.

2. Phenomenology of task specific dystonias

Focal dystonia, as with other dystonic disorders, have common characteristic features that distinguish it from other hyperkinetic movement disorders. There is co-contraction of agonists and antagonist groups of muscles and the contractions result in abnormal limb postures. The contraction is of relatively long duration and sustained as compared to that of chorea or athetosis and usually involves the same muscle groups. This involvement of the same muscle groups termed "patterned" movements may remain focal or may, in time, involve contiguous body parts. In the latter case, the term segmental dystonia may apply.

There is a directionality and predictability of the movements somehow being stereotypical in character. Variability speaks more of a psychogenic dystonia rather than an organic one.

Another special characteristic of the dystonias is the response to certain "sensory tricks" whereby doing something else apart from the task may alleviate the dystonia such as chewing a gum while playing a wind instrument relieves the lip dystonia in some musicians. There is a tendency for the movements to worsen with fatigue, stress, anxiety.

Sometimes, the dystonic contractions can occur rapidly and repeatedly mimicking a tremor. The feature that distinguishes it from the latter is the relatively irregular occurrence of the dystonic tremor, the apparent increase in the tremor when the muscles involved are pulled opposite to the direction of its contraction and activation of the muscles not required for maintenance of that particular posture(3). For this chapter, we focus our attention to task specific focal dystonias or those occurring in situations whereby repetitive skilled movements are essential to its development.

The first symptom of focal hand dystonia is usually a feeling of tightness or loss of facility with a previously easily performed action, often accompanied by fatigue and aching in the affected arm and forearm that worsens with continued use. In the case of embouchure's dystonia, there is initial feeling of tightness around the lip with somewhat difficulty in controlling lip and jaw movements. Pain, quite common in cervical dystonias, may not be as frequent in occupational dystonia. If indeed pain occurs, this could be part of muscle fatigue, myofascial pain component or corresponding joint changes. Overtime, there is involuntary posturing of the limb (or the lips, jaw or tongue in the case of embouchure's dystonia) during the performance of the task. The symptom usually disappears with discontinuation of the task or with rest.

In due course, the abnormal movements may not only appear during the task but may also occur during other movements such as buttoning clothes, typing, holding a spoon. In some, further progression may lead to the occurrence of some dystonic movements at rest however, this is not typical. Fixed dystonic postures are rare, and occurrence of "fixed posturing" puts psychogenic dystonia into the differential diagnosis.

The most common task specific focal hand dystonia is writer's cramp (4) whereby writing brings about a variety of combinations of dystonic posturing. Muscles normally not used in writing are simultaneously activated during the task and this has been demonstrated with surface EMG recordings done while writing(5). Additionally, there is lack of muscle selectivity and prolonged muscle bursts in these patients. The abnormal movements start as soon as the hand holds the pen or after having written a few words. Patients normally describe an uncontrollable force that makes them grip the pen tightly, and as a result, normal fluidity of writing is lost and patients are unable to write undisturbed. Penmanship thence becomes slow, irregular and even illegible. Symptoms stop as soon as they stop writing.

A mirror image effect(4) may occasionally be observed whereby writing with the unaffected hand simulates or produces the dystonic posture on the affected hand. This emphasizes the importance of sensory input in the pathophysiology of focal dystonia as the phenomenon impacts on central motor programming. Sensory tricks such as touching the hand during writing may ameliorate the dytonia. It appears though that, as in cervical dystonia, the sensory trick may not abolish the dystonia when the disorder has become long standing.

Patients who exhibit the dystonia only when writing are considered to have simple writer's cramp whereas those having difficulties with other tasks are considered complex forms of the latter.

As the symptoms of writer's cramp progress, it may involve more proximal forearm muscles, elbow and the shoulder causing involuntary abduction. Occasionally, the other hand may become involved.

3. Phenomenology of musician's dystonia

In musician's cramps, involuntary movements affect the limb while playing the instrument. Usually, the movements are similar as that of writer's cramp whereby pain is not as striking as the loss of control. These movements may lead to severe impairment and may result in loss of functionality and occupation. Dystonia usually begins in just one finger and eventually spreads to involve other fingers and rarely skips fingers(6). The fingers most often implicated are the two ulnar digits (fingers IV and V). These two fingers are not designed for the prolonged, rapid, highly complex movements demanded in many of those patients presenting with focal hand dystonia. Frucht (6) likewise described that there is hypermobility of these joints when ulnarly deviating to grip instruments thereby producing a mechanical susceptibility of these fingers to the development of dystonia.

Hand movement requires a degree of fine motor control which entails the precise activation of the hand area in the sensorimotor homunculus and inhibition of other uninvolved muscles. In focal hand dystonia, there is evidence of lack of inhibition at multiple levels in the central nervous system. This lack of inhibition with simultaneous contraction of both agonist and antagonist muscles are integral in the development of writer's cramp. Likewise, transcranial magnetic stimulation studies demonstrated abnormal intracortical inihibition(7). This abnormality is demonstrated bilaterally on both hemispheres despite the unilaterality of symptoms. The gaba-ergic neurotransmitter systems responsible for widespread inhibition in both direct and indirect pathways of the corticostriatothalamocortical loop in the central nervous system are found to be reduced(8).

The major contributing factor in the development of focal hand dystonia appears to be the prolonged, repetitive use of the hand (2-3). The hands are represented in the primary somatosensory cortex in high resolution, and receptive fields are small and sharply differentiated, not including more than one finger (9-10). It is known that through repeated use, this representation in the somatosensory cortex is malleable through the process of sensory learning called neuroplasticity. Among trained musicians, there is enlarged cortical representation of the hands in the somatosensory cortex and auditory domains which demonstrates this normal plasticity(11). In focal hand dystonia, repetitive sensory stimulation during the execution of the skilled manual tasks might lead to maladaptive sensorimotor plasticity in susceptible individuals. This maladaptive sensorimotor plasticity leads to changes in the representation of the digits within the somatosensory and motor cortices of the brain. As a result, the brain is unable to distinguish between near-simultaneous sensory inputs to the cortex, disrupting sensory feedback to the motor system and consequently fine motor movements. Magnetic source imaging showed that representational areas in the brain seem to fuse among these patients with this dystonia (12).

On the other hand the vibration induced illusion of movement model suggest a mechanism whereby motor subroutines become corrupted when movements are over-learned in the fatigued state (13-15). In idiopathic focal dystonia, the muscle spindles become stiff and their elastic properties vary as they are stretched or what is termed as "spindle thixotrophy"(16-17). Compared to normal individuals, the muscle spindles become stiffer in dystonia, but then become more elastic after they are over-stretched. Thus, it is the inconstancy of elastic properties of the dystonic muscle spindle that leads to the motor subroutine corruption. These peripherally-induced mechanisms may elucidate two phenomena: (a) why idiopathic focal dystonia symptoms tend to affect skilled and heavily practiced movements; (b) why sometimes dystonic symptoms evolve with time (18-19). An illustrative case at the end of the chapter will be presented to embody these phenomena.

According to previous studies (20) the correlation between peripheral trauma and hand dystonia remains controversial up to present. Even more bodies of evidence suggest a direct causal relationship. Moreover, ulnar neuropathy has been described in musician's dystonia(21). However, it is of note, that even if the relationship between injury and the development of dystonia are common, not all patients with trauma develop dystonia. Hence, trauma in an individual with a specific vulnerability is proposed. Repetitive use of the hands under extreme pressures and expectations related to the tasks may however be gleaned as a form of trauma.

The pattern of focal hand dystonia varies and may involve various combinations of distal and proximal muscles, flexors and extensors and supinators or pronators and is dependent on which groups of muscles are more often used by the sufferer. For instance, in writer's cramp, the dominant writing hand, the right, is more commonly affected. Finger flexors and wrist extension and flexion are commonly affected; Typist dystonia have variable affection of both hands; in musician's dystonia, those playing guitars, pianos or other string instruments tend to have more affection of the finger flexors. If the bowing hand is affected in a violinist, then wrist flexors are more affected. The left hand would be more involved in those playing with the violin and the flute(6). The right hand would be more vulnerable in those playing with the guitar and with the keyboard (6). Lateralization is not so prominent in musicians who use both hands like woodwind players or in keyboard typing. The dictum is, the hand which is more frequently utilized is the more frequently affected. The striking observations by Frucht and colleagues (6)showed that in musician's dystonia, the dystonic movements are stereotyped and rarely varies in a given patient.

Other task specific dystonia involving the limbs are sports related and have also been described in golfers(22) and pistol shooters(23). Among golfers, the dystonia is manifested as freezing, tremor, or an uncontrollable jerking which leads to deterioration in golf performance.

A special type of task specific dystonia involves the lips, jaws and lower cranial muscles of musicians playing brass and other wind instruments. This is termed as embouchure's dystonia. The highly specialized control of the different lower cranial muscles is required for the right production of pitch, tone and volume. Patients initially complain of lip and mouth fatigue. Rarely would pain be complained. Symptoms typically start during the fourth decade in the absence of a clear history of trauma, dental prosthesis or temporomandibular joint disease. Frucht et al described the largest group with embouchure's dystonia. Lip pulling or lip locking phenotypes(24) and other groupings such as lip tremors, jaw closure, involuntary lip movement groups have been described(25). Eventually, the dystonia not only disrupts handling of instruments but eating, chewing and speaking may also be impaired.

4. Epidemiology

According to the ESDE(26), the incidence of task specific dystonia range from1.7 to 14 and the prevalence range from 7 to 69 per million population. Usually these occur more frequently in males (2, 26-27) and typically in the third to fourth decade of life. At least 1% of professional musicians are afflicted with dystonia(28). Although other movement disorders can occur in the same patient, the true prevalence of two types of task specific dystonias occurring in the same patient is not known (2, 26). Most commonly described movement disorder occurring in the setting of task specific dystonia is the coexistence of tremor. Tremor, is present in up to 48% of patients with focal hand dystonia, usually unilateral in the affected arm, and may be task-specific(9) .

Not all patients involved in these occupations or musicians develop dystonia. Clearly there are other pathophysiologic mechanisms to consider such as environmental influences and genetics. Although most patients with musician's dystonia deny a positive family history, a report on autosomal dominant inherited forms have been made by Schmidt et al. (29). About 10 - 20% of task specific dystonias have a positive family history(30). Other risk factors such as increasing practice time, psychological stresses, anxiety, personality types have been implicated(27). At this point, the genetic underpinnings of focal hand dystonia, including that of musician's dystonia, have not yet been fully characterized. DYT1 mutation is an infrequent cause of task specific dystonia and has only been described in some cases of idiopathic dystonia and rarely in musician's cramp (2, 10).

5. Course and prognosis

In general, the course and prognosis for the different task specific dystonias are guarded. Majority of those with musician's dystonia are unable to return to their previous level of function and are forced to abandon their long passion for the instruments. In a study by Schuele et al. (31), a 13 year follow up of musicians with focal hand dystonia showed that only 38% of those who play string instruments were able to return to their careers. Those with writer's cramp, on the other hand, are rarely severely disabled. Majority of them can still continue writing despite the symptoms. The guarded prognosis of these patients also stem from the fact that only few have significant response to the different therapies available and that most of them tend to have the spasms spreading to contiguous muscle groups. Among the task specific dystonias, embouchure's dystonia is perhaps the most resistant to treatment(32).

6. Management strategies in occupationally related dystonias

Due to the high functional disability associated with these task specific dystonias, early recognition and institution of appropriate therapy is imperative. Treatment strategies are varied and include oral medications, chemodenervation, surgical approaches, limb immobilization, orthosis and physical therapy(9). Taken alone, perhaps only a handful of patients respond significantly with each of these regimen.

One non-pharmacologic intervention of interest nowadays is aimed at retraining the brain (i.e. sensorimotor retuning, SMR). Since these abnormal movements usually stem from abnormal plasticity and sensorimotor processing in the central nervous system, SMR has been devised to try to modify the cortical representation of the affected limb through immobilization. SMR is done wherein the uninvolved fingers are immobilized using splints while practicing sequential movements with their instruments at least an hour a day. This resulted in significant improvement in performance of pianists and guitarists for a 25 month follow up period(33), purportedly due to cortical remodeling. The involved side showed a much organized pattern simulating the normal side when evaluated with magnetoencephalography(34). Those playing wind instruments did not show improvement. Perhaps this is because of the anatomical constraints of muscles involved in this type of patients. A case report on one pianist (35)also showed improvement to pre-dystonia levels with SMR.

Another form of retraining is directed towards addressing abnormal sensory processing in these patients through braille reading which can improve spatial discrimination and symptoms in dystonia(36). A combination treatment with motor training and constraint induced immobilization of the dystonic hand has also been tried among musicians and showed some benefits(37). Patients with writer's cramp may also benefit from training individual fingers not involved in the dystonia (38-39). The advantage of SMR is that patients can be retrained in limiting activities that simulate the pattern which brought out the dystonia and hopefully prevent spread, thereby reducing disability. The only limitation seems to be the fact that symptoms recur as soon as they stop doing these exercises(36) and excessive retuning may again lead to maladaptive plasticity in these patients already with an inherent susceptibility. These training exercises need further validation in more large scale studies to assess long term benefits. In patients with embouchure's dystonia, Frucht (24)described some improvement when patients were asked to alter their technique by using a different mouthpiece or a different instrument. One particular problem in these training techniques in embouchure's dystonia most especially is that, retraining may push the spread of the dystonia to other contiguous muscle groups if the patient continues playing. However, studies to demonstrate this phenemenon are lacking.

The first line treatment for focal dystonia is chemodenervation with botulinum toxin. It is proposed that the peripheral action of botulinum toxin A of reducing muscle spindle signals(17, 40) could alter the balance between afferent input and motor output, thereby secondarily affecting cortical excitability(41-42). In addition, it has been shown to help in reorganizing intracortical inhibition, albeit transiently (43-44). Botulinum toxin has been shown in several randomized controlled trials to be effective in the treatment of writer's cramp (45-46). Among musicians, improvement with botulinum toxin injections has been demonstrated in 57-68% of patients (32, 47). Not infrequently, injected patients may experience weakness. Response of embouchure's dystonia, is inconsistent and disappointing. In tasks whereby fine motor control is needed, the weakness may outweigh the benefits of the improvement in dystonia and this should be discussed thoroughly with patients. Long term follow up of 10 years with botulinum toxin use in musicians show that its benefits are sustained and antibody production has not been demonstrated(48).

A variety of oral medications may be initiated in patients with task specific dystonias. Anticholinergics, gabaergics or dopaminergics have been tried with relatively inconsistent results. Trihexyphenydyl showed improvement in a third of patients (33% from 144 patients in the series) with musicians dystonia(32). Oral medications are often limited by side effects. The generally poor response probably reflects the fact that the problem is in the central nervous system (altered neuroplasticity in the somatosensory cortex) and not peripherally.

7. Illustrative case of a dual dystonia

We have had the chance to see a patient suffering from dual dystonia affecting only keyboard typing and money counting (Figures 1 and 2). Her other hand movements were unaffected by other tasks (49).

This 42 year old female bank cashier presented with two types of task specific (money counting and keyboard typing) dystonias since 8 years prior. Her right middle finger, fourth and fifth digits would hyperextend at the proximal and distal interphalangeal joints while both her thumbs hyperextend at the metacarpophalangeal joint. She has no family history of any movement disorders and has had no previous trauma. Her neurological examination was entirely normal. On work up, her cervical MRI showed cervical spondylosis at the level of C3-C4. She had normal CBC, ESR, Thyroid function tests, Anti thyroglobulin antibody, ANA panel, serum ceruloplasmin, Na, K, ionized calcium, cranial MRI and routine nerve conduction studies . Electromyography showed sustained bursts of motor unit potentials in co-contracting muscles such as the flexor and extensor carpi radialis and ulnaris on the right. The surface polymyographic analysis showed co-contraction of antagonist muscles of both arms especially when the abovementioned tasks were performed.

The following treatment options were tried but with no satisfactory results: levodopa, benzodiazepines, anticholinergics, baclofen and pregabalin. She even tried acupuncture, massage and physical therapy. Finally, botulinum toxin injection (*abobotulinumtoxinA*) was initiated as follows: To right flexor carpi radialis and flexor carpi ulnaris(100U each), extensor digitorum communis (75 units) and left extensor pollicis longus (35 units). The injections resulted in improvement on money counting but there was minimal response on keyboard typing. Prior to injection, it was the patient's wish (and thus our aim) that she sustains her job as a cashier by mainly improving her money-counting, as we were not optimistic to abolish both dystonias in one injection setting. She continued to improve in the same manner from subsequent 4-monthly injections.

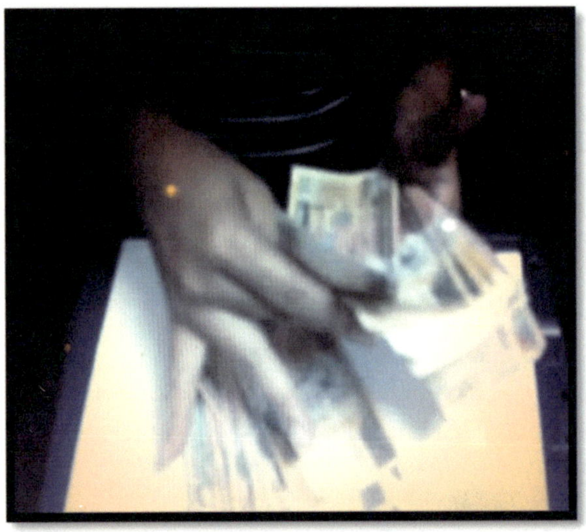

a

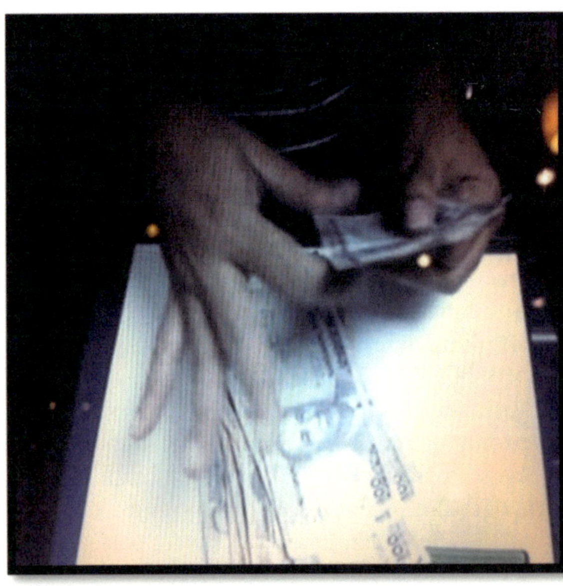

b

Fig. 1. Dystonia while counting money

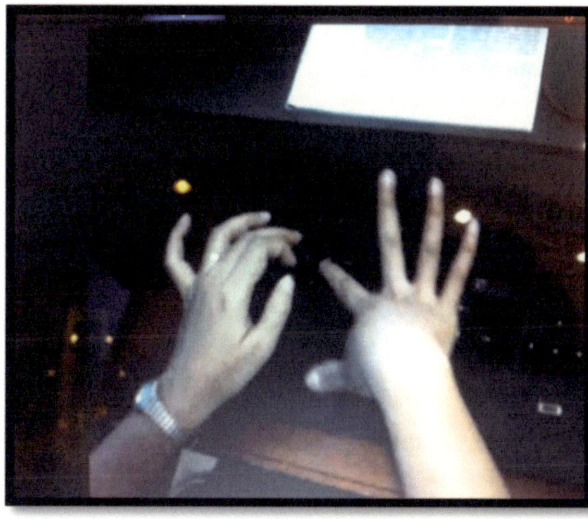

a

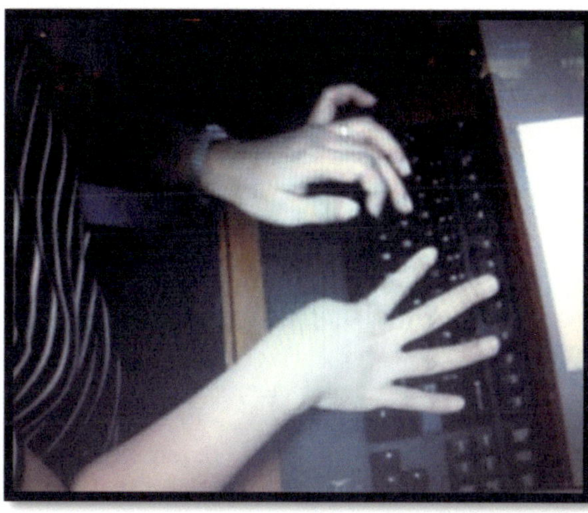

b

Fig. 2. Dystonia during keyboard typing

8. Conclusion

Task specific dystonia is phenomenologically distinct and remains to be a challenging disorder to treat. An inherent susceptibility is yet to be defined but it appears that repetitive muscle movement is the integral to the development of abnormal and maladaptive plasticity, loss of intracortical inhibition and abnormal sensory processing. Task specific dystonia tends to be disabling. Botulinum toxin remains in the first line of treatment in those presenting with focal limb dystonia. Embouchure's dystonia is even more challenging, a disorder. SMR remains an attractive management option. Multi-modal treatment approach may likely optimize outcomes.

9. References

[1] Rosales RL. Muscle Cramps In: Lisak RP, Truong DD, Carroll W, Bhidayasiri R, editors. International Neurology: A clinical approach. UK: Wiley and Blackwell 2009. p. 461-4.
[2] Soland VL, Bhatia KP, Marsden CD. Sex prevalence of focal dystonias. J Neurol Neurosurg Psychiatry. 1996 Feb;60(2):204-5.
[3] Bressman SB. Dystonia update. Clin Neuropharmacol. 2000 Sep-Oct;23(5):239-51.
[4] Torres-Russotto D, Perlmutter JS. Task-specific dystonias: a review. Ann N Y Acad Sci. 2008 Oct;1142:179-99.
[5] Cohen LG, Hallett M. Hand cramps: clinical features and electromyographic patterns in a focal dystonia. Neurology. 1988 Jul;38(7):1005-12.
[6] Frucht SJ. Focal task-specific dystonia of the musicians' hand--a practical approach for the clinician. J Hand Ther. 2009 Apr-Jun;22(2):136-42; quiz 43.
[7] Chen R, Wassermann EM, Canos M, Hallett M. Impaired inhibition in writer's cramp during voluntary muscle activation. Neurology. 1997 Oct;49(4):1054-9.
[8] Levy LM, Hallett M. Impaired brain GABA in focal dystonia. Ann Neurol. 2002 Jan;51(1):93-101.
[9] Jankovic J. Parkinson's Disease and Movement Disorders. Philadelphia: Lippincott and Williams; 2007. p. 322-4.
[10] Bara-Jimenez W, Catalan MJ, Hallett M, Gerloff C. Abnormal somatosensory homunculus in dystonia of the hand. Ann Neurol. 1998 Nov;44(5):828-31.
[11] Pantev C, Engelien A, Candia V, Elbert T. Representational cortex in musicians. Plastic alterations in response to musical practice. Ann N Y Acad Sci. 2001 Jun;930:300-14.
[12] Elbert T, Candia V, Altenmuller E, Rau H, Sterr A, Rockstroh B, et al. Alteration of digital representations in somatosensory cortex in focal hand dystonia. Neuroreport. 1998 Nov 16;9(16):3571-5.
[13] Frima N, Rome SM, Grunewald RA. The effect of fatigue on abnormal vibration induced illusion of movement in idiopathic focal dystonia. J Neurol Neurosurg Psychiatry. 2003 Aug;74(8):1154-6.
[14] Rome S, Grunewald RA. Abnormal perception of vibration-induced illusion of movement in dystonia. Neurology. 1999 Nov 10;53(8):1794-800.
[15] Grunewald RA, Yoneda Y, Shipman JM, Sagar HJ. Idiopathic focal dystonia: a disorder of muscle spindle afferent processing? Brain. 1997 Dec;120 (Pt 12)(Pt 12):2179-85.
[16] Proske U, Morgan DL, Gregory JE. Thixotropy in skeletal muscle and in muscle spindles: a review. Prog Neurobiol. 1993 Dec;41(6):705-21.
[17] Rosales RL, Dressler D. On muscle spindles, dystonia and botulinum toxin. Eur J Neurol. 2010 Jul;17 Suppl 1:71-80.
[18] Grunewald RA. Progression of dystonia: learning from distorted feedback? J Neurol Neurosurg Psychiatry. 2007 Sep;78(9):914.
[19] Rosset-Llobet J, Candia V, Fabregas S, Ray W, Pascual-Leone A. Secondary motor disturbances in 101 patients with musician's dystonia. J Neurol Neurosurg Psychiatry. 2007 Sep;78(9):949-53.
[20] Quartarone A, Bagnato S, Rizzo V, Siebner HR, Dattola V, Scalfari A, et al. Abnormal associative plasticity of the human motor cortex in writer's cramp. Brain. 2003 Dec;126(Pt 12):2586-96.

[21] Charness ME, Ross MH, Shefner JM. Ulnar neuropathy and dystonic flexion of the fourth and fifth digits: clinical correlation in musicians. Muscle Nerve. 1996 Apr;19(4):431-7.
[22] Adler CH, Crews D, Hentz JG, Smith AM, Caviness JN. Abnormal co-contraction in yips-affected but not unaffected golfers: evidence for focal dystonia. Neurology. 2005 May 24;64(10):1813-4.
[23] Sitburana O, Ondo WG. Task-specific focal hand dystonia in a professional pistol-shooter. Clin Neurol Neurosurg. 2008 Apr;110(4):423-4.
[24] Frucht SJ. Embouchure dystonia--Portrait of a task-specific cranial dystonia. Mov Disord. 2009 Sep 15;24(12):1752-62.
[25] Frucht SJ, Fahn S, Greene PE, O'Brien C, Gelb M, Truong DD, et al. The natural history of embouchure dystonia. Mov Disord. 2001 Sep;16(5):899-906.
[26] A prevalence study of primary dystonia in eight European countries. J Neurol. 2000 Oct;247(10):787-92.
[27] Altenmuller E, Jabusch HC. Focal dystonia in musicians: phenomenology, pathophysiology and triggering factors. Eur J Neurol. 2010 Jul;17 Suppl 1:31-6.
[28] Altenmuller E. Focal dystonia: advances in brain imaging and understanding of fine motor control in musicians. Hand Clin. 2003 Aug;19(3):523-38, xi.
[29] Schmidt A, Jabusch HC, Altenmuller E, Hagenah J, Bruggemann N, Hedrich K, et al. Dominantly transmitted focal dystonia in families of patients with musician's cramp. Neurology. 2006 Aug 22;67(4):691-3.
[30] Waddy HM, Fletcher NA, Harding AE, Marsden CD. A genetic study of idiopathic focal dystonias. Ann Neurol. 1991 Mar;29(3):320-4.
[31] Schuele S, Lederman RJ. Long-term outcome of focal dystonia in string instrumentalists. Mov Disord. 2004 Jan;19(1):43-8.
[32] Jabusch HC, Zschucke D, Schmidt A, Schuele S, Altenmuller E. Focal dystonia in musicians: treatment strategies and long-term outcome in 144 patients. Mov Disord. 2005 Dec;20(12):1623-6.
[33] Candia V, Schafer T, Taub E, Rau H, Altenmuller E, Rockstroh B, et al. Sensory motor retuning: a behavioral treatment for focal hand dystonia of pianists and guitarists. Arch Phys Med Rehabil. 2002 Oct;83(10):1342-8.
[34] Candia V, Rosset-Llobet J, Elbert T, Pascual-Leone A. Changing the brain through therapy for musicians' hand dystonia. Ann N Y Acad Sci. 2005 Dec;1060:335-42.
[35] Rosset-Llobet J, Fabregas-Molas S. Long-term treatment effects of sensory motor retuning in a pianist with focal dystonia. Med Probl Perform Art. 2011 Jun;26(2):106-7.
[36] Zeuner KE, Bara-Jimenez W, Noguchi PS, Goldstein SR, Dambrosia JM, Hallett M. Sensory training for patients with focal hand dystonia. Ann Neurol. 2002 May;51(5):593-8.
[37] Berque P, Gray H, Harkness C, McFadyen A. A combination of constraint-induced therapy and motor control retraining in the treatment of focal hand dystonia in musicians. Med Probl Perform Art. 2010 Dec;25(4):149-61.
[38] Zeuner KE, Shill HA, Sohn YH, Molloy FM, Thornton BC, Dambrosia JM, et al. Motor training as treatment in focal hand dystonia. Mov Disord. 2005 Mar;20(3):335-41.

[39] Zeuner KE, Molloy FM. Abnormal reorganization in focal hand dystonia--sensory and motor training programs to retrain cortical function. NeuroRehabilitation. 2008;23(1):43-53.

[40] Rosales RL, Arimura K, Takenaga S, Osame M. Extrafusal and intrafusal muscle effects in experimental botulinum toxin-A injection. Muscle Nerve. 1996 Apr;19(4):488-96.

[41] Curra A, Trompetto C, Abbruzzese G, Berardelli A. Central effects of botulinum toxin type A: evidence and supposition. Mov Disord. 2004 Mar;19 Suppl 8(8):S60-4.

[42] Pickett A, Rosales RL. New trends in the science of botulinum toxin-A as applied in dystonia. Int J Neurosci. 2011;121 Suppl 1:22-34.

[43] Gilio F, Curra A, Lorenzano C, Modugno N, Manfredi M, Berardelli A. Effects of botulinum toxin type A on intracortical inhibition in patients with dystonia. Ann Neurol. 2000 Jul;48(1):20-6.

[44] Kanovsky P, Rosales RL. The pathophysiologic puzzle of dystonia in relation to botulinum toxin therapy. Parkinsonism and Related Disorders. 2011, in press

[45] Tsui JK, Bhatt M, Calne S, Calne DB. Botulinum toxin in the treatment of writer's cramp: a double-blind study. Neurology. 1993 Jan;43(1):183-5.

[46] Kruisdijk JJ, Koelman JH, Ongerboer de Visser BW, de Haan RJ, Speelman JD. Botulinum toxin for writer's cramp: a randomised, placebo-controlled trial and 1-year follow-up. J Neurol Neurosurg Psychiatry. 2007 Mar;78(3):264-70.

[47] Schuele S, Jabusch HC, Lederman RJ, Altenmuller E. Botulinum toxin injections in the treatment of musician's dystonia. Neurology. 2005 Jan 25;64(2):341-3.

[48] Lungu C, Karp BI, Alter K, Zolbrod R, Hallett M. Long-term follow-up of botulinum toxin therapy for focal hand dystonia: outcome at 10 years or more. Mov Disord. 2011 Mar;26(4):750-3.

[49] Go CL, Rosales RL. Money Counting and Keyboard Typing Dual Dystonia in an Adult Filipino Female: A CASE REPORT. Movement Disorders 15th International congress final program. June 2011; 629: 107

5

Dystonia Secondary to Use of Antipsychotic Agents

Nobutomo Yamamoto and Toshiya Inada
Seiwa Hospital, Institute of Neuropsychiatry, Tokyo, Japan

1. Introduction

Following the introduction of first-generation antipsychotics (FGAs) in the early 1950s, there was a radical change in the therapeutic regimens for schizophrenia. However, it soon became apparent that these antipsychotic agents produced serious side effects including distressing and often debilitating movement disorders known as extrapyramidal symptoms (EPS). To prevent EPS, second-generation antipsychotics (SGAs) were developed and introduced, including risperidone in 1996, quetiapine, perospirone, and olanzapine in 2001, aripiprazole in 2006, and blonanserin in 2008. Clozapine was approved in 2010 in Japan with strict regulation of its use. These newer medications differ from FGAs, primarily on the basis of their reduced risk of inducing EPS. EPS lie at the interface of neurology and psychiatry and have generated a vast literature in both disciplines. EPS can be categorized as acute (dystonia, akathisia and parkinsonism) and tardive (tardive dyskinesia, tardive akathisia and tardive dystonia). Acute EPS has often been reported as an early sign of predisposition to tardive dyskinesia. Acute and tardive EPS may also adversely influence a patient's motor and mental performance and reduce compliance to treatment. Poor compliance leads to high relapse rates, with both ethical and economic consequences. Acute dystonic reaction is a common side effect of antipsychotics, but can be caused by any agents that block dopamine receptors, such as the antidepressant amoxapine and anti-emetic drugs such as metoclopramide.

Dystonia is characterized by prolonged muscle contraction provoking slow, repetitive, involuntary, often twisting, movements that result in sustained abnormal, and at times bizarre, postures, which eventually become fixed. Patients who have developed dystonic reactions often feel extremely uncomfortable, or suffer chronic pain. Dystonia is a symptom rather than a specific disease, and has many causes. This article reviews antipsychotic-induced acute and tardive dystonia (Inada et al, 1990).

2. Acute dystonic reaction

Antipsychotic-induced acute dystonic reaction often occurs within the first few days of antipsychotic treatment or when the dosage is increased. It has been reported that approximately 90% of these reactions occur within the first three to five days (Ayd, 1961; Lehan et al, 2004). If untreated, acute dystonic reaction may last hours or days. When the cause is a long-acting depot injection, the duration of the acute dystonic reaction may be particularly long. This is often distressing and frightening for the patient, and may even be dangerous, possibly causing loss of drug adherence. Thus, acute dystonia continues to be a serious problem in the treatment of psychotic disorders. FGAs, such as butyrophenones, are the antipsychotics with the greatest likelihood of producing these complications (Lehan et al, 2004). As a result of the gradual increase in the use of SGAs in Japan, the incidence of antipsychotic-induced acute dystonic reaction has gradually decreased. Among all patients treated with antipsychotics, acute dystonic reactions occur in 2-10%, among whom the symptoms appear within days of therapy initiation in approximately 2-3% (Ayd, 1961). In Japan, there have been several reports on the prevalence of acute dystonic reactions. Kondo et al. (1999) reported that acute dystonic reactions developed in 51% of schizophrenic patients treated with nemonapride, and that 90% of them occurred within 3 days of therapy initiation. Yasui-Furukori et al. (2002) reported that acute dystonic reactions developed in 10 of 33 patients with acute schizophrenia treated with bromperidol. In a recent double blind study comparing the efficacy of blonanserin, an SGA developed in Japan, with that of risperidone, dystonia occurred in 2.8% of patients treated with risperidone and 4.5% of patients treated with blonanserin (Miura, 2008). Long-acting depot injections, such as haloperidol decanoate and fluphenazine decanoate, usually produce dystonic reactions within 72 hours after delivery (Tarsy, 1984). Data showed that the occurrence of acute dystonia could be lower in patients with schizophrenia receiving long-acting depot antipsychotics than in those receiving oral agents (Inada & Sasada, 2004). Miller and Jankovic (1990) reported that 24% of patients with antipsychotic-induced movement disorders had dystonia, but that such disorders were relatively rare in patients who received SGAs. Risperidone long-acting injectable (RLAI) was first approved in Japan as a long-acting depot SGA antipsychotic for the treatment of schizophrenia in 2009. Kamishima et al. (2009) reported that there was no significant difference between oral risperidone and RLAI. Kamishima et al. (2009) reported that dystonic reactions developed in 7.2% of patients with schizophrenia treated with RLAI within 48 weeks. In addition to the use of high-potency conventional antipsychotics, other risk factors for acute dystonic reactions include young age, male gender, high doses and intramuscular administration. A history of acute dystonic reaction has been identified as the most powerful predictor of a patient developing the condition. In a prospective study, cocaine use was also found to be a risk factor (Van Harten et al, 1998). The psychiatric aspects of acute dystonic reaction are related to the fear and anxiety associated with the unpredictable, sudden onset of involuntary movements and the loss of control of specific muscle groups. This can be particularly intimidating to psychotic patients with paranoid delusions about external forces attempting to control them.

Drug-induced dystonic movements are caused mainly by blockade of dopamine receptors. Dopamine is one of several transmitters that act on the central nervous system, and numerous dopamine receptor subtypes have been found in the extrapyramidal system. Dopamine D2 receptors are those most strongly associated with the efficacy of antipsychotics, and their blockade is at least partially responsible for the movement disorders like those in acute dystonia. Although also known to block other receptors, FGAs exert their therapeutic action primarily by blocking D2 receptors in the central nervous system, and have a high risk of inducing such side effects. SGAs are effective against psychosis and, at therapeutic doses, seldom cause EPS including acute dystonic reaction. Their therapeutic effects are attributable to central antagonism of both serotonin and dopamine receptors, and also possibly to relatively loose binding to D2 receptors (Lehan et al., 2004). However, the exact mechanism responsible for acute dystonic reactions is not entirely understood. Although they are related to blockade of the D2 receptor, in common with all antipsychotics, the delay between receptor blockade and onset of clinical symptomatology suggests involvement of additional mechanisms, possibly secondary dopamine receptor hypersensitivity (Mazurek & Rosebush, 1996).

	Test compound		Haloperidol			Risk Ratio
Study or Subgroup	Events	Total	Events	Total	Weight	M-H, Random, 95% CI
PerphenazineKurihara	0	95	0	94		Not estimable
Fluphenazine/Kaneno	0	127	2	132	3.0%	0.21 [0.01, 4.29]
Quetiapine/Murasaki	2	100	8	97	10.9%	0.24 [0.05, 1.11]
Sultopride/Mori	2	105	6	100	10.3%	0.32 [0.07, 1.54]
Haloperidol.D/Ookuma	3	141	7	142	13.8%	0.43 [0.11, 1.64]
Risperidone/Murasaki	4	97	7	95	16.5%	0.56 [0.17, 1.85]
Bromperidol/Onodera	1	67	1	63	3.7%	0.94 [0.06, 14.71]
Perospirone/Murasaki	4	70	3	75	11.7%	1.43 [0.33, 6.16]
Nemonapride/Mori	9	81	6	86	22.2%	1.59 [0.59, 4.27]
Sultopride/Kudou	2	44	1	49	4.9%	2.23 [0.21, 23.72]
ClocapramineKurihara	2	97	0	94	3.1%	4.85 [0.24, 99.64]
Total (95% CI)		**1024**		**1027**	**100.0%**	**0.74 [0.43, 1.27]**
Total events	29		41			

Heterogeneity: Tau² = 0.08; Chi² = 10.14, df = 9 (P = 0.34); I² = 11%
Test for overall effect: Z = 1.10 (P = 0.27)

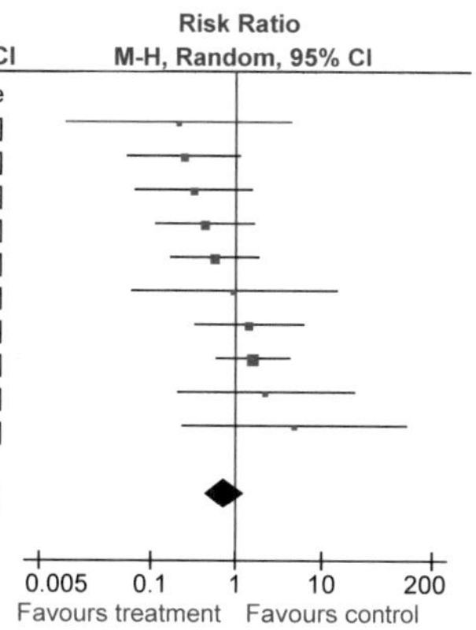

Fig. 1. Comparison of the occurrence of acute dystonic reactions in double-blind randomized controlled trials with haloperidol conducted in Japan (Inada T & Sasada K: Comparison of the efficacy of psychotropic drug at a glance Vol 3 Evidence of side effect and adverse events. Jiho Inc., Tokyo, 16-17 (Article in Japanese).

Acute dystonic reactions are sudden in onset and typically consist of bizarre movements involving tonic contractions of skeletal muscles. Common symptoms include intermittent or sustained muscular spasms. These dystonic reactions are most often localized in the face, neck and upper part of the body, while rarely involving the lower limbs. Laryngeal dystonia occurs only rarely, but may be life-threatening. The specific name of the reaction is derived from the specific anatomic region that is affected. Hence, the terms "torticollis," "laryngospasm," "oculogyric crisis," and "opisthotonos" are used to describe dystonic reactions in the specific body regions. Although oculogyric crisis used to be seen most commonly in postencephalitic parkinsonism, it is now almost entirely attributable to neuroleptic exposure.

3. Tardive dystonia

Tardive dystonia has been considered a late-onset subtype of dystonic reaction characterized by a state of muscle hypertonus, seen in patients who have been receiving antipsychotic treatment for a prolonged period. Tardive dystonia has been considered a rare movement disorder. Although the prevalence of this condition in Japan has been estimated to be only 0.5-2.1% of all schizophrenic patients receiving long-term antipsychotic treatment (Harada 1989; Inada et al., 1991a: Inada et al., 1991b), the development of this condition still remains a potential treatment limitation factor. Van Harten and Kahn (1999) conducted a meta-analysis of 13 studies on the prevalence of tardive dystonia. The estimated prevalence, based on the mean value for all 13 studies, was 5.3%. However, they reported that these data may have been inappropriate because not all of the studies had used the same criteria for defining tardive dystonia.

Tardive dystonia was first thought to be a subtype of tardive dyskinesia, since it often develops simultaneously with the latter. Burke et al. (1982a) demonstrated that it was correlated with frequent use of antipsychotics, and thereafter it became regarded as an entity independent of tardive dyskinesia. Inada et al. (1990) conducted a statistical trial in order to distinguish between tardive dyskinesia and tardive dystonia. The clinical features of tardive dystonia are usually divided into four categories: 1) focal (only a single body part affected), 2) segmental (two or more segments of a body part), 3) multifocal (two or more non-contiguous body parts), and 4) generalized (combined involvement of at least one leg, trunk and body part) (Fahn et al., 1987). Tardive dystonia often develops insidiously, and in about two-thirds of cases onset is observed in the face, neck, or both. Onset in an arm is less common, and onset in a leg is rare. In about three-quarters of patients, the dystonia progresses to a segmental state, but progression to a generalized state is uncommon. Patients with generalized dystonia are reportedly younger than those with focal dystonia (Van Harten and Kahn, 1999). Tardive dystonia can affect every body area, including twisting of the neck musculature in all directions, blepharospasm and oromandibular, laryngeal, arm, trunk and leg dystonia. The neck regions are most commonly involved, but arm involvement is also common. Blepharospasm is a common focal dystonia of the eyelids. Meige's syndrome is a segmental dystonia involving the eyelids, facial muscles and lower jaw. Both of these two forms are considered to belong to tardive dystonia, but are thought to be less severe than the typical neck or arm dystonia. "Pisa syndrome" is also a subtype of tardive dystonia, characterized by twisting and bending the neck and head to one side of the upper thorax. Oculogyric crisis is a common symptom of acute dystonic reaction, but a tardive form has also been reported (Sachdev, 1993). Tardive myoclonus has been considered a variant of tardive dystonia.

Tardive dystonia is a rare extrapyramidal adverse effect, and many studies have not distinguished it from tardive dyskinesia. Older age is the most firmly established risk factor for tardive dyskinesia. Other risk factors include mood disorders, organic brain dysfunction, diabetes mellitus, alcohol abuse, occurrence of extrapyramidal adverse effects during treatment, and use of high dosages of antipsychotics (Raja, 1998). Gender has also been considered a possible risk factor. Some studies have reported a male predominance whereas others have reported no gender difference. The onset of tardive dystonia seems to occur earlier in males than in females (Van Hatten and Kahn, 1999). In a study of the natural history of tardive dystonia in 107 patients, Kiriakakis et al. (1998) found that males were significantly younger than females at onset, and that the condition developed after a shorter period of drug exposure in men. Fatigue and stress exacerbate the severity of tardive dystonia or the subjective discomfort of affected patients. Relaxation and sleep can alleviate these to some extent. In some patients with bipolar disorder who develop tardive dystonia, their dystonia has been reported to become exacerbated during the depressive phase and to improve or disappear during the manic phase (Sacdev, 1989; Sandyk & Pardeshi, 1990; Yazici et al, 1991).

The pathophysiological background of tardive dystonia is unclear. It is thought to result from hypersensitivity of post-synaptic receptors associated with continuous blockade of dopaminergic neuronal transmission due to antipsychotic drugs (LeWitt, 1995). An anti-noradrenergic action may play an important role because the amount of noradrenaline has been shown to be reduced in the hypothalamus, mammillary body, and other areas

(Hornykiewicz et al., 1986). Go et al. (2009) reported that the prevalence rate of tardive dyskinesia was 20.3% (46 out of 277 patients) in a Filipino cohort of schizophrenia patients receiving SGA. In a recent double blind study comparing the efficacy of blonanserin, an SGA developed in Japan, with that of risperidone, dystonia occurred in 2.8% of patients treated with risperidone and 4.5% of patients treated with blonanserin (Miura, 2008).

4. Diagnosis of dystonia

The differential diagnosis of drug-induced acute dystonic reactions must include cramps, contractures, tetany, acute dystonic reactions to non-antipsychotic agents, catatonia and restless legs syndrome. Catatonia, which is sometimes associated with mood disorder or schizophrenia, can be distinguished by a transient relationship with antipsychotic exposure and response to pharmacological intervention. Neuroleptic malignant syndrome can produce dystonia, but this differs in being also accompanied by fever and generalized rigidity. Acute dystonic reaction may sometimes be misdiagnosed as hysteria or related disorders. These reactions are distinguishable from tardive dystonia or tardive dyskinesia by their sudden onset. Lack of response to anticholinergic agents suggests an alternative diagnosis (Raja, 1998).

Tardive dystonia was first reported by Keegan and Rajput (1973). Burke et al. (1982a) demonstrated that it was correlated with frequent use of antipsychotics, and established the following four criteria for diagnosis of tardive dystonia: 1) presence of dystonic movements or postures; 2) their development during treatment with D2 receptor blockers or within 2 months of treatment discontinuation; 3) a negative family history for dystonia; 4) exclusion of other secondary dystonias, such as Wilson's disease, etc. Tardive dystonia may sometimes coexist with tardive dyskinesia or tardive akathisia. In such cases, the diagnosis should be made on the basis of the most predominant disturbance (Raja, 1998).

The differential diagnosis of tardive dystonia must include acute dystonic reactions, idiopathic dystonia, dystonia induced by other non-antipsychotic agents, Wilson's disease, tardive dyskinesia, etc. A progressive course and possibly a family history of dystonia would suggest idiopathic dystonia. Wilson's disease, an inborn error of copper metabolism, can be manifested as dystonia, but can be ruled out by the presence of a normal serum ceruloplasmin level and absence of a Kayser-Fleischer ring. Acute dystonic reaction almost always occurs within the first day of antipsychotic treatment and usually responds to anticholinergic agents, thus allowing distinction from tardive dystonia. Tardive dystonia, like the other dystonias, is involuntary and cannot be inhibited, thus differing from stereotypes, habit spasms or tics. Secondary dystonia resulting from infections, metabolic disorders, or structured lesions of the brain should be distinguished on clinical grounds (Raja, 1998). Although tardive dystonia can often be confused with tardive dyskinesia, it can be differentiated by the following features: 1) it has different phenomenological manifestations, 2) it has different demographic features: patients with tardive dystonia are younger at onset and lack the female predominance seen with tardive dyskinesia, and 3) it has reactions from those of anticholinergics: they can alleviate tardive dystonia but can exacerbate tardive dyskinesia (Burke, 1992; Greene 1997; van Harten and Kahn, 1999).

Dystonia can also be elicited by compounds other than antipsychotics, such as levodopa, carbamazepine, phenytoin, dextroamphetamine and diphenylhydantoin. Dystonia generally disappears after reduction of the dose or withdrawal of the causative drug. Idiopathic or primary dystonia can often be differentiated from tardive dystonia by taking a careful medical history at onset of the dystonia in relation to the initiation of antipsychotics. Furthermore, the prevalence of idiopathic dystonia in the general population is only 0.03%, which is much lower than that of antipsychotic-induced dystonia (Van Hatten and Kahn, 1999).

The diagnosis and symptom severity of dystonia have been evaluated using the Drug-induced Extrapyramidal Symptoms Scale (DIEPSS), a standardized rating scale for evaluating antipsychotic-induced EPS in Japan. The DIEPSS was developed in Japan (Inada & Yagi, 1995, 1996; Inada, 2009) and has been used widely for the assessment of EPS in Japan. The DIEPSS is designed to evaluate the severity of drug-induced EPS occurring during treatment with antipsychotics, and consists of 8 individual items (gait, bradykinesia, sialorrhea, muscle rigidity, tremor, akathisia, dystonia and dyskinesia) and one global item. The scale measures the severity of drug-induced EPS on a five-point scale (0-4). Raters should receive basic evaluation training on how to rate the severity of each DIEPSS item by attending DIEPSS workshops so that they can reproduce the stable data (Inada, 1996). Once an increase in muscle tone has been observed and the existence of dystonia has been confirmed, the severity of dystonia can be evaluated depending on the degree of impairment of daily living activity and the distress resulting from this painful condition during the observation period. The degree of abnormal movements resulting from the dystonia should be rated using the dyskinesia item of the scale.

5. Treatment of acute dystonic reaction

The first approach for treating acute dystonic reactions, i.e., the therapeutic strategy initially considered for these conditions, has been reduction of the dosage, or withdrawal, of antipsychotics. Treatment strategies may include switching from a FGA to a SGA. Anticholinergic agents, dopamine agonists and benzodiazepines may often reduce the severity of the acute dystonic reaction.

5.1 Switching to a SGA

The prevalence of acute dystonic reactions is lower in patients receiving SGAs than in those receiving FGAs at clinically effective doses. To date, the SGAs that have been released in Japan are risperidone, perospirone, quetiapine, olanzapine, aripiprazole, blonanserin and clozapine. As EPS, such as dystonia, may result in treatment refusal or non-compliance, the use of, or switching to a SGA with a significantly lower risk of EPS is very important. However, the risk of EPS cannot be ignored; emergence of EPS with risperidone at a dosage of over 6 mg per day has been reported (Lehan et al., 2004).

5.2 Anticholinergic agents

Anticholinergic agents, which have central anticholinergic properties, are often used for the treatment of dystonic reactions. These agents, which are useful not only for curative but also diagnostic applications, usually result in improvement within 10 minutes of parenteral administration, and the peak benefit is evident at 30 minutes. The standard parenteral anticholinergic employed in Japan is intramuscular injection of biperiden 1 vial (5 mg). Intravenous injection of these agents may be considered for relief of life-threatening dystonias, such as laryngospasm. Improvement and peak benefit typically occur within 10 and 30 minutes, respectively, after oral administration. Once an acute dystonic reaction has been controlled, prophylactic use of oral anticholinergic agents is recommended for at least 4 weeks, especially in patients with a history of susceptibility to EPS and patients for whom antipsychotics are known to induce these effects (e.g., first-generation agents, high-dose risperidone) (Lehan et al., 2004). Biperiden and trihexyphenidyl have been released, but benztropine, commonly used for treating acute dystonic reactions in the USA, has not yet been approved in Japan.

The peripheral adverse effects of anticholinergic agents include dry mouth, constipation, blurred vision and urine retention. Anticholinergic agents may also impair memory, and thus worsen cognitive deficits in elderly patients, especially those with pre-existing symptoms of dementia. Anticholinergic agents should be avoided, if possible, in patients with prostatic hypertrophy, urine retention and narrow-angle glaucoma. If a patient cannot tolerate the anticholinergic adverse effects, the lowest effective dosage should be used, or the drug be replaced with a benzodiazepine.

5.3 Benzodiazepines

Benzodiazepines are an alternative therapeutic option for patients with acute dystonic reactions in whom anticholinergic agents are contraindicated. Representative benzodiazepines used in Japan include lorazepam, diazepam and clonazepam. Intravenous injection of 5-10 mg diazepam, the only available injectable benzodiazepine for this indication in Japan, can be used in especially severe cases.

5.4 Antihistaminic agents

Diphenhydramine, commonly used for treating acute dystonic reactions in the USA, is rarely used for this purpose in Japan. Instead, promethazine (15-50 mg 2-3 times per day) is sometimes used.

6. Treatment of tardive dystonia

There is no established therapy for tardive dystonia. Treatment of this condition has been considered even more difficult than that for tardive dyskinesia. Tardive dystonia shows a lower incidence of spontaneous remission than tardive dystonia (Raja, 1998).

The first approach for treating tardive dystonia is to evaluate the need for antipsychotics and to reduce their doses, if possible, because antipsychotics are often prescribed for non-psychotic conditions (Burke et al., 1982a, 1982b). Switching from a FGA to a SGA has been recommended in patients receiving FGAs, based on the clinical guidelines for the treatment of schizophrenia. Yamamoto (2005) reported a schizophrenic patient whose antipsychotic-induced Pisa syndrome improved after switching from olanzapine and risperidone to quetiapine. Imai and Ikawa (2011) also reported a case of antipsychotic-induced tardive oromandibular dystonia that improved after switching from sulpiride to aripiprazole. Clozapine, which has been reported to be effective for treatment-resistant schizophrenia, and has been available since 2009, may be the only antipsychotic with an established minimal risk of inducing tardive dyskinesia. Switching to clozapine may be potentially the first choice for patients showing tardive dystonia (Raja, 1998). In humans, clozapine can produce bradykinesia and mild akathisia, but no acute creaction or rigidity has been reported, and tremor has only rarely. Clozapine has been approved for treatment-resistant or treatment-intolerant patients with schizophrenia. It can be used for treatment-intolerant schizophrenic patients with dystonia showing severity of 3or higher in the dystonia item of the DIEPSS, after they have received two or more second-generation antipsychotics.

Tetrabenazine has been approved for the treatment of tardive dyskinesia in the United Kingdom. Fahn and Eldridge (1976) and others have reported that it may also be effective for tardive dystonia. However, tetrabenazine has yet to be released in Japan.

High dosages of anticholinergics, such as biperiden and trihexyphenidyl, are reportedly effective in some patients with tardive dystonia. Sugiyama et al. (1996) have reported that tardive dystonia was improved by treatment with trihexyphenidyl 18 mg/day in schizophrenic patients receiving antipsychotics. Benzodiazepines may also exert some benefits in patients with tardive dystonia. Yamamoto et al. (2007) reported a case of methamphetamine psychosis in which tardive dystonia was successfully treated with clonazepam. Treatment with dantrolene sodium is reserved for alternative situations in cases where clonazepam is not effective (Otsuki et al., 1991). Clonazepam should be administered carefully to avoid any adverse effects such as hepatotoxicity.

When tardive dystonia is relatively localized, as is the case for focal or mild segmental forms, botulinum toxin, which blocks release of acetylcholine at the neurotransmitter junction, can be considered. Local injections of botulinum toxin are reportedly very effective for treatment of focal dystonia (Jancovic & Brin, 1991). Injection of botulinum toxin in minute quantities into the contorted muscles induces prolonged muscle weakness without systemic toxicity. The therapeutic effects of botulinum toxin last on average 2-6 months as new nerve terminals develop. Excessive weakness of the injected muscle, which is the main adverse effect, is usually mild and transitory. Over 15% of patients may develop neutralizing antibodies in response to botulinum toxin treatment and become non-responders (Raja, 1998). In Japan, botulinum toxin A has been released, but other types of botulinum toxin have not. Kimura et al. (2005) have reported improvement of tardive dystonia in a schizophrenic patient after treatment with botulinum A toxin.

7. References

Burke RE, Fahn S, Jankovic J, et al: Tardive dystonia: late-onset and persistent dystonia caused by antipsychotic drugs. Neurology 32: 1335-1346, 1982a.

Ayd FJ Jr: A survey of drug-induces extrapyramidal reactions. JAMA 175: 1054-1060，1961.

Inada T, Ichikawa T, Kamizima K, et al: A statistical trial of subclassification for tardive dyskinesia. Acta PsychistStand 82 404-407, 1990.

Lehan AF, Lieberman JA, Dixon JA, et al: Practice guideline for the treatment of schizophrenia, 2nd edition. American Psychiatric Association, Washington D.C., 2004.

Kondo T, Otani K, Tokinaga N, et al: Characteristics and risk factors of acute dystonia in schizophrenic patients treated with nemonapride, a selective dopamine antagonist. J Clin Psychopharmacol 19: 45-50, 1999.

Yasui-Furukori N, Kondo T, Ishida M, et al: The characteristics of side-effects of bromperidol in schizophrenic patients. Psychiatry Clin Neurosci 56: 103-106, 2002.

Miura S: Clinical evaluation of blonanserin for schizophrenia - A randomized controlled study comparing blonanserin with risperidone. Jpn J Clin Psychopharmacol 11: 297-314, 2008. (Article in Japanese)

Keegan DL, Rajput AH: Drug induced dystonia tarda: Treatment with 1-dopa. Dis Nerv Syst 34: 167–169, 1973.

Tarsy D: Movement disorders with neuroleptic drug treatment. Psychiatr North Am 7:435-471, 1984

Inada T, Sasada K: Comparison of the efficasy of psychotropic drugs at a glance: Evidence graphic version Vol 3: Evidence of side effects and adverse events. Jiho Inc., Tokyo, pp16-17, 2004. (Article in Japanese)

Inada T, Sasada K: Comparison of the efficasy of psychotropic drugs at a glance: Evidence graphic version Vol 3: Evidence of side effects and adverse events. Jiho Inc., Tokyo, pp16-17, 2004. (Article in Japanese)

Kamishima K, Ishigooka J, Komada Y: Long term .treatment with risperidone long-acting injectable in patients with schizophrenia. Jpn J Psychiatr Treat 12: 1223-1244, 2009. (Article in Japanese)

Miller LG, Jankovic J: Neurogenic approach to drug induced movement disorders: a study of 125 patients. South Med J 8: 525-532, 1990.

Kamishima K, Ishigooka J, Komada Y: Comparison study between risperidone long-acting injectable and risperidone tablets in patients with schizophrenia. Jpn J Psychiatr Treat 12: 1199-1222, 2009. (Article in Japanese)

Van Harten PN, van Trier JC, Horwitz EH, et al: Cocaine as a risk factor for neuroleptic-induced acute dystonia. J Clin Psychiatry 59: 128-130, 1998.

Mazurek MF, Rosebush PI: Circadian pattern of acute, neuroleptic-induced dystonic reactions. Am J Psychiatry 153: 708-710, 196.

Inada T, Yagi G, Kamijima K, Ohnishi K, Kamisada M, Takamiya M, Nakajima S, Rockhold RW: A statistical trial of subclassification for tardive dyskinesia. Acta Psychiatr Scand 82: 404-407, 1990.

Fahn S, Marsden CD, Calne DB: Classification and investigation of dystonia. In Marsden CD & Fahn S eds. Movement Disorders 2. Butterworth & Co, London, pp332-358, 1987.

Inada T, Ohnishi K, Kamisada M, Matsuda G, Tajima O, Yanagisawa Y, Hashiguchi K, Shima S, Oh-e Y, Masuda Y, Chiba T, Kamijima K, Rockhold RW, Yagi G: A prospective study of tardive dyskinesia in Japan. Euro Arch Psychiatry Clin Neurosci 240: 250-254, 1991a.

Inada T, Yagi G, Kamijima K, Ohnishi K, Kamisada M, Rockhold RW: Clinical variants of tardive dyskinesia in Japan. Jpn J Psychiatr Neurol 45: 67-71, 1991b.

Harada T: Neuroleptic-induced tardive dystonia. Seishin Igaku 32: 237-243, 1990. (Article in Japanese)

Sachdev P: Clinical characteristics of 15 patients with tardive dystonia. Am J Psychiatry 150: 498-500, 1993.

Van Harten PN, Kahn RS: Tardive dystonia. Schizophr Bull 25: 741-748, 1999.

Raja M: Managing antipsychotic-induced acute and tardive dystonia. Drug Saf 19: 57-72, 1998.

Kiriakakis V, Bhatia KP, Quinn NP, et al: The natural history of tardive dystonia: A long-term follow up study of 107 cases. Brain 121: 2053-2066, 1998.

Sachdev PS: Depression-dependent exacerbation of tardive dyskinesia. Br J Psychiatry 155: 253-255, 1989.

Sandyk R, Pardeshi R. Mood-dependent fluctuations in the severity of tardive dyskinesia and psoriasis vulgaris in a patient with schizoaffective disorder: possible role of melatonin. Int J Neurosci 50: 215-221

Yazici O, Kantemir E, Taştaban Y, et al: Spontaneous improvement of tardive dystonia during mania. Br J Psychiatry 158: 847-850, 1991.

LeWitt PA. Dystonia caused by drugs. In: Tsui JKC, King J, Calne DB ed. Handbook of Dystonia. Marcel Dekker Inc, New York, 227-240, 1995.

Hornykiewicz O, Kish SJ, Becker LE, et al: Brain neurotransmitters in dystonia musculorum deformans, N Engl J Med 315: 347-353, 1986.

Walker JM, Matsumoto RR, Bowen WD, et al: Evidence for a role of haloperidol-sensitive sigma-'opiate' receptors in the motor effects of antipsychotic drugs. Neurology 38: 961-965, 1988.

GO CL, Rosales RL, Caraos RJ, et al: The current prevalence and factors assosiated with tardive dyskinesia among Filipino schzophtrnic patients. Parkinsonisn and Relatd Disorders 15: 655-659, 2009.

Keegan DL, Rajupt AH: Drug induced dystonia tarda: treatment with 1-dopa. Dis \nerv Syst 34: 167-169, 1973.

Burke RE, Fahn S, Jancovic J, et al: Tardive dystonia and inappropriate use of neuroleptic drugs. Lancet 1: 1299, 1982b.

Burke RE: Neuroleptic-tardive dyskinesia variants. In: Lang AE and Weiner WJ eds. Drug-Induced Movement Disorders. Futura Publishing, New York, pp167-198, 1992.

Greene P: Tardive dystonia in neuroleptic induced movement disorders, In Yassa R, Nair NPV, Jeste DV eds. Neuroleptic Induced Movement Disorders. Cambridge University Press, Cambridge, pp395-408, 1997.

Inada T, Yagi G: Current topics in tardive dyskinesia in Japan. Psychiatr Clin Neurosci 49: 239-244, 1995.

Inada T, Yagi G: Current topics in neuroleptic-induced extrapyramidal symptoms in Japan. Keio J Med 95-99, 1996.

Inada T: DIEPSS A second-generation rating scale for antipsychjotic-induced extrapyramidal symptoms: Drug-induced Extrapyramidal Symptom Scale. Seiwa Shoten Publishers INC, Tokyo, 2009.

Yamamoto N: A schizophrenic patients with Pisa syndrome treated successfully with quetiapine. Seishin-Igaku 47: 1323-1325, 2005. (Article in Japanese)

Imai N, Ikawa M: Efficacy of aripiprazole in sulpiride-induced tardive oromandibular dystonia. Intern Med 50: 635-637, 2011.

Fahn S, Eldridge R: Definition of dystonia and classification of the dystonic states. Adv Neurol 14: 1-5, 1976.

Sugiyama H, Asada T, Kariya T: A case of the antipsychotic-induced tardive dystonia treated successfully with high dose of trihexyphenidil. Jpn J Psychiatr Treat 11: 845-850, 1996. (Article in Japanese)

Yamamoto N, Oda T, Inada T: Methamphetamine psychosis in which tardive dystonia was successfully treated with clonazepam. Psychiatry Clin Neurosci 61: 691-694, 2007.

Otsuki K, Nagano T, Harada T, et al: The efficacy of dantrolene on the neuroleptic-induced tardive dystonia: A case report. Jpn J Psychiatr Treat 6: 207-209, 1991. (Article in Japanese)

Jancovic J, Brin MF: Therapeutic uses of botulinum toxin. N Engl J Med 324: 1186-1194, 1991

Kimura T, Iwara K, Nagahashi T, et al: Clinical experience of botulinum toxin A in the treatment of tardive dystonia. Jpn J Clin Psychopharmacol 8: 507-514, 2005. (Article in Japanese)

6

Dystonia in Parkinsonian Syndromes

Ramon Lugo and Hubert H. Fernandez
Cleveland Clinic
USA

1. Introduction

Dystonia is a common feature in parkinsonian syndromes. In one Brazilian study, dystonia was observed in up to 50% of patients with "atypical parkinsonism" (1). It is also a prominent feature in various hereditary and neurodegenerative conditions implicating the basal ganglia such as Huntington's disease, Wilson's disease, familial basal ganglia calcifications and neurodegeneration with brain iron accumulation (NBAI) (2). Moreover, we have to keep in mind that a proportion of patient thought to have idiopathic Parkinson's disease (PD) may later be found to have a different parkinsonian syndrome. In this chapter, the features of dystonia in parkinsonian syndromes will be discussed, with an emphasis on PD, progressive supranuclear palsy (PSP), multiple systems atrophy (MSA), with a brief discussion about other parkinsonian syndromes where dystonia can present. A general treatment algorithm is proposed for parkinsonian disorders that present with dystonia (see Figure 1).

2. Parkinson's disease

The most common presentation of dystonia in PD is in the context of levodopa exposure, experienced by approximately 30% of patients (3-5). Several dystonic conditions exist: pre-treatment dystonia, peak dose dystonia, early morning dystonia and off period dystonia (3). Of which, the most common dystonic condition is off-state lower extremity painful dystonia (2,5). With regards to the area of involvement, Sheffield et al reported a frequency of 10% for facial dystonia, 10% for cervical, 30% for leg, 17.5% for arm and 7.5% for trunk dystonia (5). One common feature is that the dystonia is often ipsilateral to the initially affected (and therefore more affected) side in PD (2). The age of onset seems to be a major factor in the development of dystonia. It has been reported in up to 53%-60% of PD patients with onset before age 40 (2,5). As mentioned above we can classify the dystonic phenomenology in PD in relation to the exposure to levodopa: pre-treatment dystonia, peak dose dystonia, early morning dystonia and off period dystonia.

It was previously assumed that early onset primary torsion dystonia (PTD) and early onset PD shared common DYT1 gene mutations since both conditions seems to have dopamine dysfunction. However, a study have shown the association of DYT1 with early onset PTD but not early onset PD (6).

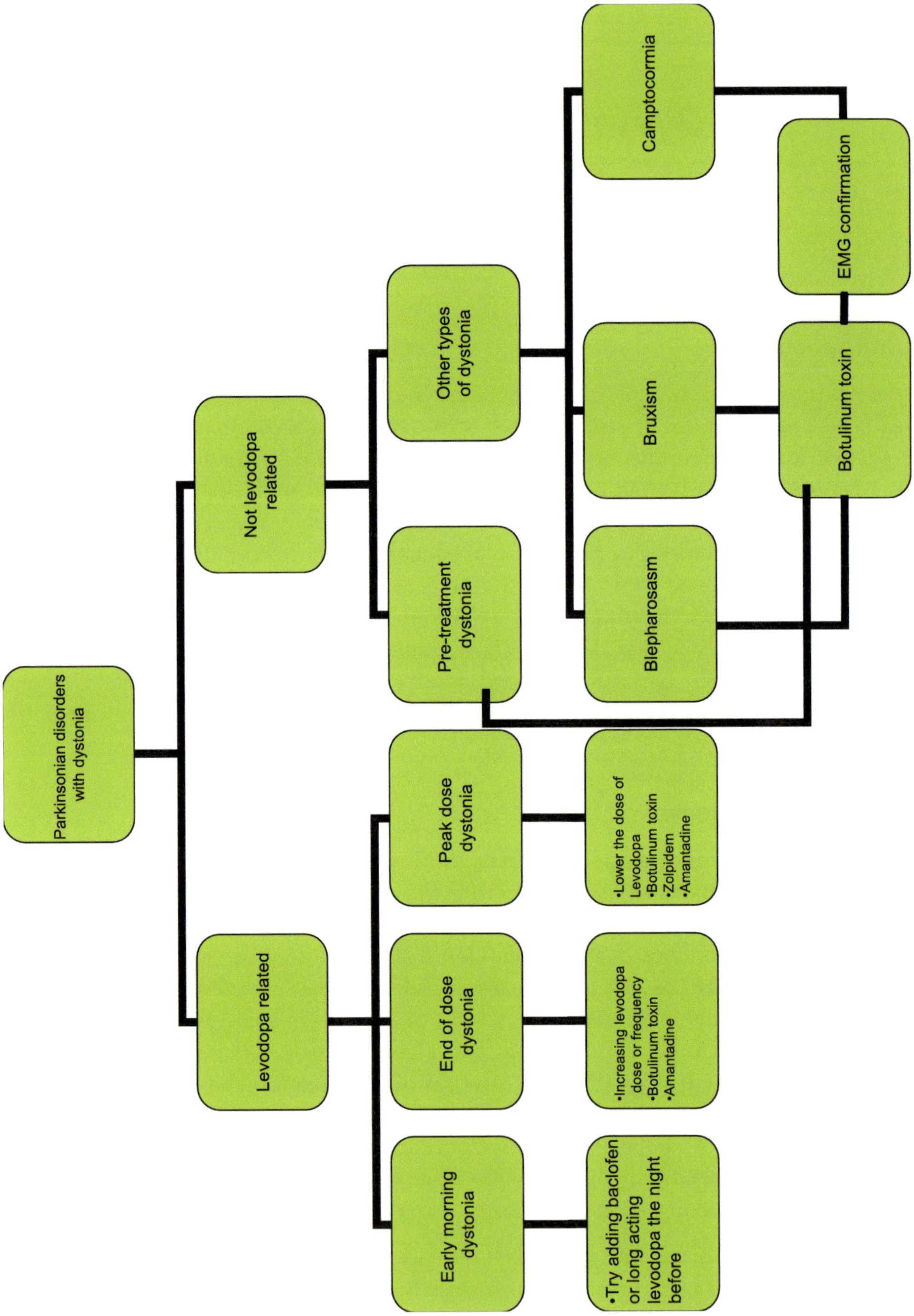
Parkinsonian disorders with dystonia
Not levodopa related
Levodopa related
Other types of dystonia
Pre-treatment dystonia
Camptocormia
Bruxism
Blepharosasm
EMG confirmation
Botulinum toxin
Peak dose dystonia
End of dose dystonia
Early morning dystonia
•Lower the dose of Levodopa
•Botulinum toxin
•Zolpidem
•Amantadine
•Increasing levodopa dose or frequency
•Botulinum toxin
•Amantadine
•Try adding baclofen or long acting levodopa the night before

Fig. 1.

2.1 Pretreatment dystonia

This is generally defined as dystonia before exposure to levodopa. Kidron et al, reported the frequency of this type of dystonia to be 2.4% in their population (3). It typically involved the feet, was induced by volitional activity and usually involved the most parkinsonian side. Laryngeal dystonia has also been reported to precede the diagnosis of PD (7). This was effectively treated with botulinum toxin (BoNT) injections.

2.2 Peak dose dystonia

This is generally defined as dystonia occurring during the "on" period following levodopa dosing. Usually it is present in the midst of generalized dyskinesia, occurring in about 7% of patients (8). It appears mostly after long term exposure of levodopa. It affects mostly the extremities but it can also affect the trunk or the neck. Typically, it appears after 30 minutes to two hours of taking levodopa and stops after 15 minutes to 2 hours. It may not appear with every levodopa dose, nor does it have followed a particular pattern. The treatment is typically to decrease the dose of levodopa. However, PD symptoms may worsen with this approach. BoNT has been used effectively for treatment of this focal dystonia (5). Zolpidem has been reported to be effective in treating not only peak dose dystonia but also dyskinesia in PD patients (8), supposedly due to its GABA-ergic activity.

2.3 Early morning dystonia

This dystonia often appears upon awakening, before the first dose of levodopa, in up to 16% of patients (3,19). It also appears after long exposure to levodopa. It usually affects the lower extremities only, either unilaterally or bilaterally. This time, the most parkinsonian side is not always the affected side. It can happen when they still in bed or after trying to walk. It is mostly a painful dystonia lasting up to 2 hours. It usually subsides spontaneously without any relation to levodopa dosing. Changing or adding more levodopa may have little to no benefit in the treatment of this kind of dystonia. However, one study showed that adding baclofen the night prior, helped to shorten the duration of the dystonia in half of patients (3).

2.4 Off period dystonia

This type of dystonia develops when the benefits of levodopa on PD symptoms wears off. In one study, 10% was found to have off period dystonia (3). It can occur at rest or during activity, and it can be quite severe. In one case, the patient suffered a left metatarsal fracture in the setting of an off period dystonia (10). Also it appears after long exposure of levodopa. It has a tendency to appear ipsilaterally to the most parkinsonian side. In one study, off period dystonia appeared regardless of stopping levodopa abruptly or slowly. Dystonia appeared when the concentrations of levodopa in the blood dropped to a 30% from its optimal antiparkinsonian effect. This dystonia can respond to either increase in the daily levodopa dose or the number of doses. In one case series, 41% of patients with off period dystonia resolved immediately after implantation of bilateral subthalamic nucleus (STN), presumably from its lesioning effect (11). BoNT has also been used to treat this phenomenon effectively (5). Continuous levodopa duodenal infusion has also been reported to be beneficial in treating the dystonia (12).

2.5 Other types of dystonia

2.5.1 Blepharospasm

This is characterized by involuntary forceful eyelid closure. It is rarely present in idiopathic PD, especially in its pure form. More often than not, when is present, it is associated with apraxia of eyelid opening—characterized by difficulty in voluntarily opening the eyes, sometimes with the patients needing to use their thumb and index finger to open their eyes. In both instances, BoNT is the treatment of choice.

2.5.2 Bruxism

This can be classified as a form of oromandibular dyskinesia, and can lead to headache, teeth destruction and temporomandibular joint disease. Long term use of levodopa is known to cause this. This phenomenon has also been successfully treated with BoNT.

2.5.3 Camptocormia

This characterized by involuntary and often forceful forward bending of the trunk. Patients often feel like something is pulling them to bend forward. This responds poorly to levodopa or dopamine agonist (DA). However there is a report of camptocormia responsive to levodopa treatment (13). Unfortunately, anti-spasticity medications have shown no benefit on this challenging condition (5). If there is EMG evidence of abdominal rectus contraction, BoNT has proven to be an effective treatment (5).

2.5.4 Pisa syndrome

This refers to the forceful lateral flexion of the trunk. It can involve the head and neck as well. It can be idiopathic, related to antipsychotic treatment, and more recently described in neurodegenerative disorders, especially in the setting of cholinesterase inhibitor, selective serotonin reuptake inhibitor or antiparkinsonian treatment (14). Improvement of this condition has been reported with treatment with BoNT alone or in conjunction with physical therapy/rehabilitation treatment (14,15). Walking aids that accentuate trunk extension and minimize flexion may provide as a sensory aid (that can transiently improve the condition while using the walker) as well as assist in gait and mobility in this condition. In one study, Pisa syndrome was most often observed in relation to changes in Parkinsonian regimens (16). This can occur when increasing or decreasing dopaminergic stimulation by either increasing or decreasing dosages or adding or eliminating medications. In this particular seriese, prompt recognition that ledd to the undoing of the changes made (whenever possible) resulted in the improvement or even resolution of Pisa syndrome. The authors emphasized the importance of recognizing the onset of this syndrome before it becomes a chronic and possibly irreversible problem.

2.5.5 Anterocollis

This refers to the forward flexion of the neck and is a sign most commonly seen in MSA. However, Kashihara et al, published that anterocollis can happen in 15 out of 252 (6%) patients with PD (17).

3. Multiple system atrophy

More recently, MSA has been officially sub-classified as MSA-P if the predominant symptoms are parkinsonian, or MSA-C if the most predominant symptoms are cerebellar. Autonomic disturbance can occur in 73% of patients with this syndrome (2, 18). The dystonic features of this syndrome can affect the axial muscles and neck. They can also have dystonic movement of the toes. In one case series, they found that the frequency of dystonia in MSA was between 30.4%- 42% (1,19). Dystonia can manifest 2 to 4 years after clinical onset (2). Severe anterocollis has been associated with this syndrome and being the most common form of dystonia. It has been observed in about 25-50% of cases. However, there are some doubts as to whether this severe anterocollis is dystonic in nature. Some argue that the nature of the anterocollis could be severe and disproportionate rigidity affecting the anterior neck (1). Another possibility is that the nature of the anterocollis in MSA can be due to myopathy affecting the neck extensors (19,20). The lack of meaningful response to BoNT when injecting both sternocleidomastoid muscles (SCM) which tend to support these alternate hypotheses. The presence of dystonia in MSA has been associated with lesions in the contralateral head of the caudate. In one study,dystonia was present in 46% of MSA patients. All of the patients had focal dystonia (19). In all patients dystonia developed in the same side where the initial symptoms presented. All of these patients were exposed to levodopa, however, their response depended in part on their MSA subtype. Approximately 38% of them did not have benefit with escalating dose of levodopa up to 1200 mg/day and therapy was withdrawn. Most of these patients had MSA-C. Moreover, none of these patients developed dyskinesias. On the other hand, motor fluctuations developed in all the patients with MSA-P that responded to levodopa and 80% developed dyskinesia approximately 2 years after levodopa exposure. Dystonia developed in all but one patient with dyskinesia (19).

4. Progressive supranuclear palsy

This condition, described more than 25 years ago, often involving the geriatric population, is characterized by parkinsonism associated with early gait instability and significant, early onset ophthalmoplegia affecting mostly the vertical axis. This can be manifested by the inability of the patient to perform saccades or in pursuing a target. However, this ophthalmoplegia can be overcoeme with oculocephalics thus making it "supranuclear". While often early in onset, this feature may not appear for up to 9 years into the disease (2). Another feature is retrocollis (involuntary extension of the neck). This also has been debated whether it is a form of dystonia or severe rigidity. The typical characteristics of dystonia are absent in the axial dystonia seen in PSP, such as: worsening during walking, when there is stress to the musculature; having a diurnal fluctuation; and, responding to sensory tricks. In one study "axial dystonia in extension" was found 17% of patients (2). None of these patients, however, presented the typical dystonic features mentioned above. For these reasons the term dystonia should be avoided in these cases. Instead, "nuchal rigidity in extension" should be adopted (21).

Blepharospasm has also been associated with PSP. It can occur as reflex blepharospasm or spontaneous blepharospasm. The frequency has been reported to be from 8% to 23%. Some scholars argue that apraxia of eye lid opening has been confused with blepharospasm. Around 50% of patients may have an associated apraxia of eyelid opening. In one study the frequency of blepharospasm was 24% (21). There is a discrepancy when reviewing limb dystonia in pathologically confirmed cases versus clinical observation. In the former, limb dystonia seems to be a rare occurrence. In contrast, numerous clinical reports support its common occurrence (1). One study showed that the rate of dystonia in PSP was 46%, while another reported that dystonia, of any type, occurred in 62.5% of patients with PSP, with equal distribution of retrocollis and limb dystonia (1). Just one patient in this series had blepharospasm. Another study showed that limb dystonia occurred at a rate of 27% (21). Among those patients 11% had hemidystonic distribution. One unusual pattern noted was the "pointing gun" posture-- when the index finger and thumb were extended (21). Only in 10% of patients did the dystonia involve a single limb (21). However, it should also be noted that in this series, most all of these patients with limb dystonia that had autopsies actually had concurrent brain diseases, the most common being cerebrovascular disease. Only 3 were shown to pathologically fulfill PSP criteria. Given these findings the authors suggested that some cases of PSP can be misdiagnosed as CBGD and vascular parkinsonism.

5. Corticobasalganlionic degeneration

The clinical features of corticobasalganlionic degeneration (CBGD) include akinesia, postural instability, limb dystonia, rigidity, tremors (postural and kinetic), cortical myoclonus, in addition of cortical sensory loss, ideomotor limb apraxia, alien hand syndrome, typically presenting (and often remaining) asymmetrically. One of the dystonic manifestations of CBGD is severe hand dystonia with some fingers extended and some flexed. However this may not be as frequent (1). Action-induced or reflex myoclonus usually accompanies dystonic posturing. In one series, all the patients with CBGD developed limb dystonia (2). Asymmetric cortical atrophy is typically seen contralateral to the most affected, dystonic side (22).

6. Miscellaneous

6.1 Dopamine transporter dysfunction

In one study Blackstone reported a mutation in the dopamine transporter (DAT) as the cause of infantile parkinsonism-dystonia syndrome (23). This syndrome is usually present in infancy with slowness of movement, rigidity and rest tremor. Dystonia accompanies the parkinsonism. This protein is involved in the reuptake of dopamine from the synaptic cleft to the presynaptic neuron. This mutation is associated to a loss of function thereby impairing dopamine reuptake. In this study, the affected patients showed increased levels of dopamine metabolites such as homovanillic acid in the cerebrospinal fluid (CSF). This drove the conclusion that the excess of dopamine in the synaptic left can 1) deplete intracellular stores of dopamine, 2) down regulate the postsynaptic receptors and 3) activate D2 presynaptic receptors to further decrease the synthesis of dopamine (23).

However there have been other cases of infantile parkinsonism-dystonia where no mutations in the DAT have been identified. There is a wide range of presentation of the disease. Ocular flutter (involuntary burst of eye movement around a point of fixation), and saccade initiation failure have also been reported (23,24).

6.2 Dopamine responsive dystonia

The cause of dopamine responsive dystonia (DRD) is a hereditary deficiency in the dopamine pathway. These patients tend to have a brisk response to low dose levodopa. Two mutations will be mentione--one affecting the enzyme GTP cyclo-hydrolase (GTPCH) or DYT5a. This mutation is inherited in an autosomal dominant pattern. The other is tyrosine hydroxylase (TH) or DYT5b, which seems to be inherited recessively. These also are more severe and more complex than the typical DRD.

One characteristic feature is the diurnal fluctuations, with symptoms getting worse as the day progresses, and improving after sleep. It most commonly presents in the first decade of life, typically involving the legs first, then gradually generalizing. However, when presenting later, parkinsonian symptoms may be observed. The presentation of children with TH mutations are more complex. These patients can have mental retardation, oculogyric crisis and hypotonia (25).

6.3 Wilson's disease

This is a recessively inherited condition due to mutations in the *ATP7B* gene. It can present mostly in the first decade of life but later presentations, usually before the age of 50, have been reported. It is often associated with liver disease and psychiatric disorders. Movement disorder presentations include: dystonia, ataxia, tremors, chorea, and parkinsonism. Cooper studies are necessary for the diagnosis. Serum cooper is unreliable in Wilson's disease. The more reliable work up includes: 24 hour urine copper, serum ceruloplasmin, and a slit lamp examination looking for Kayser-Fleischer rings. MRI of the brain can show variety of abnormalities that affect the basal ganglia, brainstem, white matter and thalamus. Genetic testing is available but can be complicated by individual mutations specific to a family (25).

6.4 PARK2-Parkin

Mutations in this gene cause autosomal recessive young-onset parkinsonism. The symptomatology of PARK2 patients is very similar to idiopathic PD. However there is the thought that PARK2 patients have intact sense of smell (25). Dystonia can be present and can be the presenting symptom in about 40% of patients. It typically affects the lower extremities.

6.5 PARK6- PTEN-induced putative kinase 1 (PINK1)

Mutations in this gene can also cause autosomal recessive inherited parkinsonism. It is of slow progression and typically with a sustained response to levodopa. Foot dystonia, urinary urgency, orthostatic hypotension, cognitive disorders and psychiatric disorders have also been described (25).

6.6 X-lined dystonia and parkinsonism (Lubag)

As the name implies this is an X-linked inherited syndrome characterized by the onset of dystonia affecting the craniocervical region, trunk, or the distal limbs and later progressing to develop parkinsonism (26). The dystonic manifestations are diverse, including oromandibular, lingual, cervical, truncal, foot and limb dystonia. (27,28). It is minimally responsive to medication. It is very prominent in Philippines, particular among inhabitants and descendants from the Island of Panay (29). Within 5 years it can progress to generalized dystonia. Parkinsonism may not be the only accompanied symptoms but myoclonus, chorea, focal tremor, and myorhythmia may be present. Females may also be affected but in a much milder form (25). MRI may show signal abnormalities in and mild atrophy of the caudate and putamen during the beginning of the disease. However when parkinsonian symptoms develops there is much more striking atrophy and signal abnormalities in those structures.

Treatment can be challenging since antipsychotics, anticholinergic and antiparkinsonian drugs are not consistently effective (30). However BoNT may give temporary relief of the dystonia (25,27,28). There is one report of Zolpidem to be effective in treating the dyskinesia, dystonia and akinesia in a patient with XDP. There are some reports that DBS implantation in bilateral globus pallidus internus improved the dystonia in this syndrome (26,30). However one of this reports showed no benefit in the patient's parkinsonism (26).

6.7 Other disorders that can present with dystonia-parkinsonism

1. PARK7- DJ1
2. Neurodegenration with Brain Iron Accumulation (NBA)1-Pantothenate Kinase-associated Neurodegenration (PKAN)
3. NBIA 2 Associated with PLA2G6 gene mutation/PARK 14
4. PARK 9- Kufor-Rakeb Disease
5. SENDA syndrome
6. Neuroferritinopathy
7. PARK15-FBXO7-associated neurodegeneration
8. DYT16
9. Rapid onset dystonia Parkinsonism (DYT12)
10. Spatacsin (SPG11)

7. Conclusions

Dystonia in parkinsonian disorders is a well-recognized entity. For the most part the diagnosis of a parkinsonian syndrome is largely clinical. This makes the classification of patients challenging at times. Symptoms can overlap between different parkinsonian disorders. Complicating this picture is that dystonia can occur in primary parkinsonian conditions, and parkinsonism can occur in primay dystonic conditions. Recent advancements on genetics have challenged our traditional classification of parkinsonian and dystonic conditions based on clinical presentation. Organized data of pathologically-confirmed cases are wanting. More extensive studies with larger patient cohorts with pathological and/or genetic confirmation are needed. Finally, treatment of dystonia in parkinsonian conditions remain challenging, despite the growing utilization of BoNT and the promise of DBS surgery.

8. References

[1] Godeiro C., Felicio A.C., et al. (2008). Clinical features of dystonia in atypical Parkinsonism. *Arq. Neuropsiaquiatr.* Vol. 66, 4, pp 800-804

[2] Rivest J., Quinn N. (1990). Dystonia in Parkinson's Disease, multiple system atrophy, and progressive supranuclear palsy. *Neurology.* Vol. 40, pp. 1571-1578 Print ISSN 0028-3878 Online ISSN 1526-632X

[3] Kindron D., Melamed E. (1987). Forms of Dystonia in patients with Parkinson's disease. *Neurology.* Vol. 37, pp. 1009-1011 Print ISSN 0028-3878 Online ISSN 1526-632X

[4] Bravi D., Moudradian M.M., et al. (1993). End of dose dystonia in Parkinson's disease. *Neurology.* Vol. 43 pp 2130-2131

[5] Sheffield J.K., Jankovick J. (2007). Botulinum toxin in the treatment of tremors, dystonias, sialorrhea and other symptoms associated with Parkinson's disease. *Expert Revision Neurotherapeutics.* Vol. 7, 6, pp 637-647. ISSN 1473-7175

[6] Yang J., Wu T., et al. (2009). DYT1 mutations in early onset primary torsion dystonia and Parkinson disease in Chinese populations. *Neuroscience letters.* Vol. 450, pp 117-121

[7] Papapetropoulos S., Lundy D.S., et al (2007). Laryngeal Dystonia as a Presenting Symptom of Young Onset Parkinson's Disease. *Movement disorders.* Vol. 22, pp 1670-1671

[8] Chen ,Y. (2008). Zolpidem improves akinesia, dystonia and dyskinesia in advance Parkinson's disease. *Journal of Clinical Neuroscience.* Vol. 15, pp 955-956

[9] Currie L.J., Harrison J.M., et al. (1997). Early morning dystonia in Parkinson's disease. *Neurology.* Vol. 51, pp 283

[10] Mcdade E., Weiner W.J., (2007). Metatarsal fracture as a consequence of foot dystonia in Parkinson's disease. *Parkinsonism and Related disorders.* Vol. 14 pp 353-355

[11] Derrey S., Lefaucheur R., et al. (2010). Alleviation of off-period dystonia in Parkinson's disease by microlesion following subthalamic implantation. *Journal of Neurosurgery.* Vol. 112, pp 1263-1266

[12] Sage J.I., McHale. (1989). Continuous Levodopa infusion to treat complex dystonia in Parkinson's disease. *Neurology.* Vol. 39 pp 888-891

[13] Ho B., Parkash R., et al. (2007). A case of levodopa-responsive camptocormia associated with advance Parkinson's disease. *Nature Clinical Practice.* Vol. 3, 9, pp 526-530

[14] Santamato A., Ranieri M., et al. (2010). Botulinum toxin Type A and rehabilitation program in the treatment of Pisa syndrome in Parkinson's disease. *Journal of Neurology.* Vol. 257, pp 139-141

[15] Bonanni L., Thomas A., et al. (2007). Botulinum toxin treatment of lateral axial dystonia in Parkinsonism. *Movement disorders.* Vol. 22, 14, pp 2097-2103

[16] Cannas A., Solla P., et al. (2009). Reversible Pisa syndrome in patients with Parkinson's disease on dopaminergic therapy. *Journal of Neurology.* Vol. 256, pp 390-395

[17] Geser F., Kashihara K. (2007). Disproportionate Anterocollis: A warning sign for Multiple System Atrophy. *Movements disorders.* Vol. 22, 13, pp

[18] Jellinger K.A. (2002). Neuropathological findings in multiple system atrophy with dystonia. *Journal of Neurology Neurosurgery and Psychiatry.* Vol. 73, pp 460-464

[19] Boesch S.M., Wenning G.K., et al. (2002). Dystonia in multiple system atrophy. *Journal of Neurology Neurosurgery and Psychiatry.* Vol. 72 pp 300-303

[20] Riley D.E. (2002). Dystonia in multiple system atrophy. *Journal of Neurology Neurosurgery and Psychiatry.* Vol. 72 p 286

[21] Barclay C. L., Lang A. E. (1997). Dystonia in progressive supranuclear palsy. *Journal of Neurology, Neurosurgery, and Psychiatry.* Vol. 62, pp. 352-356

[22] Riley D.E., Lang A.E., et al. (1990). Cortical-basal ganglionic degeneration.*eurology.* Vol. 40, pp1203-1212

[23] Blackstone C. (2009). Infantile Parkinsonism- dystonia a dopamine "transportopathy". *The Journal of Clinical Investigation.* Vol. 119, 6, pp 1455-1458

[24] Blackstone C. (2010). Infantile parkinsonism-dystonia due to dopamine transporter gene mutation: another genetic twist. *The Lancet.* Vol. 10, pp 24-25

[25] Schneider S.A., Bhatia K.P. (2010). Rare causes of Dystonia Parkinsonism. *Current Neurological and Neurosurgical Report.*ol. 10, pp 431-439

[26] Oyama G., Fernandez H.H. (2010). Differential Response of Dystonia and Parkinsonism following Globus Pallidus Internus Deep Brain Stimulation in X-Linked Dystonia-Parkinsonism (Lubag). *Stereotactic Functional Neurosurgery.* Vol. 88, pp 329-333

[27] Rosales RL, Santos MM, Ng AR, Teleg R, Dantes M, Lee LV, Fernandez HH. The broadening application of chemodenervation in X-linked dystonia-parkinsonism (Part I): Muscle Afferent Block versus Botulinum Toxin-A in Cervical and Limb Dystonia. *Int J Neurosci* 2011; 121 Suppl 1: 34-43

[28] Rosalez RL, Ng AR, Santoss MM, Fernandez HH. The broadening application of chemodenervation in X-linked dystonia-parkinsonism (Part II): An open-label experience3 with botulinum toxin-A (dysport) injection for oromandubular, lingual and truncal-axial dystonias. *Int J Neurosci* 2011; 121 Suppl 1:44-56)

[29] Fernandez HH, Rosales RL. Uncovering the Mystery from the Philippine Island of Panay. Int J Neurosci 2011; 121 Suppl 1:1-2

[30] Wadia P.M., Lim S., et al. (2010). Bilateral Pallidal stimulation for X-linked dystonia Parkinsonism. *Archives Neurology.* Vol. 67, 8, pp 1012-1015

7

Dystonia with Tremors: A Clinical Approach

Young Eun Kim and Beom Seok Jeon
Seoul National University Hospital
Korea

1. Introduction

Dystonia commonly accompanies tremors but the prevalence of the association is controversial. Oppenheim had already described that tremors were associated with dystonic symptoms in "Dystonia Musculorum Deformans" in the early 20th century (Oppenheim et al, 1911, as cited in Jedynak et al., 1991). Yanagisawa analyzed idiopathic dystonia with electromyography and found that dystonia was associated with rhythmic activity in all of the patients (Yanagisawa & Goto, 1971). In a genetic and clinical population study on dystonia, 80% of the population had tremors for generalized dystonia (Larsson and Sjogren, 1966). Marsden reported that 14% of patients with generalized nonfamilial idiopathic dystonia presented with tremors (Marsden, 1974). In addition, 68% of patients with cervical dystonia had head tremors (Pal et al., 2000). However, Rondot examined 132 patients with cervical dystonia, which revealed rhythmic activity and upper limb tremors in 40% and 21% of the patients, respectively (Rondot et al., 1981, as cited in Jedynak et al., 1991). In a survey on writer`s cramp, hand tremors were reported in almost half of the subjects (Sheehy, 1982). In addition, Jankovic investigated 350 patients diagnosed with Essential tremor (ET), based on the presence of tremors in the head, hand, or voice in the absence of any other diseases that may cause tremors. Forty-seven percent of these subjects also had dystonia (Lou and Jankovic, 1991). Therefore, the prevalence of dystonia with tremors varies greatly depending on the reports.

Dystonic tremor syndrome has been under-recognized and sometimes mistaken as ET or even Parkinson`s disease (Elble and Deuschl, 2011). However, dystonic tremor syndrome is not just ET but also a distinct clinical entity, and has the possibility of having a secondary cause (Bain, 2009; Cho et al., 2000; Jankovic & Linden, 1988; Kim & Lee, 2007; Oyama et al, 2011; Schneider et al., 2007; Vidailhet et al., 1998; Yoon et al., 2009). Moreover, the progress and treatment of dystonic tremors are different from other tremor disorders (Gironell & Kulisevsky, 2009).

However, dystonic tremor syndrome is still under debate and different definitions have been proposed (Deuschl et al., 1998).

This chapter will focus on the clinical criteria and differential characteristics of dystonic tremor syndrome.

2. Clinical criteria of dystonic tremor syndrome: According to the involved site

Dystonic tremor is a relatively new classification of tremor. The Movement Disorder Society (MDS) proposed a consensus statement for the tremor in 1998 (Deuschl et al, 1998).

According to these criteria, dystonic tremor syndromes were divided into three types: dystonic tremor, tremor associated with dystonia, and dystonia gene-associated tremor.

2.1 Dystonic tremor

Dystonic tremor means tremor in a body part affected by dystonia. That is to say, the tremor and dystonia occur simultaneously in the same body part such as the arm or neck. This is usually a focal, postural, or kinetic tremor but usually not seen during complete rest (Deuschl et al, 1998). Typical examples of this type are a dystonic head tremor, which is a head tremor in patients with cervical dystonia, and a dystonic writing tremor, which is a writing tremor in patients with writer`s cramp.

2.2 Tremor associated with dystonia

This tremor occurs in a body part not affected by dystonia, but the patient has dystonia elsewhere (Deuschl et al, 1998). It is uncertain whether this type of tremor is the cormorbid occurrence of ET along with dystonia (Lou & Jankovic, 1991) or is a distinct entity (Deuschl et al., 1997; Munchanu., 2001; Shaikh et al., 2008). A typical type is an upper limb postural tremor in patients with cervical dystonia.

2.3 Dystonia gene-associated tremor

This type of tremor is an isolated finding in patients with a dystonia pedigree. A typical example of this type is an isolated tremor occurring in a patient with first-degree relatives with spasmodic torticollis (Deuschl et al, 1997; Yanagisawa et al., 1972).

2.4 Variability in the definition of dystonic tremor

Quinn reported that in the absence of any alternative causes for their tremor, dystonic tremor and tremor associated with dystonia should be called dystonic tremor (Quinn et al., 2011). The prevalence and other clinical details of dystonic tremor are variously reported since the clinical criteria of dystonic tremor are not clearly defined. This chapter describes dystonic tremor syndrome following the MDS criteria.

3. Differential characteristics of dystonic tremor syndrome

The dystonic tremor is significantly different from disorders with pure tremors. In addition, the tremor associated with dystonia has also been reported recently to be different from other pure forms of tremors combined with dystonia. However, the clinical significance of the dystonia gene-associated tremor is not known.

3.1 Dystonic tremor

In a study on idiopathic dystonia with electromyography, Yanagisawa described that dystonia was stimulated by postural effort, and that, largely irregular, sometimes regular, tremulous muscle activity was observed during a dystonic posture (Yanagisawa & Goto, 1971). In a study on dystonic tremors with electromyography, the dystonic tremor was shown to be postural, localized, and irregular in amplitude and periodicity; and absent during muscle relaxation, exacerbated by smooth muscle contraction, and associated frequently with myoclonus (Jedynak et al., 1991). The frequency of the dystonic tremor is mostly below 7Hz, and very rarely, rest tremors may occur (Deuschl, 1998, 2001). The dystonic tremor may have some specific features of dystonia such as "geste antagoniste" (sensory trick) (Jahanshahi, 2000).

3.2 Tremor associated with dystonia

Tremors of the hands can be seen often in patients with cervical dystonia (Couch, 1976). There were some controversies whether this type of tremor is the same as ET or not. ET and cervical dystonia may be physiologically and possibly also genetically related. Cervical dystonia has been reported in 0.6~30% of patients with ET (Critchley, 1972; Baxter and Lal, 1979; Martinelli and Gabellini, 1982; Rajput et al., 1984; Lou and Jankovic, 1991; Koller et al., 1994; Tallon-Barranco et al.,1997, as cited in Munchau et al., 2001). Additionally, postural and kinetic tremors are found in 4-55% of patients with cervical dystonia (Patterson and Little, 1943; Couch, 1976; Chan et al., 1991; Lang et al., 1992; Dubinski et al., 1993; Deuschl et al., 1997, 1998, as cited in Munchau et al., 2001). In 1991, Lou and Jankovic reported 47% of patients with ET had dystonia, but this analysis found no support for the differentiation of ET subtypes although it was heterogenous in its clinical presentation (Lou and Jankovic, 1991).

However, in a study on tremors with 55 cervical dystonia patients, hand tremors in patients with cervical dystonia more closely resembled an enhanced physiological tremor than a dystonic tremor or ET (Deuschl et al 1997). In addition, arm tremors in patients with cervical dystonia was found to develop either before or simultaneously with the onset of torticollis; such a temporal relationship does not correspond to a dystonic tremor either (Munchanu et al., 2001). Besides, the temporal relationship and physiological quantity is also different. The irregularity of the tremor was significantly greater (~50%) in hand tremors associated with cervical dystonia than that of ET (Shaikh et al., 2008). Moreover, the latency of the second agonist EMG burst was later in ET than in CD patients during ballistic wrist flexion movement (Munchau et al., 2001). These findings suggest that the mechanism for the tremor associated with dystonia may differ from that of ET.

3.3 Dystonia gene-associated tremor

This type of tremor was reported in a large pedigree of "Dystonia Musculorum Deformans" of Japanese descent with autosomal dominant inheritance (Yanagisawa et al., 1972).

4. The clinical approach to dystonic tremors

It is difficult to discriminate a dystonic tremor from ET and myoclonic dystonia and from psychogenic and Parkinsonian tremors. There are some observations that help to differentiate these features.

4.1 Dystonic tremor versus Essential tremor

As mentioned above, a dystonic tremor has an irregular, broader range of frequency than that of ET. Myoclonus sometimes can present in a dystonic tremor, but it is never seen in ET. The dystonic tremor is more localized and less symmetric, that is, it occurs in one arm and hand (Yanagisawa & Goto, 1971).

There may be diagnostic ambiguity in cases of head tremors only. How can this type of tremor be differentiated? A dystonic head tremor has a sensory trick (Deuschl et al., 1992). The occurrence of the sensory trick is useful in the differential diagnosis of a head tremor because the sensory trick is found in as many as 90% of the patients with cervical dystonia but not in patients with ET (Jahanshahi, 2000; Elble & Deuschl, 2011). In addition, the dystonic head tremor appears in large amplitude when the affected body part is placed in a position opposite to the major direction of pulling by the dystonia, but the tremor disappears or decreases when the body part is positioned where the dystonia wants to place it (Fahn, 2009). Moreover, cervical dystonia can have hypertrophy of the affected muscles (Jankovic, 2007) and 75% of patients with cervical dystonia have neck pain (Chan et al., 1991) but never in ET.

Less regular,
Asymmetric
Myoclonic component
Sensory tricks
Aggravation for specific posture or null point
Muscle hypertrophy
Pain

Table 1. Clinical features indicative of a dystonic tremor in an isolated head tremor

4.2 Dystonic tremor versus myoclonic tremor

A dystonic tremor has rhythmic activity and appears when a posture is assumed. However, in myoclonic dystonia, a burst of muscular activity can be recorded even at rest although it is facilitated by postures and movements, and the burst of muscular activity can recur at irregular intervals. Myoclonus can present in addition to the dystonic tremor (Jedynak et al, 1991). However, if myoclonus occurs consecutively, it is difficult to draw a line between a dystonic tremor and myoclonic dystonia (Jedynak et al, 1991).

4.3 Dystonic tremor versus psychogenic tremor

A psychogenic tremor can be confused with a dystonic tremor since the duration of the tremor burst in the dystonic tremor is widely variable reflecting its jerky nature and is similar to some psychogenic tremors (McAuley and Rothwell, 2004). However, the psychogenic tremor has psychogenic signs, multiple somatizations, secondary gain, or is related to an injury or event (Elble, 2000).

4.4 Dystonic tremor versus Parkinsonian tremor

A dystonic tremor may present with Parkinsonism, which can lead to a misdiagnosis of PD. SWEDD (Scan Without Evidence of Dopaminergic Deficit) means there can be cases in which some patients with Parkinson-like tremors have no dopaminergic deficit and therefore, do not have Parkinson`s disease (Schwingenschuh et al., 2010). Adult-onset dystonic tremor is one of the causes of SWEDD (Schneider et al., 2007). However, the two conditions are distinguishable by the presence of a jerky tremor, head tremor, dystonic voice, rapid emergence of a postural tremor, normal olfaction, lack of response to dopaminergic medication, relatively stable natural history, and no progression towards developing features other than the tremor and dystonia suggesting a dystonic tremor rather than PD (Schneider et al., 2007; Bain, 2009).

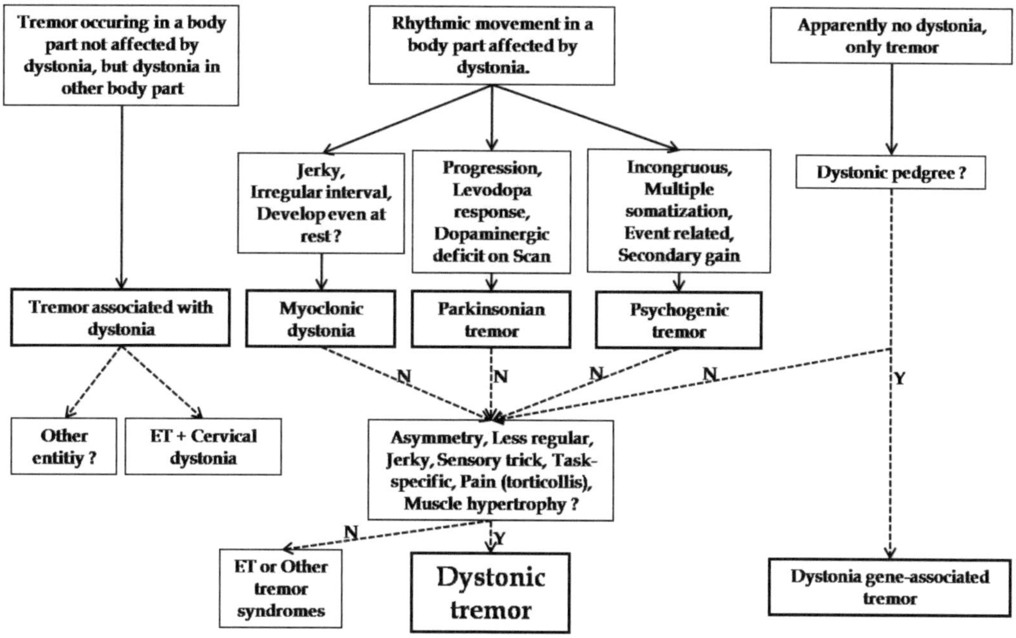

Fig. 1. Clinical approach to dystonic tremor syndrome (Y: yes, N: no)

5. The etiology of dystonic tremor syndrome

Typical primary dystonic tremors are dystonic head tremors and hand tremors in patients with writer`s cramp. However, there are many non-primary causes of dystonic tremor syndrome including Parkinsonism, SWEDD, Wilson disease, NBIA (neurodegeneration in brain iron accumulation), and peripheral trauma and following brain lesions such as thalamus and parietal lesions (Bain, 2009; Cho et al., 2000; Jankovic & Linden, 1988; Kim & Lee, 2007; Oyama et al, 2011; Schneider et al., 2007; Vidailhet et al., 1998; Yoon et al., 2009).

6. The mechanism of dystonic tremor syndrome

The underlying mechanism of dystonic tremor syndrome is not well known. Hallet has proposed that the sensory tricks in dystonic tremors are related to the basic mechanisms underlying the dystonia rather than being a specific feature of the dystonic tremor (Hallet, 1995). Moreover, one widespread notion is that it may be related to the mechanism of dystonia most likely generated within the basal ganglia loop (Deuschl & Bergman., 2002). However, dystonic tremors may also be caused by peripheral mechanisms (Jankovic & Linden, 1988).

7. Conclusion

Dystonic tremor syndrome is distinct clinical entity. Knowing the clinical characteristics of dystonic tremor syndrome is important to help discriminate it from other tremor disorders and to manage it.

8. Acknowledgments

We would like to express our gratitude to the members of the Movement Disorder Center at Seoul National University Hospital for the helpful discussion.

9. References

Bain, PG. (2009). Dystonic tremor presenting as Parkinsonism: long term follow-up of SWEDDs. *Neurology*, Vol.72, pp.1443, ISSN 0028-3878

Baxter, DW. & Lal, S. (1979). Essential tremor and dystonic syndromes. *Advanced Neurology* Vol.24, pp. 373-377

Chan, J., Brin, MF. & Fahn, S. (1991). Idiopathic cervical dystonia: clinical characteristics. *Movement Disorders*, Vol.6, No.2, pp.119-126, ISSN 0885-3185

Cho,C., Lawrence, BS. & Samkoff, (2000). M. A Lesion of the Anterior Thalamus Producing Dystonic Tremor of the Hand *Archives of Neurology*, (2000), Vol.57, pp.1353-1355

Couch, JR. (1976). Dystonia and tremor in spasmodic torticollis. *Advanced Neurology*, Vol.14, (1976), pp.245-258, ISSN 0091-3952

Critchley, E. (1972). Clinical manifestation of essential tremor. *Journal of Neurology, Neurosurgery, and Psychiatry*, Vol.35, pp.365-372, ISSN 0022-3050

Deuschl, G., Heinen, F., Guschlbauer, B., Schneider, S., Clocker, FX & Lucking, SH. (1997). Hand Tremor in Patients with Spasmodic Torticollis. *Movement Disorders*, Vol. 12, No. 4, pp. 547-552, ISSN 0885-3185

Deuschl, G., Bain, P.,Brin, M. & an Ad Hoc Scientific Committee. (1998). Consensus Statement of the Movement Disorder Society on Tremor. *Movement Disorders*, Vol.13, Suppl.3, pp.2-23, ISSN 0885-3185

Deuschl, G., Raethjen, J., Lindemann., M., Krack, M. & Krack, P. (2001). The pathophysiology of tremor. *Muscle Nerve*, Vol.24, Issue 6, pp.716–735, ISSN 0148-639X

Dueschl, G. & Bergman, H. (2002). Pathophysiology of Nonparkinsonian Tremors. *Movement Disorders*, Vol.17, Suppl.3, (2002), pp.S41-S48, ISSN 0885-3185

Dubinsky, RM., Gray, CS. & Koller, WC. (1993). Essential tremor and dystonia. *Neurology*. Vol.43, No.11, (November 1993), pp.2382-2384, ISSN 0028-3878

Elble, RJ.(2000). Diagnostic criteria for essential tremor and differential diagnosis. *Neurology*, Vol.54, No.11, Suppl. 4, pp.S2-6, ISSN 0028-3878

Elble, R. & Deuschl, G. (2011). Milestones in Tremor Research. *Movement Disorders*, Vol.26, No.6, (2011), pp.1096-1105, ISSN 0885-3185

Fahn, S. & Jankovic, J. (September, 2007). *Principles and practice of movement disorders*. Churchill Livingstone, ISBN: 978-0-443-07941-2,

Gironell, A. & Kulisevsky, J. (2009). Diagnosis and management of essential tremor and dystonic tremor. *Therapeutic Advances in Neurological Disorders*, Vol.2, No.4, pp.215-222, ISSN 1756-2856

Jahanshahi, M. (2000). Factors that ameliorate or aggravate spasmodic torticollis. *Journal of Neurology, Neurosurgery, and Psychiatry*, Vol.68, (2000), pp.227-229, ISSN 0022-3050

Jankovic, J. & Tolosa, E. (2007). *Parkinsons disease & movement disorders*, Lippincott Williams & Wilkins, ISBN 13: 978-0-7827-7882-7, Philadelphia, USA

Jankovic, J. & Liden, CD. (1988). Dystonia and tremor induced by peripheral trauma: predisposing factors *Journal of Neurology, Neurosurgery, and Psychiatry,*Vol.51, No.12, (1988), pp.1512-1519, ISSN 0022-3050

Jedynak, CP., Bonnet, AM. & Agid, Y. (1991). Tremor and Idiopathic Dystonia. *Movement Disorders,* Vol.6, No.3, (1991), pp. 230-236, ISSN 0885-3185

Kim, JW & Lee, PH. (2007). Dystonic head tremor associated with a parietal lesion, *European Journal of Neurology,* Vol.14, No.1,(2007), pp.e32–e33, ISSN 1351-5101

Koller, WC., Busenbark, K. & Miner, K. (1994). The relationship of essential tremor to other movement disorders: report on 678 patients. Essential Tremor Study Group. *Annals of Neurology,* Vol.35, No.6, (June 1994), pp.717-723, ISSN 0364-5134

Lang, A., Quinn, N., Marsden, CD., Findley, L., Koller, W., Brin, M. & Fahn, S. (1992). Essential tremor. *Neurology,* Vol.42, No.7, (July 1992), pp.1432-1434, ISSN 0028-3878

Larsson, T. & Sjogren, T. (1966). Dystonia musculorum deformans. A genetic and clinical population study of 121 cases. *Acta Neurologica Scandinavia* Vol.42, suppl.17, pp. 1-233, ISSN 0065-1427

Lou, JS. & Jankovic, J. (1991). Essential tremor: Clinical correlates in 350 patients. *Neurology,* Vol.41, pp.234-238, ISSN 0028-3878

McAuley, J. & Rothwell, J. (2004). Identification of psychogenic, dystonic, and other organic tremor by a coherence entrainment test. *Movement Disorders,* Vol.19, pp.253–267, ISSN 0885-3185

Marsden, CD. & Harrison, MJG. (1974). Idiopathic torsion dystonia (dystonia musculorum deformans). A review of forty-two patients. *Brain,* Vol.97, No.4, pp.793-810 ISSN 0006-8950

Martinelli, P. & Gabellini, AS. (1982). Essential tremor and buccolinguofacial dystonias. *Acta Neurologica Scandinavia,* Vol.66, No.6, pp. 705-708, ISSN 0001-6314

Munchau, A., Schrag, A., Chuang, C., Colum, DM., Bhatia, KP., Quinn, NP., & Rothwell, JC. (2001). Arm tremor in cervical dystonia differs from essential tremor and can be classifies by onset age and spread of symptoms. *Brain* Vol.124, pp.1765-1776, ISSN 0006-8950

Oppenheim, H. (1911). Uber eine eigenartige Krampfkrankheit des kindlichen und jungendichen Alters (dysbasia lordotica progressiva, dystonia musculorum deformans). *Neurol. Centralbl,* Vol.30, (1911), pp.1090-1107

Oyama, G., Rodriguez, RL., Fernandez, HH., Jacobson IV, CE., Ong, TL., Hwynn, N., Malaty, IA. & Okun, MS. (2011). The distal partial trisomy 1q syndrome and dystonic tremor. *Parkinsonism and Related Disorders* (2011), Vol.17, No.2, pp.128–129, ISSN 1353-8020

Pal, PK., Samii, A., Schulzer, E., Mak, E. & Tsui, JKC. (2000). Head tremor in Cervical dystonia. *The Canadian Journal of Neurological Sciences* (May 2000), Vol.27, No.2, pp.137-142, ISSN 0317-1671

Patterson, RM. & Little, SC. (1943). Spasmodic torticollis. *J Nerv Ment dis,* Vol.98, pp. 571-599

Quinn, NP., Schneider, SA., Schwingenschuh, P. & Bhatia, KP. (2011). Tremor—Some Controversial Aspects. *Movement Disorders,* Vol.26, No.1, pp.18-23, ISSN 0885-3185

Rajput, AH., Offord, KP., Beard, CM. & Kurland, LT. (1984). Essential tremor in Rochester, Minnesota: a 45-year study. *Journal of Neurology, Neurosurgery, and Psychiatry,* Vol.47, No.5, (May, 1984), pp.466-470, ISSN 0022-3050

Rondot, P., Jedynak, CP. & Ferrey, G., eds. (1981). Le torticolis spasmodique. *Rapport de neurologie. In: CongrPs de psychiatrie et de neurologie de langue francaise,* (1981), pp.1-57. ISBN Paris, Masson

Rivest, J. & Marsden, CD. (1990). Turnk and head tremor as Isolated manifestations of dystonia. *Movement Disorders,* Vol.5, No.1, (1990), pp.60-65, ISSN 0885-3185

Schneider, SA., Edwards, MJ, Mir, P., Cordivari, C., Hooker, J., Dickson, J., Quinn, N.& Bhatia, KP. (2007). Patients With Adult-Onset Dystonic Tremor Resembling Parkinsonian Tremor Have Scans Without Evidence of Dopaminergic Deficit (SWEDDs) *Movement Disorders,* Vol.22, No.15, (2007), pp.2210–2215, ISSN 0885-3185

Schwingenschuh, P., Ruge, D., Edwards, MJ., Terranova, C., Katschnig, P., Carrillo, F., Silveira-Moriyama, L., Schneider, SA., Kägi, G, Dickson, J, Lees, AJ., Quinn, N., Mir, P., Rothwell, JC. & Bhatia, KP.(2010). Distinguishing SWEDDs patients with asymmetric resting tremor from Parkinson's disease: a clinical and electrophysiological study. *Movement Disorders,* Vol.25, No.5, (April 2010), pp. 560-569, ISSN 0885-3185

Shaikh, AG., Jinnah, HA., Tripp, RM., Optican, LM., Ramat, S., Lenz, FA. & Zee, DS. (2008). Irregularity distinguishes limb tremor in cervical dystonia from essential tremor. *Journal of Neurology, Neurosurgery, and Psychiatry,* (2008), Vol.79, No.2, pp.187–189, ISSN 0022-3050

Sheehy, MP. & Marsden, CD. (1982). Writer's cramp. A focal dystonia. *Brain,* Vol.105, pp.461-480, ISSN 0006-8950

Tallón-Barranco, A., Vázquez, A ., Javier, JF., Ortí-Pareja, M., Gasalla, T., Cabrera-Valdivia, F., Benito-León, J. & Molina, JA. (1997). Clinical features of essential tremor seen in neurology practice: a study of 357 patients. *Parkinsonism and Related Disorders,* Vol.3, No.4, (December 1997), pp.187-190, ISSN 1353-8020

Vidailhet, M., Jedynak, C., Pollak, P. & Agid, Y. (1998). Pathology of symptomatic tremors. *Movement Disorders,* Vol.13, Suppl. 3, (1998), ISSN 0885-3185

Yanagisawa, N. & Goto, A. (1971). Dystonia musculorum deformans: Analysis with electromyography. *Journal of the Neurological Sciences,* Vol.13, No.1, (May 1971), pp.39-65, ISSN 0022-510X

Yanagisawa, N., Goto, A. & Narabayashi, H. (1972). Familial Dystonia Musculorum Deformans and Tremor. *Journal of the Neurological Sciences,* Vol.16, No.2, (June 1972), pp.125-136, ISSN 0022-510X

Yoon, JH. & Yong, SW. (2009). Dystonic hand tremor in a patient with Wernicke encephalopathy *Parkinsonism and Related Disorders,* Vol.15, (2009), pp.479–481, ISSN 1353-8020

8

Dystonia, Spasticity and Botulinum Toxin Therapy: Rationale, Evidences and Clinical Context

Raymond L. Rosales[1,2]
[1]*Department of Neurology and Psychiatry, University of Santo Tomas and Hospital, Manila,*
[2]*Center for Neurodiagnostic and Therapeutic Services, Metropolitan Medical Center, Manila, Sections of Neuromuscular and Movement Disorders Philippines*

1. Introduction

Perhaps among the central nervous system (CNS) conditions with muscle hyperactivity, dystonia and spasticity figure as those that are disabling and requiring therapeutic intervention. Dystonia is a neurological syndrome characterized by sustained muscle contractions usually producing twisting and repetitive movements or abnormal postures. The sustained movements of dystonia may have overlying spasms similar to tremor but have a directional preponderance. Three other important clinical features of dystonia are occurrences of pain, sensory trick phenomenon (i.e. touching "hot spots" in body surface that abolishes the dystonia), and changes in severity depending on activity and posture . Spasticity is typified by a velocity-dependent occurrence of a "catch" following passive limb movement. Recently, the scope of spasticity has been broadened in its definition as a disordered sensori-motor control resulting from an upper motor neuron (UMN) lesion presenting as intermittent or sustained involuntary activation of muscles(1-2) . Although their etiopathogenesis differ, both conditions overlap as regard the following: [a] occurrence of muscle co-contractions; [b] Overactivity involves not only extrafusal but also intrafusal muscles(3-4) [c] Intrinsic muscle changes in size and visceco-elastic properties (5-6); [d] contractures if left unattended (7);[e] muscular spread in synergy, "overflow" and compensatory muscles; [f] loss of dexterity; [g] occurrence of pain to varying degrees; [h] secondary bone and joint abnormalities; [i] may lead to "compensatory circuitry changes" at segmental and suprasegmental levels (4) ; [j] May lead to posturing and cosmesis issues, and [k] hygiene, quality of life and social impact . Another common thread between dystonia and spasticity is the reduction in muscle tone following botulinum neurotoxin therapy (BoNT), and effectively addressing the disordered sensori-motor control in both conditions. Intuitively, BoNT will be most efficacious in cases with a combination of spasticity and dystonia (i.e. spastic dystonia), such as in childhood spasticity(8). This chapter summarizes the clinical efficacy of BoNT in both dystonia and spasticity.

2. BoNT: Peripheral blockade and beyond

There are two kinds of BoNT (type A [BoNT-A: *onabotulinumtoxinA* or Botox®, *abobotulinumtoxinA* or Dysport ® and *incobotulinumtoxinA* or Xeomin®], and type B [BoNT-B: *rimabotulinumtoxinB* or Neurobloc®/Myobloc®]) that have been proven to be safe and effective in treating various hyperfunctional cholinergic states. Their therapeutic applications range from various forms of muscle hyperactivity (e.g. dystonia, spasticity, spasms, tremors, and tics), autonomic hyperactivity (e.g. drooling, hyperhidrosis and bladder overactivity) and cosmesis (e.g. frown lines and "crow's feet). BoNT is more effective in blocking active neuromuscular junctions(9), and this effect can be enhanced by electric stimulation of the peripheral nerve(10). This toxin disrupts neurotransmission by cleavage of pre-synaptic vesicle fusion proteins; SNAP-25 for BoNT-A and synaptobrevin for BoNT-B, effectively blocking release of acetylcholine to the neuromuscular junctions and induce chemodenervation. The BoNT-A initially binds presynaptically (via the heavy chain attachment domain) and enters neurons by binding to the synaptic vesicle protein SV2(11). The toxin then undergoes internalization by vesicle endocytosis and translocation into the cytosol, to eventually exert its light chain proteolytic activity(12). After injection, the BoNT complex dissociates and diffuses into the target tissues. Toxin spread is a fast and active phenomenon that is driven by BoNT dose, dilution, needle size, and injection technique among others(13) . Subclinical effects of BoNT on endplates far away from the injected sites can be demonstrated by increased jitter in single-fiber electromyography (SFEMG) in animals(3,14) and humans(15-16). Clinically not relevant for the moment and taken with a cautious stand because of the high animal doses applied, BoNT may undergo retrograde axonal transport, possibly transcytosed to afferent neurons, in which it cleaves its substrate SNAP-25. BoNT-truncated SNAP-25 appears not only at the injection site but also in distant regions that project to the infusion area. This retrograde spread was blocked by colchicine, pointing to a likely involvement of microtubule-dependent axonal transport(17). BoNTalso affects the cholinergically mediated intrafusal fibers of muscle spindles, parallel to that of extrafusal fibers , implying an important functional effect (see a review on the subject by Rosales and Dressler, 2010[4]). In healthy, dystonic or spastic adults, the effect on muscle spindles appear to be more prolonged than that in extrafusal fibers, and whether one applies studies using the tonic vibration reflex (TVR)(18-19); or the transcranial magnetic stimulation(20). Since the gamma-motor-neurons are unable to activate the intrafusal fibers with BoNT-A, the muscle spindle output via the afferent axons will be reduced, and because muscle activity is supported by afferent feedback, there may be reduced alpha-motor-neuron drive(3). These events imply that there could be potential modulation of central motor programs following BoNT-A(21). In fact, recent BoNT-A studies in dystonia and spasticity have shown evidences of modifications in the cortical and subcortical levels(22-24); including plasticity changes(25).

3. BoNT for dystonia

3.1 Rationale

Dystonia is a multi-level system disorder where involvement spans from the peripheral (muscular) to the segmental and suprasegmental levels (brainstem, basal ganglia and cortex)(4,26). Muscle hypertonus/spasms in dystonia are relieved by chemodenervation procedures that include muscle-based injections (i.e. muscle afferent block [MAB] and

BoNT) and near nerve injections (i.e. phenol block). Although useful in near large nerve injections (e.g. obturator and femoral nerves), phenol has not been encouraging because of pain associated with the procedure and its unpredictable response (27) . Hinged on the abolition of abnormal muscle spasms with "sensory trick" and MAB in dystonia (i.e. applying TVR[28]), it is believed that the BoNT does have sensory modulatory effects, apart from pure muscle relaxation (see a recent review on the subject by Kanovsky and Rosales[26]). In addition, BoNT-A may reduce pain comorbidity that occur in dystonia (see a recent review by Rawicki and cohorts[29]). The fact that BoNT injections are able to improve an individual's occupational function and quality of life elevates the rationale for its applications. The latter is best exemplified by occupational dystonias (A separate chapter is dedicated to this end). Figure-1 depicts cases of focal hand dystonias with task-specificity and those with complex regional pain syndrome, being prepared for BoNT-A injections.

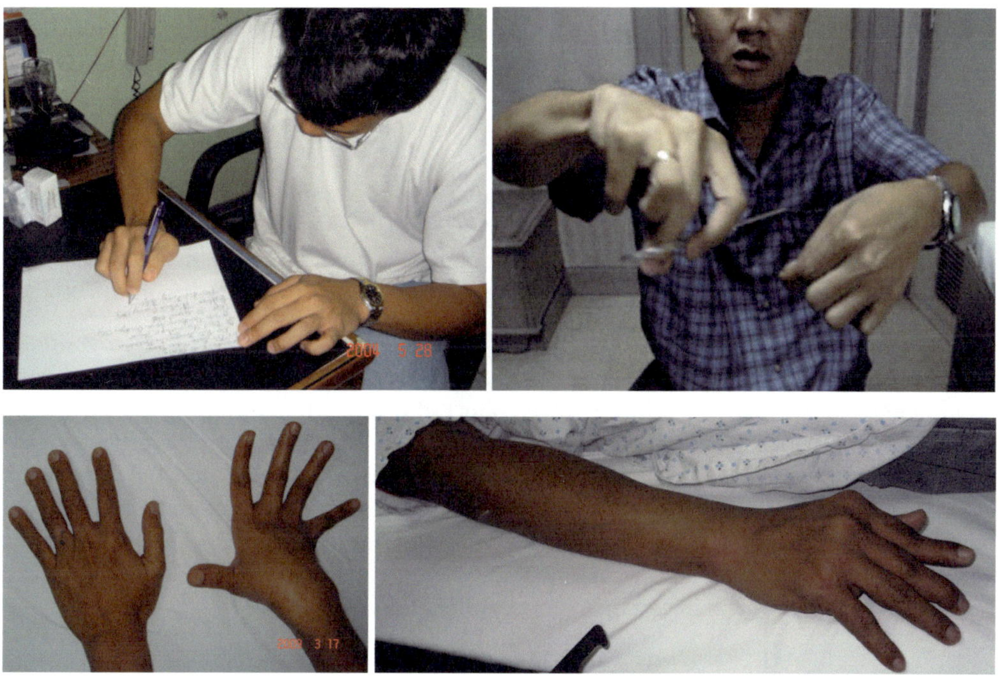

Fig. 1. Focal hand dystonias (upper panel: with task-specificity [Writer's cramp and Barber's cramp]); (lower panel: with complex regional pain syndrome)

3.2 Evidence-based medicine

Cochrane reviews summarized the evidences of BoNT superiority as a therapy for blepharospasm(30) and cervical dystonia(31). The American Academy of Neurology (AAN)(32) recommended that BoNT injections should be offered as a treatment option for cervical dystonia (established as effective) and may be offered for blepharospasm, focal upper extremity dystonia, adductor laryngeal dystonia (probably effective). A lower level of evidence was detected for focal lower limb dystonia (possibly effective). According to the European Federation of Neurological Societies [EFNS] version(33), BoNT-A is considered the first-line treatment for primary cranial (except oromandibular) or cervical dystonia; it is also effective for writing dystonia; BoNT-B is not inferior to BNT-A in cervical dystonia. Despite the variety of trial formats, virtually all the trials individually, and each outcome measure (objective and subjective) separately, suggested that a single injection cycle of BoNT-A is effective and safe for treating cervical dystonia. Enriched trials (using patients previously treated with BoNT-A), suggest that further injection cycles continue to work for most patients. Appropriate injections of BoNT-A into cervical muscles at therapeutic doses are well tolerated, and although adverse effects occur these are transient and rarely severe(31). Furthermore, the available evidence suggests that BoNT-A injections provide more objective and subjective benefits than an anticholinergic drug (i.e. trihexyphenidyl) to patients with cervical dystonia(34).

An international consensus on the aftercare for cervical dystonia and other causes of hypertonia of the neck stated that the benefits following BoNT injection include increased range of movement at the neck for head turning, decreased pain, and increased functional capacity (Class I evidence, level A recommendation). The evidence for efficacy and safety in patients with secondary dystonia in the neck is unclear based on the lack of rigorous research conducted in this heterogeneous population (level U recommendation). Psychometrically sound assessments and outcome measures exist to guide decision-making (Class I evidence, level A recommendation). Much less is known about the effectiveness of therapy to augment the effects of the injection (Class IV, level U recommendation). More research is needed to answer questions about safety and efficacy in secondary neck dystonia, effective adjunctive therapy, dosing and favourable injection techniques(35).

On the issues of BoNT-A application in secondary dystonia as well as for oromandibular dystonia, an applied example is the case of x-linked dystonia-partkinsonism (XDP), a type of heredo-degenerative disorder . In the large cohort of oromandibular and lingual dystonias found in XDP, BoNT-A was shown to be safe and effective as one carefully navigates through recommended technical considerations(36). In XDP as well, BoNT-A targeted in cervical and limb dystonias, indicated its superiority over MAB(37). Interestingly, BoNT-A may also be combined with pallidal deep brain stimulation (DBS) in XDP(38), when the former eventually fails as the only treatment, or when toxin doses increase due to body area spread of dystonia, or even in certain instances after DBS .

3.3 Clinical context

BoNT is a safe and targeted treatment approach suited for focal dystonia where certain muscles are clearly involved during co-contraction and in which injections can be modified for the changing dystonia patterns, including segmental and overflow muscles involved (4,13,26). Depending upon factors such as muscle bulk, severity of muscle spasm and whether one may want/avoid contiguous muscles in a clinical context, BoNT-A in dystonia may be tailored in certain instances. A "high potency, low dilution" of BoNT-A may best be applied in the cranio-cervical (i.e. injections in the peri-ocular, facial, oromandibular, lingual, laryngeal and neck muscles) and distal limb regions, where BoNT-A is expected to be maximized in a targeted (usually smaller) muscles through 1–2 injection sites, and where spread is best avoided. Whereas, in dystonias of the abdominal, paraspinal, and proximal limb muscles, a "low potency, high dilution" BoNT-A injection protocol could best be applied, since spread may be desirable for very large muscles, when multipoint muscle injections is utilized (36). In view of its "dual effects" on the extrafusal and intrafusal muscles, the clinical benefit in practice may "outstrip" the weakness induced by the BoNT(4,39) . Interestingly in cervical dystonia, discrepant and time-related effects vary between relief of muscle hypertonus, associated pain and head posture(31) . These findings underscore the BoNT effects far beyond simply blocking muscle spasms in dystonia. For instance, the head posture may be related to muscle spindle changes among other factors(4) and the associated pain relief having perhaps an independent mechanism(29) . The role of BoNT-A in pain pathophysiology is beginning to be understood, however, larger studies in neuropathic pain, joint pain, and myofascial pain syndrome are needed to fully ascertain robustness of BoNT therapy in those areas(40-41).

4. BNT for spasticity

4.1 Rationale

Arguably only one component of UMN, spasticity in both children (e.g. cerebral palsy, see Figure-2) and adults (e.g. post-stroke, traumatic brain/spinal injuries and multiple sclerosis; see Figure-3), may impair one's motor control, quality of life and may eventually lead to economic and care-giver burden. More than one third of patients develop spasticity within

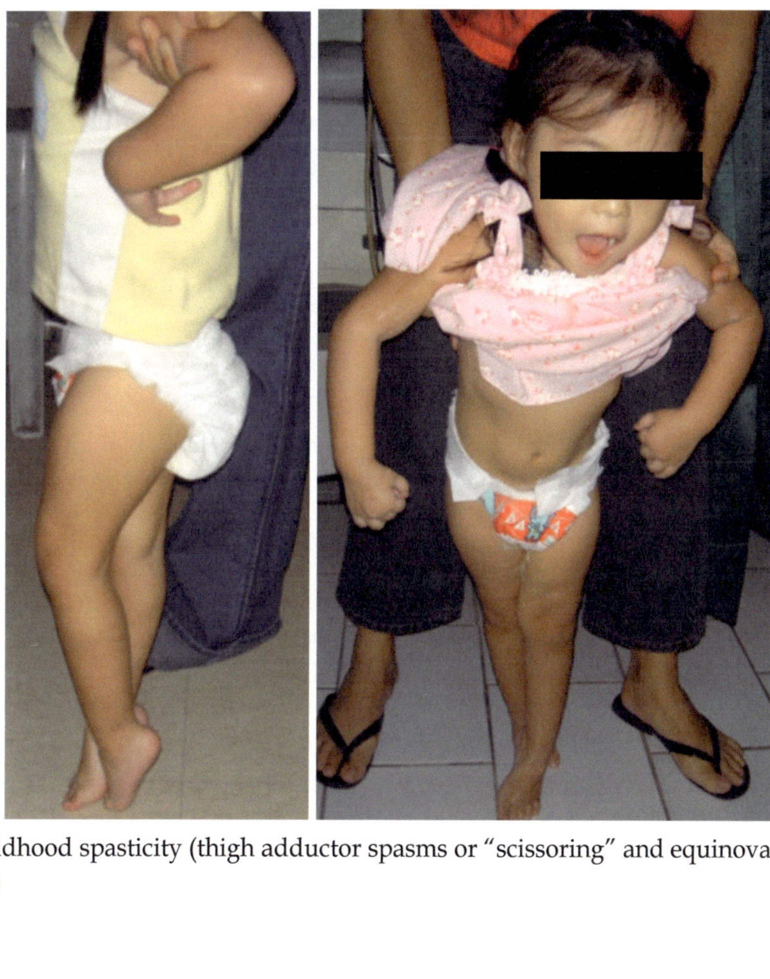

Fig. 2. Childhood spasticity (thigh adductor spasms or "scissoring" and equinovarus foot deformity)

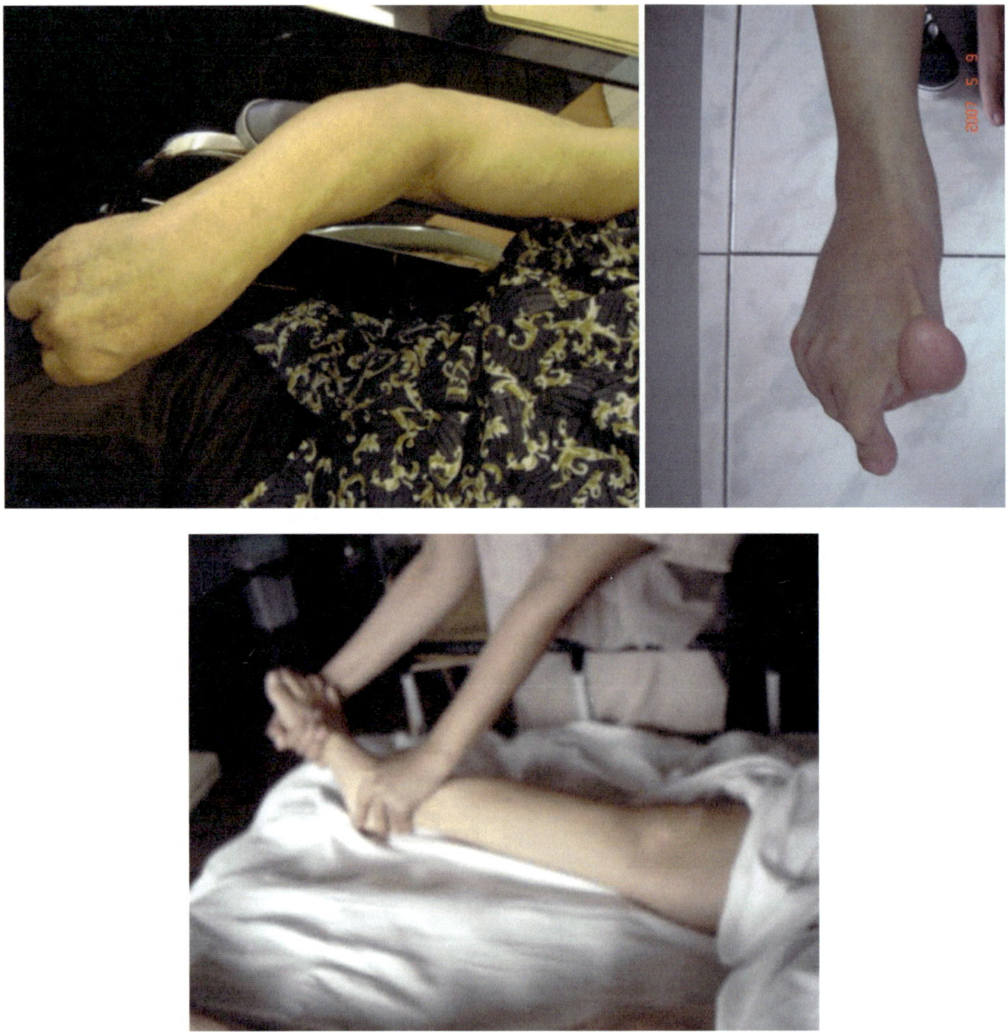

Fig. 3. Spasticity "plus"(Post-stroke with spastic dystonia-left panel; Multiple Sclerosis with spastic dystonia-middle panel; Traumatic brain injury with spasticity and dynamic contracture-right panel)

12 months after stroke(42-43) and a proportion of these patients will develop disabling spasticity requiring intervention(44). Even in the early phases of stroke ("evolving spasticity"[45]) about 19% of patients(46) or possibly more(47), develop spasticity within 3 months after the ictus. In fact, as many as 80% of patients without useful functional arm movement after the ictus, develop spasticity (measured by muscle activation recording) within 6 weeks of first stroke(48).

Strokes in the middle cerebral artery region occur in three quarters of patients, hence, the upper limb is affected in a large number of them. In regard to therapeutic intervention, differences may arise between the hemiplegic upper and lower limbs, and these are(49): (a) functional recovery of an arm that enables grasping, holding, and manipulating objects, requires the recruitment and complex integration of muscle activity from the shoulder to the fingers. In contrast, a minimal (or less complex) amount of recovery of a hemiplegic leg may be sufficient to obtain functional ambulation; (b) the ability to reach and grasp is a necessary component of many daily life functional tasks, hence reduced upper limb function is likely to reduce independence and increase burden of care. Moreover, muscles in the affected ankle cannot be efficiently recruited in a timely manner to overcome reaching task impairment in stroke patients (50); (c) left uncorrected, secondary complications such as inferior subluxation of the glenohumeral joint, shoulder-hand syndrome, soft tissue lesions, and painful shoulder further hinder rehabilitation of the hemiplegic arm; (d) there is a lack of spontaneous stimulation when performing upper limb functional activities that "assist" in recovery, compared to lower limb activities. Bilateral activity in the legs is often required whenever a patient attempts to transfer, stand or walk, whereas, in performing upper limb activities, the patient may opt to simply use the non-affected side exclusively(51); and, (e) the "protective effect" of spasticity applies more to the lower limbs, and not necessarily for the upper limbs. For example, lower limb spasticity may be beneficial by enabling patients to stand despite the co-occurrence of lower limb weakness. When it does cause harm, however, treatment is required(51-52). Spasticity in the upper limbs (ULS), with these inherent characteristics, may lead to compensatory central nervous system adaptations and changes after stroke such as the "learned non-use" of the affected upper limb. As a form of maladaptive plasticity, the frequent assistance of the non-affected limb may prove to be disadvantageous in the efforts to improve functional recovery(45). Not all patients with ULS will have spasticity-related symptoms (i.e. *symptomatic spasticity*), but those with functional impairment can be categorized into: (a) those relating to passive function, e.g. hand hygiene, wearing of upper garment, application of splints; (b) pain; (c) associated reaction, and (d) those relating to impaired active function(53). Therefore, it is not unusual that a large majority of BoNT randomized and systematic spasticity intervention studies have been performed on the upper limbs(54). Having its effect in the neural component of spasticity(2,55), the rationale for BoNT-A use is hinged on its reduction of muscle tone via chemodenervation of injected overactive muscles, and potentially prevent, through early injection protocols, eventual complications brought about by the non-neural components (e.g. contracture in spasticity, Fig-3)(45). In fact, BoNT-A is likewise able to address muscle overactivity in spasticity with associated reactions and dystonia (spastic dystonia; Fig-3) (45). The current state of knowledge on the application of BoNT-A in the management of spasticity is depicted in Figure-4.

4.2 Evidence-based medicine

Based on meta-analysis derived from well-conducted, randomized controlled clinical trials(54) BoNT-A proved to be safe and efficacious in treating upper and lower limb spasticity, as measured by lowering the Modified Ashworth Score (MAS) that clinically assesses hypertonicity during passive range of motion across a joint(56). A contemporary review on ULS also indicated robust efficacy of BoNT-A, over other pharmacologic therapies(57). Systematic reviews from the AAN (58), Royal College of Physicians (UK-RCP)(59), European Consensus (60) and Movement Disorders Society (MDS)(61) lead to formulation of therapeutic guidelines for the application of BoNT-A in the over-all

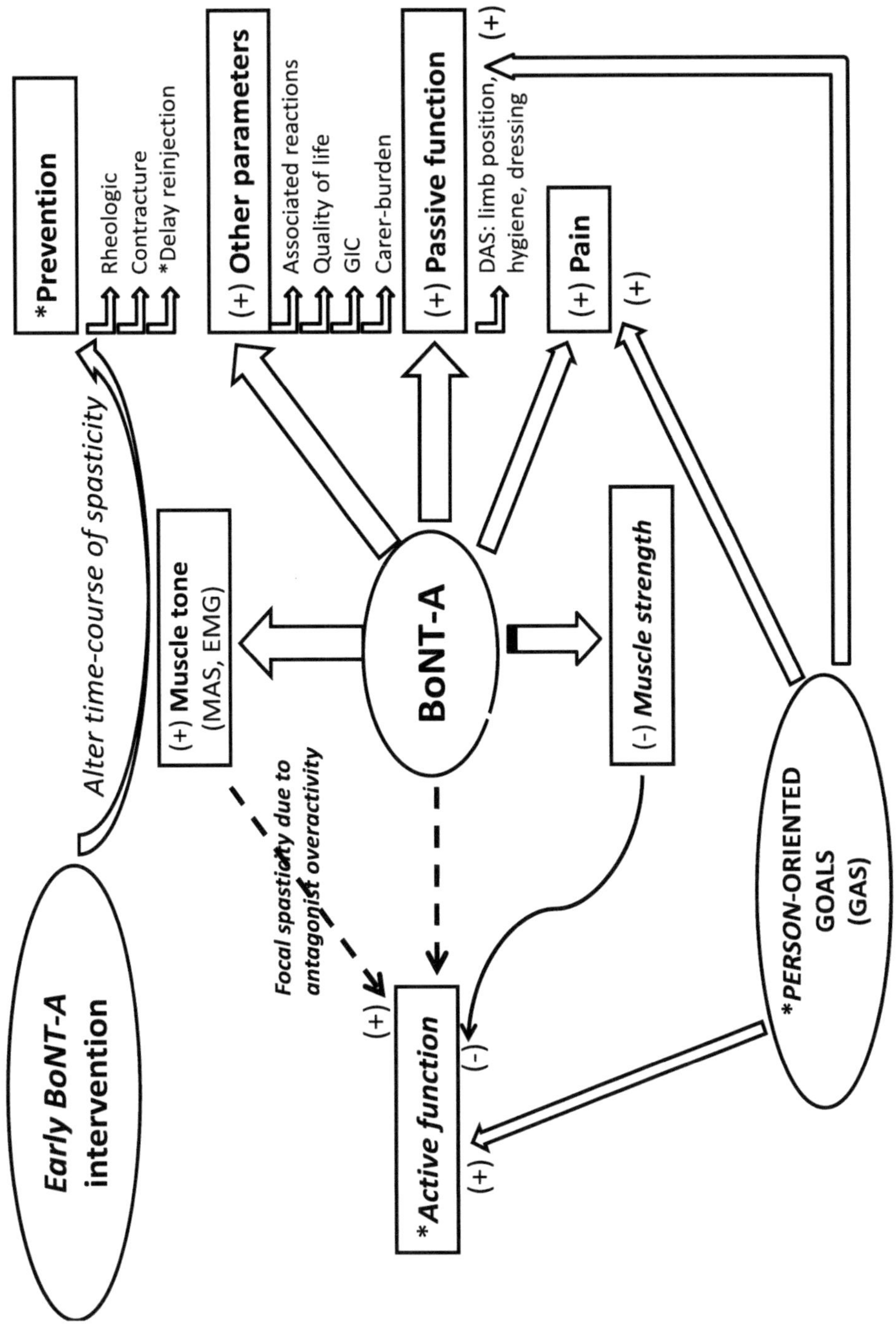

Fig. 4. A schematic diagram on the current state of knowledge on the roles of botulinum neurotoxin injections type A (BoNT-A) in spasticity management; MAS-Modified Ashworth Scale; EMG-Electromyography; GIC-Global impression of change; DAS-Disability Assessment Scale; GAS-Goal Attainment Scaling

management of spasticity. In parallel, international consensus statements were made on the use of BoNT-A over a wide range of indications for adult and childhood spasticity(62-65). The benefit from BoNT-A is maintained after repeated treatment cycles(66-67) and thus, BoNT-A has been thought to be a first line treatment in focal/multifocal spasticity(68). In addition, BoNT treatment has been shown to improve associated reactions in ULS(69) reduce predetermined disability parameters (including pain) (70-73), reduce carer burden(70,73-74), improve person-centered goals(75) and self-reported efficacy with safety(76). However, efficacy of BoNT-A for improvement of motor control and active functions have not been attained(77). While spasticity is an important component of reduced upper limb function, Shaw and colleagues(71) argue that motor weakness is the most important factor. Likewise, their study did not demonstrate improved active function (despite an improvement in muscle tone in favor of intervention), arguably suggesting that spasticity is of less importance . To date, most of the studies show that BoNT-A injection has been applied in the chronic stage(78-80) (i.e.more than 6 months after stroke; average of 2.5 years) wherein spasticity has been established(45) and wherein non-neural, rheologic changes have set-in. Early intervention with BoNT-A (i.e. less than 3 months post-stroke) has been performed in two Phase II trials (designed to estimate sample sizes)(81-82) and in a Phase III trial(83). The first Phase II study by Cousins and associates(81) indicated some functional recovery at 20 weeks in the groups that received *onabotulinumtoxinA*, following a subanalysis of patients with no arm function (employing Action Research Arm Test) in the baseline assessment (i.e. 3 weeks post-stroke). Interestingly, the second Phase II study by the German group(82) failed to demonstrate improvement in motor control with the Fugl-Meyer arm score, despite a reduction in finger flexor stiffness, 6 months after injecting *incobotulinumtoxinA*. The Asian Botulinum Toxin Clinical Trial Designed for Early Post-Stroke Spasticity (ABCDE-S) was a Phase III study (83) that demonstrated reduction in muscle tone (MAS) at week 4, and which was sustained to 24 weeks, despite a single cycle, uniform injection of 500units *abobotulinumtoxinA*. In the latter cohort of patients that enrolled patients 2 -12 weeks post- stroke, significant pain reduction (i.e. weeks 4 and 24) was demonstrated among those that had initial spasticity-related pain, but showed no motor control improvement (using the Motor Assessment Scale).

4.3 Clinical context

Spasticity has been shown to inhibit active upper limb function(84) mainly because the prime mover is not fully able to overcome the resistance of the spastic (antagonist) muscle. BoNT-A should be used to address specific functional limitations resulting from focal spasticity (i.e . muscle over-activity confined to one or a group of muscles that contribute to a specific functional problem). However, BoNT-A is not always expected to fully or partially recover lost function, except perhaps when that function has been lost primarily due to antagonist muscle over-activity(59) The effect of BoNT-A on muscle tone and muscle strength is dose-dependent (85). It is therefore important to titrate the dose in patients with an "incomplete" UMN lesion to reduce muscle tone sufficiently without inducing excessive weakness (and loss of function)(86). The appropriate time to initiate BoNT-A therapy in ULS should not be dependent on post- stroke duration, but rather on the goals initially set forth. In established spasticity, treatment should be based on the occurrence of impediments to occupational therapy or physiotherapy, or when the disability has reached a plateau or when the disability continues to worsen despite such therapies (62). Predefined goals are ideally smart, achievable and person-centered, in order to optimize BoNT-A effects in areas of muscle tone, pain, active/passive functions, burden of care, cosmesis, among others(87). However, in early BoNT-A injection protocols, when spasticity is evolving, goals are likely different, as these are largely for prevention of contracture or possibly improvement in arm function in the long run. Finally, there are generally a couple of ways for which improvements in function can occur . Pre-morbid movement patterns may be regained first because of true motor recovery, and second, because of the redundancy in the number of degrees of freedom of the body(88). In the latter, actions can be accompanied by substitution of other degrees of freedom for movements of impaired joints. Such alternative movements or motor compensations(89) have also been observed in primates recovering from experimental stroke(90). Therefore, targeting specific muscle groups with BoNT-A, without affecting others, has the theoretical potential to unmask selective voluntary movement in situations where this is over-ridden by mass patterns of spasticity in antagonistic muscle groups(91). This underscores the interaction and complexity of proper (or improper) selection/targeting and accidental (or intentional) spread in achieving treatment goals. Last but not least, BoNT should not be administered alone, and its effects are best optimized in concert with a good rehabilitation program and an inter-disciplinary team.

5. Conclusion

Backed by robust clinical trials, we have undoubtedly reached a stage where the roles of BoNT in the management of dystonia and spasticity have been historically etched. This is paralleled by a BoNT safety profile that withstood the test of time over 20 years of application in hypertonic muscular disorders. The clinician is placed in a state to choose the best individualized approach to patients with dystonia and spasticity, bearing in mind that for BoNT, the evidences exist, as one negotiates through management issues related to benefit, harm and cost.

6. Acknowledgment

Michelle Joya-Tanglao, PTRP, provided bibliography search support and assisted in the manuscript preparation. The CNS staff of Metropolitan Medical Center (Manila) were behind the author in every stage of this chapter preparation.

7. References

[1] Pandyan AD, Gregoric M, Barnes MP, Wood D, Van Wijck F, Burridge J, et al. Spasticity: clinical perceptions, neurological realities and meaningful measurement. Disabil Rehabil. 2005;27:2-6.
[2] Esquenazi A, Novak I, Sheean G, Singer BJ, Ward AB. International consensus statement for the use of botulinum toxin treatment in adults and children with neurological impairments–introduction. Eur J Neurol. 2010;17 Suppl 2:1-8.
[3] Rosales RL, Arimura K, Takenaga S, Osame M. Extrafusal and intrafusal muscle effects in experimental botulinum toxin-A injection. Muscle Nerve. 1996;19:488-96
[4] Rosales RL, Dressler D. On muscle spindles, dystonia and botulinum toxin. Eur J Neurol. 2010;17 Suppl 1:71-80.

[5] Lieber RL, Steinman S, Barash IA, Chambers H. Structural and functional changes in spastic skeletal muscle. *Muscle Nerve* 2004;29:615-27 .
[6] Welmer AK, Widen HL, Sommerfeld DK. Location and severity of spasticity in the first 1-2 weeks and at 3 and 18 months after stroke. *Eur J Neurol* 2010;17:720-5.)
[7] O'Dwyer NJ, Ada L, Neilson PD. Spasticity and muscle contracture following stroke. *Brain* 1996;119:1737–49).
[8] Lukban MB, Rosales RL, Dressler D. Effectiveness of botulinum toxin A for upper and lower limb spasticity in children with cerebral palsy: a summary of evidence. J Neural Transm. 2009;116:319-31.
[9] Hallett M, Glocker FX, Deuschl G. Mechanism of action of botulinum toxin. Ann Neurol. 1994;36:449-50.
[10] Eleopora R, Tugnoli V, De Grandis D. The variability in the clinical effect induced by botulinum toxin type A: the role of muscle activity in humans. Mov Disord. 1997;12:89-94.
[11] Dong M, Yeh F, Tepp W, Dean C, Johnson EA, Janz R, et al. SV2 is the protein receptor for botulinum neurotoxin A. Sci Exp. 2006;312:592-6.
[12] Rossetto O, Morbiato L, Caccin P, Rigoni M, Montecucco C. Presynaptic enzymatic neurotoxins. J Neurochem. 2006;97: 1534-45.
[13] Pickett A, Rosales RL. New trends in the science of botulinum toxin-A as applied in dystonia. Int J Neuroscience. 2011;121:22-34.
[14] Rosales RL, Bigalke H, Dressler D. Pharmacology of botulinum toxin: differences between type A preparations. Eur J Neurol. 2006;13 Suppl 1:2-10.
[15] Garner CG, Straube A, Witt TN, Oertel WH. Time course of distant effects of local injections of botulinum toxin. Mov Disord. 1993;8:33-7.
[16] Rosales RL, Arimura K, Gamez G, Osame M. X-linked dystonia-parkinsonism: botulinum toxin therapy and stimulation single-fiber electromyography. Electroencephalogr Clin Neurophysiol. 1995;97 Suppl:S234-5.
[17] Antonucci F, Rossi C, Gianfranceschi L, Rossetto O, Caleo M. Long distance retrograde effects of botulinum neurotoxin A. J Neurosci. 2008;28:3689-96.
[18] Trompetto C, Curra A, Buccolieri A, Suppa A, Abbruzzese G, Berardelli A. Botulinum toxin changes intrafusal feedback in dystonia: a study with the tonic vibration reflex. Mov Disord. 2006;21:777-82.
[19] Trompetto C, Bove M, Avanzino L, Francavilla G, Berardelli A, Abbruzzese G. Intrafusal effects of botulinum toxin in post-stroke upper limb spasticity. Eur J Neurol. 2008;15:367-70.
[20] Kim D, Oh B, Paik N. Central effect of botulinum toxin type A in humans. Int J Neurosci. 2006;116:667-80.
[21] Curra A, Trompetto C, Abbruzzese G, Berardelli A. Central effects of botulinum toxin A. Evidence and supposition. Mov Disord. 2004;19 Suppl 8:S60-4.
[22] Senkarova Z, Hlustik P, Otruba P, Herzig R, Kanovsky P. Modulation of cortical activity in patients suffering from upper arm spasticity following stroke and treated with Botulinum Toxin A: an fMRI study. J Neuroimaging. 2009;20:9-15.
[23] Opavsky R, Hlustik P, Otruba P, Kanovsky P. Sensorimotor network in cervical dystonia and the effect of botulinum toxin treatment: a functional MRI study. J Neurol Sci. 2011;306:71-5.

[24] Dresel C, Bayer F, Castrop F, Rimpau C, Zimmer C, Haslinger B. Botulinum Toxin Modulates Basal Ganglia But Not Deficient Somatosensory Activation in Orofacial Dystonia. Mov Disord. 2011;DOI:10.1002/mds.23497.
[25] Kojovic M, Caronni A, Bologna M, Rothwell JC, Bhatia KP, Edwards MJ . Botulinum toxin injections reduce associative plasticity in patients with primary dystonia. Mov Disord. 2011;DOI: 10.1002/mds.23681.
[26] Kanovský P, Rosales RL. Debunking the pathophysiological puzzle of dystonia: with special reference to botulinum toxin therapy. Parkinsonism Rel Disord. 2011;17:S11-4.
[27] Massey JM. Electromyography-guided chemodenervation with phenol in cervical dystonia (Spasmodic torticollis). In: Brin MF, Jankovic J, Hallett M, editors. Scientific and Therapeutic Aspects of Botulinum Toxin. Philadelphia, PA: Lippincott, Williams & Wilkins; 2002.
[28] Kaji R, Rothwell JC, Katayama M, Ikeda T, Kubori T, Kohara N, et al. Tonic vibration reflex and muscle afferent block in writer's cramp. Ann Neurol. 1995;38:155-62.
[29] Rawicki B, Sheean G, Fung VSC, Goldsmith S, Morgan C, Novak I. Botulinum toxin assessment, intervention and aftercare for paediatric and adult niche indications including pain: international consensus statement. Eur J Neurol. 2010;17:S122-34.
[30] Costa J, Espirito-Santo C, Borges A, Ferreira JJ, Coelho M, Moore P, et al. Botulinum toxin type A therapy for blepharospasm. Cochrane Database Syst Rev. 2005;CD004900.
[31] Costa J, Espírito-Santo CC, Borges AA, Ferreira J, Coelho MM, Moore P, et al. Botulinum toxin type A therapy for cervical dystonia. Cochrane Database Sys Rev. 2005;Issue 1. Art.No.:CD003633.
[32] Simpson DM, Blitzer A, Brashear A, Comella C, Dubinsky R, Hallett M, et al. Assessment: botulinum neurotoxin for the treatment of movement disorders (an evidence-based review): report of the Therapeutics and Technology Assessment Subcommittee of the American Academy of Neurology. Neurology. 2008;70(19):1699-1706.
[33] Albanese A, Asmus F, Bhatia KP, Elia AE, Elibol B, Filippini G, et al . EFNS guidelines on diagnosis and treatment of primary dystonias. Eur J Neurol. 2010;doi:10.1111/j.1468-1331.2010.03042.x.
[34] Costa J, Espírito-Santo CC, Borges AA, Moore P, Ferreira J, Coelho MM, et al. Botulinum toxin type A versus anticholinergics for cervical dystonia. Cochrane Database Sys Rev. 2005; Issue 1. Art. No.: CD004312.DOI: 10.1002/14651858.CD004312.pub2.
[35] Novak I, Campbell L, Boycec M, Fung VSC. Botulinum toxin assessment, intervention and aftercare for cervical dystonia and other causes of hypertonia of the neck: international consensus statement. Eur J of Neurol. 2010;17:S94-108.
[36] Rosales RL , Ng AR, Delos Santos MM, Fernandez HH. The broadening application of chemodenervation in x-linked dystonia-parkinsonism (part II): an open-label experience with botulinum toxin-A (Dysport®) injections for oromandibular, lingual, and truncal-axial dystonias. Int J Neuroscience. 2011;21:44-56.
[37] Rosales RL, Delos Santos MM, Ng AR, Teleg R, Dantes M, Lee LV, et al. The broadening application of chemodenervation in x-linked dystonia-parkinsonism (part I): muscle afferent block versus botulinum toxin-A in cervical and limb dystonias. Int J Neuroscience. 2011;121:35-43.

[38] Aguilar J, Vesagas TS, Jamora RD, Teleg R, Ledesma L, Rosales RL, at al. The promise of deep brain stimulation in x-linked dystonia parkinsonism. Int J Neuroscience. 2011;121:57–63.

[39] Hallett M. Effects of botulinum toxin at the neuromuscularjunction. In: Brin MF, Jankovic J, Hallett M, editors. Scientific and Therapeutic Aspects of Botulinum Toxin. Philadelphia, PA: Lippincott, Williams & Wilkins; 2002.p.167-70.

[40] Qerama E, Fuglsang-Frederiksen A, Jensen T. The role of botulinum toxin in management of pain: an evidence based review. Curr Opin Anaesthesiol. 2010;23:602-610.

[41] Finnerup N, Sindrup S , Jensen T. The evidence for pharmacological treatment of neuropathic pain. Pain. 2010;150: 573-81.

[42] Watkins CL, Leathley MJ, Gregson JM, Moore AP, Smith TL, Sharma AK. Prevalence of spasticity post stroke. Clin Rehabil. 2002;16:515-22.

[43] Leathley MJ, Gregson JM, Moore AP, Smith TL, Sharma AK, Watkins CL. Predicting spasticity after stroke in those surviving to 12 months. Clin Rehabil. 2004;18:438-43.

[44] Lundström E, Terént A, Borg J. Prevalence of disabling spasticity 1 year after first-ever stroke. Eur J Neurol. 2008;15:533-9.

[45] Rosales RL, Kanovsky P, Fernandez HH. What's the "catch" in upper-limb post-stroke spasticity: Expanding the role of botulinum toxin applications. Parkinsonism and Rel Disord. 2011;17: S3-10.

[46] Sommerfeld DK, Eek EU, Svensson AK, Holmqvist LW, von Arbin MH. Spasticity after stroke: its occurrence and association with motor impairments and activity limitations. Stroke. 2004;35:134-9.

[47] Lao A, Rosales RL, Po P, Salazar G, Reyes RV, Magsino R, et al. Spasticity among stroke patients: time of occurrence and predictive factors. Neurorehabil Neural Repair. 2008;22:207.

[48] Malhotra S, Cousins E, Ward A, Day C, Jones P, Roffe C, et al. An investigation into the agreement between clinical, biomechanical and neurophysiological measures of spasticity. Clin Rehabil. 2008;22:1105-15.

[49] Feys HM, De Weerdt WJ, Selz BE, Cox Steck GA, Spichiger R, Vereeck LE, et al. Effect of a therapeutic intervention for the hemiplegic upper limb in the acute phase after stroke: A single blind, randomized, controlled multicenter trial. Stroke. 1998;29:785-92.

[50] Hsu WL, Yang YR, Hong CT, Wang RV. Ankle muscle activation during functional reach in hemi-paretic and healthy subjects. Am J Phys Med Rehabil. 2005;84(10):749-55.

[51] Hyman N, Barnes M, Bhakta B, Cozens A, Bakheit M, Kreczy-Kleedorfer B, et al. Botulinum toxin (Dysport®) treatment of hip adductor spasticity in multiple sclerosis: a prospective, randomised, double-blind, placebo controlled dose ranging study. J Neurol Neurosurg Psychiatry. 2000;68:707-12.

[52] Ward AB. A summary of spasticity management - a treatment algorithm. Eur J Neurol. 2002;1 Suppl 1:S48-52

[53] Kong KH, Chua KSG, Lee J. Symptomatic upper limb spasticity in patients with chronic stroke attending a rehabilitation clinic: frequency, clinical correlates and predictors. Rehabil Med. 2010;42:453-7.

[54] Rosales RL, Chua-Yap AS. Evidence based systematic review on the efficacy and safety of BoNT-A in post-stroke spasticity. J Neural Transm. 2008;115(4): 617-23.

[55] Alhusaini A, Crosbie J, Shepherd R, Dean C, Scheinberg A . No change in calf muscle passive stiffness after botulinum toxin injection in children with cerebral palsy. Dev Med Child Neurol. 2011;53:553-8.

[56] Bohannon RW, Smith MB. Inter rater reliability of a modified Ashworth scale of muscle spasticity. Phys Ther . 1987;67:206-7.

[57] Olvey EL, Armstrong EP, Grizzle AJ. Contemporary pharmacologic treatments for spasticity of the upper limb after stroke: a systematic review. Clin Ther. 2010;32:2282-303.

[58] Simpson DM, Gracies JM, Graham HK, Miyasaki JM, Naumann M, Russman B, et al. Botulinum neurotoxin for the treatment of spasticity (an evidence based review): report of the Therapeutics and Technology Assessment Subcommittee of the American Academy of Neurology. Neurology. 2008;70:1691-8.

[59] Turner-Stokes L, Ashford S, Bhakta B, Heward K, Moore AP, Robertson A, et al. Spasticity in adults: management using botulinum toxin: national guidelines. London: Royal College of Physicians 2009.

[60] Wissel J, Ward AB, Erztgaard P, Bensmail D, Hecht MJ, Lejeune TM, et al. European consensus table on the use of botulinum toxin type A in adult spasticity. J Rehabil Med. 2009;4:113-25.

[61] Elia AE, Filippini G, Calandrella D, Albanese A. Botulinum neurotoxins for post-stroke spasticity in adults: A systematic review. Mov Disord. 2009;24:801-12.

[62] Sheean G, Lannin NA, Turner-Stokes L, Rawicki B, Snow BJ. Botulinum toxin assessment, intervention and after-care for upper limb hypertonicity in adults: international consensus statement. Eur J Neurol. 2010;17:74-93.

[63] Olver J, Esquenazi A, Fung VSC, Singer BJ, Ward AB. Botulinum toxin assessment, intervention and aftercare for lower limb disorders of movement and muscle tone in adults: international consensus statement. Eur J Neurol. 2010;17 Suppl 2: 57-73.

[64] Fehlings D, Novak I, Berweck S, Hoare B, Stott NS, Russo RN. Botulinum toxin assessment, intervention and follow-up for paediatric upper limb hypertonicity: international consensus statement. Eur J Neurol. 2010;17 Suppl 2: 38-56.

[65] Love SC, Novak I, Kentish M, Desloovere K, Heinen F, Molenaers G, et al. Botulinum toxin assessment, intervention and after-care for lower limb spasticity in children with cerebral palsy: international consensus statement. Eur J Neurol. 2010;17 Suppl 2: 9-37.

[66] Bakheit AMO, Fedorova NV, Skoromets AA, Timerbaeva SL, Bhakta BB, Coxon L. The beneficial antispasticity effect of botulinum toxin type A is maintained after repeated treatment cycles. J Neurol Neurosurg Psychiatry. 2004;75: 1558-61.

[67] Lagalla G, Danni M, Reiter F, Ceravolo MG, Provinciali L. Post-stroke spasticity management with repeated botulinum toxin injections in the upper limb. Am J Phys Med Rehabil. 2000;79:377-84.

[68] Sheean G. Botulinum toxin should be first-line treatment for poststroke spasticity. J Neurol Neurosurg Psychiatry. 2009;80:359.

[69] Bhakta BB, O'Connor RJ, Cozens JA. Associated reactions after stroke: a randomized controlled trial of the effect of botulinum toxin type A. J Rehabil Med. 2008;40(1):36-41.

[70] Brashear A, Gordon MF, Elovic E, Kassicieh VD, Marciniak C, Do M, et al. Intramuscular injection of botulinum toxin for the treatment of wrist and finger spasticity after stroke. N Eng J Med. 2002;347:395-400.
[71] Shaw LC, Price CI, van Wijck FM, Shackley P, Steen N, Barnes MP, et al. Botulinum toxin for the upper limb after stroke (BoTULS) trial: effect on impairment, activity limitation, and pain. Stroke. 2011;42:1371-9.
[72] Kaji R, Osako Y, Suyama K, Maeda T, Uechi Y, Iwasaki M, et al. Botulinum toxin type A in post-stroke upper limb spasticity. Curr Med Res Opin. 2010;26:1983-92.
[73] Kanovsky P, Slawek J, Denes Z, Platz T, Sassin I, Comes G, et al. Efficacy and safety of botulinum neurotoxin NT 201 in poststroke upper limb spasticity. Clin Neuropharmacol. 2009;32:259-65.
[74] Bhakta BB, Cozens JA, Chamberlain MA, Bamford JM. Impact of botulinum toxin type a on disability and carer burden due to arm spasticity after stroke: a randomised double blind placebo controlled trial. J Neurol Neurosurg Psychiatry. 2000;69: 217-21.
[75] McCrory P, Turner-Stokes L, Baguley IJ, De Graaff S, Katrak P, Sandanam J, et al. Botulinum toxin A for treatment of upper limb spasticity following stroke: a multi-centre randomized placebo-controlled study of the effects on quality of life and other person-centred outcomes. J Rehabil Med. 2009;41: 536-44.
[76] Muller F, Cugy E, Ducerf C, Delleci C, Guehl D, Joseph PA, et al. Of botulinum toxin for adult spasticity in current clinical practice: a prospective observational study. Clin Rehabil. 2011;DOI: 10.1177/0269215511412799.
[77] Shaw L, Rodgers H, Price C, van Wijck F, Shackley P, Steen N. et al. BoTULS: a multicentre randomised controlled trial to evaluate the clinical effectiveness and cost-effectiveness of treating upper limb spasticity due to stroke with botulinum toxin type A. Health Technol Assess. 2010;14(26).
[78] Kreisel SH, Bazner H, Hennerici MG. Pathophysiology of stroke rehabilitation: temporal aspects of neuro-functional recovery. Cerebrovasc Dis. 2006; 21:6-17.
[79] Kreisel SH, Hennerici MG, Bazner H. Pathophysiology of stroke rehabilitation: the natural course of clinical recovery, use-dependent plasticity and rehabilitative outcome. Cerebrovasc Dis. 2007;23:243-55.
[80] Ozcakir S, Sivrioglu K. Botulinum toxin in poststroke spasticity. Clin Med Res. 2007;5:132-8.
[81] Cousins E, Ward A, Roffe C, Rimington L, Pandyan A. Does low-dose botulinum toxin help the recovery of arm function when given early after stroke? A phase II randomized controlled pilot study to estimate effect size. Clin Rehabil. 2010;24: 501-13.
[82] Hesse S, Mach H, Fro hlich S, Behrend S, Werner C, Melzer I. An early botulinum toxin A treatment in subacute stroke patients may prevent a disabling finger flexor stiffness six months later: a randomized controlled trial. Clin Rehabil. 2011;DOI: 10.1177/0269215511421355.
[83] Rosales RL, He KK, Goh KJ, Kumthornthip W, Mok VCT, Delgado-De Los Santos MM, MD, Chua KSG, Abdullah SJF, Zakine B, Maisonobe P, Magis A, Wong KSL. Botulinum toxin injection for hypertonicity of the upper extremity within 12 weeks after stroke: A randomized controlled trial. Neurorehabil Neural Repair, *in press*
[84] Mizrahi EM, Angel RW. Impairment of voluntary movement by spasticity. Ann Neurol. 1979;5:494-5.

[85] Sloop RR, Escutin RO, Matus JA, Cole BA, Peterson GW. Dose-response curve of human extensor digitorum brevis muscle function to intramuscularly injected botulinum toxin type A. Neurology. 1995;46:1382-6.
[86] Bakheit AMO, Zakine B, Maisonobe P, Aymard C, Fheodoroff K, Hefter H, et al. The profile of patients and current practice of treatment of upper limb muscle spasticity with botulinum toxin type a: an international survey. Int J Rehabil Res. 2010;33(3):199-204.
[87] Turner-Stokes L. Goal attainment scaling and its relationship with standardized outcome measures: a commentary. J Rehabil Med. 2011;43:70-2.
[88] Bernstein NA. The coordination and regulation of movements. Oxford: Pergamon Press; 1967.
[89] Cristea MC, Levin MF. Compensatory Strategies for Reaching in Stroke. Brain. 2000;123(5):940-53.
[90] Friel KM, Nudo RJ. Recovery of motor function after cortical injury in primates: compensatory movement patterns used during rehabilitative training. Somatosensory and Motor Research 1998;15(3):173-89.
[91] Esquenazi A, Mayer N. Botulinum toxin for the management of muscle overactivity and spasticity after stroke. Curr Atheroscler Rep. 2001;3:295-8.

9

Dystonia and Dopaminergic Therapy: Rationale Derived from Pediatric Neurotransmitter Diseases

Hiroki Fujioka
Osaka City University
Japan

1. Introduction

The paucity of literature in pediatric neurotransmitter diseases indicates a gap in our understanding of neurochemistry and the clinical phenomenology. However, the dramatic clinical responses to dopaminergic therapy in dopa-responsive dystonias opened avenues for rationalizing this therapeutic approach in other pediatric neurotransmitter disorders. This chapter aims to link up dopaminergic therapy, dystonia and other pediatric neurotransmitter diseases. It was in 1971 that Segawa (Segawa et al., 1971, 1976) reported patients with child-onset periodic dystonia, whose dystonia had diurnal variation, with towards evening being worse with walking. The symptom was recovered in the morning. Unlike other dystonic disorders, levodopa was effective to alleviate involuntary movements in those patients. (Tarsy et al., 2006) This disease was later named as Dopa responsive dystonia (DRD), DYT-5, or Segawa disease. (Nygaard et al., 1988)

In 1994, Ichinose et al. detected that the cause of Segawa disease was heterozygous defect of guanosine triphosphate cyclohydrolase I (GTPCH) located at 14q22-q22.2. (Ichinose et al., 1994) GTPCH is a rate-limiting enzyme of tetrahydrobiopterin (BH4) synthesis from guanosine triphosphate (GTP). (Shintaku, 2002) BH4 is co-factor of aromatic amino acids hydroxylase. Tyrosine hydroxylase (TH) is one of aromatic amino acids hydroxylase and it is a rate-limiting enzyme of dopamine synthesis. In Segawa disease, decrease of BH4 is considered to suppress the activity of TH and dopamine production. Dopamine begins to be used up after waking up and the individual becomes active. In effect, the total amount of dopamine in terminals of dopaminergic neurons decrease in the evening, when dystonic symptoms occur. At night, during sleep as one rests, dopamine is recharged such that upon waking up, no dystonia is noted (Furukawa et al., 1999, 2002; Segawa et al., 2003).

It was reported that other diseases showed symptoms of dystonia and other movement disorders that were responsive for L-dopa. There were tyrosine hydroxylase deficiency and sepiapterin reductase (SR) deficiency. Defect of several other enzymes that were related BH4 metabolism, that is, 6-pyruvoyl tetrahydropterin synthase deficiency, dihydropteridine reductase deficiency, and autosomal recessive GTPCH deficiency also demonstrate dopa-responsive involuntary movements. However, those disorders have been considered as diseases related phenylketonuria, for those diseases showed hyperphenylalaninemia and it is important to reduce phenylalanine concentration in central nervous system (CNS) in patients with those diseases. Some patients with familial parkinsonism also indicated dopa-responsive movement disorder that was resemble for Segawa disease. (Tassin et al., 2000) However, those diseases were considered as a parkinsonism and were not considered as PNDs.

2. Pediatric neurotransmitter diseases

In addition to Segawa disease, several disorders related to dopamine/serotonin metabolism have been reported. Disorders of gamma amino butyric acid (GABA) metabolism were also rare metabolic diseases. They were all rare inherited metabolic diseases. Those disorders were called as pediatric neurotransmitter diseases (PND) (Swoboda et al., 2002; Pearl et al., 2007), for they showed involuntary movements due to defect or excess of neurotransmitters from childhood. In this report, the author described summary of clinical manifestations and current treatments of those diseases.

2.1 Disease of BH4 metabolism

BH4 is constructed from GTP by several enzymes. Defect of these enzymes decrease the amount of BH4. As BH4 work as co-factor of each aromatic amino acids hydroxylase, suppression of BH4 production affect the synthesis of neurotransmitters. As kinetics of each aromatic amino acids hydroxylase was different, degree of suppression of BH4 synthesis is important to decide the manifestation of each patient. Complete defect of BH4 causes hyperphenylalaninemia, for all of each aromatic amino acids hydroxylase. Those diseases are usually classified as disorders related phenylketonuria and are not considered as PNDs. Two disorders, Segawa disease and Sepiapterin reductase (SR) deficiency, are classified as PNDs, for these diseases indicate normal serum phenylalanine concentration.

In this section, the author described about those two diseases.

However no essential difference was existed between the two diseases and other BH4 deficiency. Plasma phenylalanine level of Segawa disease was significantly higher than those of controls. (See Fig.1) However the values of plasma phenylalanine were within the normal range (less than 2 mg/dl or 121 μmol/l). (Fujioka et al., 2009) Activity of phenylalanine hydroxylase was slightly suppressed in Segawa disease patients. In this chapter, diseases of BH4 deficiency with hyperphenylalaninemia are also described simply.

2.1.1 Segawa disease

Segawa disease was first reported PNDs and caused by partial defect of GTPCH. (Segawa et al., 1971; Ichinose et al., 1994) This disorder is autosomal dominant inheritance with incomplete penetrance. (Furukawa et al., 1998) Most of patients showed dystonic symptoms before 7 year-old. Adult-onset Segawa disease was also reported. (Turjanski et al., 1993) Number of female patients was reported to 2 to 6 times higher than those of male patients. (Furukawa et al., 1998) The most popular symptom of Segawa disease is postural dystonia. (Segawa et al., 2003) In these patients, often dystonia in one side of legs was observed. The dystonic symptoms were often spread to both sides of upper and lower limbs around 15 year-old. Muscle rigidity progressed around 20 year-old. After that, most of their symptoms were fixed. In a part of these patients, postural tremor was also observed. In other patients, action dystonia was observed. Those patients often showed involuntary movements after 8 year-old.

Their symptoms were often upper-limb dystonia, cervical dystonia, or oculogyric crisis. After the age of young adult, they also showed spasmodic torticollis, or writer's cramp. Some patients with action type Segawa disease showed paroxysmal kinesigenic dyskinesia or restless leg syndrome-like symptoms. Adult-onset type Segawa disease patients showed spasmodic torticollis, or writer's cramp, parkinsonism-like symptoms.

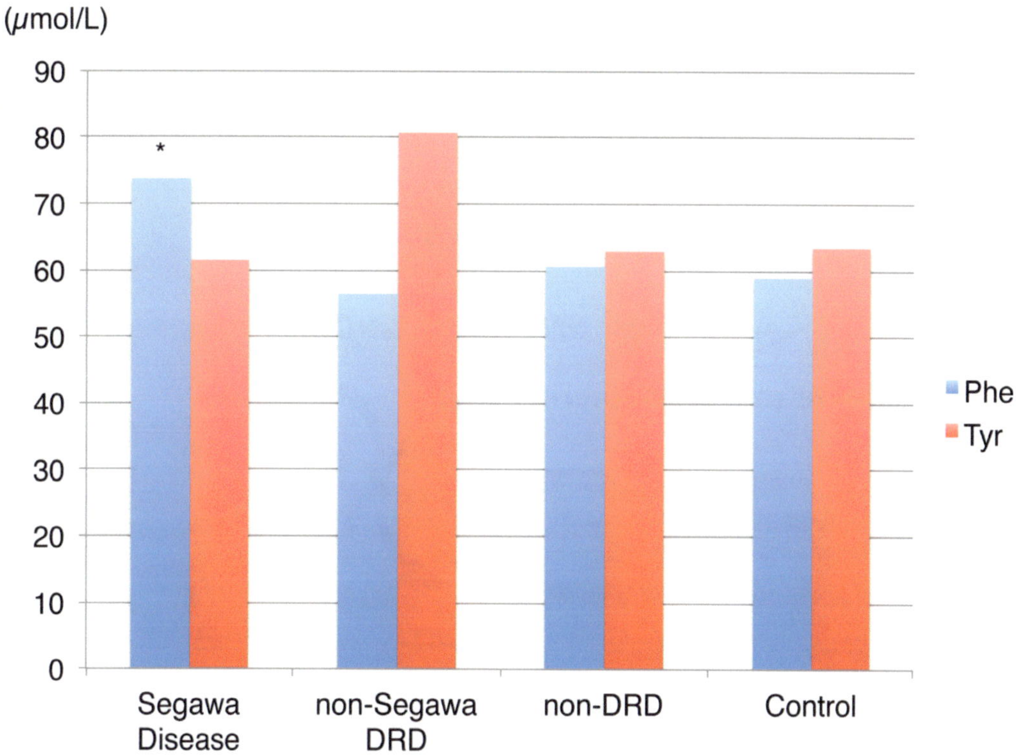

Fig. 1. Comparison of plasma phenylalanine (Phe) and Tyrosine (Tyr) concentration. (Modified from Fujioka et al., 2009)

Analysis of variance indicated that plasma phenylalanine concentration of Segawa disease was higher than those of other group (asterisk: $p<0.05$). However, the value was within the normal range (less than 121μmol/l). No significant difference was observed in plasma tyrosine concentration.

Usually patients of Segawa disease did not show psychomotor delay or convulsion. Their locomotion was also normal. However some Action type patients showed depression. Several patients who occurred symptoms during infantile periods often showed autistic tendency, depression, obsessive-compulsive disorders, or headache that suggested shortage of serotonin. In those patients, decrease of muscle tonus or abnormality of locomotion was also observed.

To diagnose Segawa disease is difficult, for its symptom is broad. (Chaila et al., 2006) Gene analysis of GTPCH enzyme is one of good method to diagnose Segawa disease, however, mutation of GCH1 gene, which is coding GTPCH, has been reported various. Some reports described that a part of patients with dopa-responsive dystonia and clinically diagnosed as Segawa disease did not have any mutation in GCH1 gene. (Zirn et al., 2008) Biochemical diagnose of Segawa disease has also been reported. One method is oral phenylalanine loading test. (Hyland et al., 1997; Bandmann et al., 2003; Opladen et al., 2010) As activity of GTPCH of Segawa disease patients is lower than that of control, amount of neopterin, a metabolite of biopterin synthesis pathway (Fig. 2) in cerebrospinal fluids (CSF) is expected to decrease. (Fujita et al., 1990; Furukawa et al., 1993; Bandmann et al., 1996) Amount of BH4 in CNS of patient with Segawa disease also decreased. (Furukawa et al., 1999)

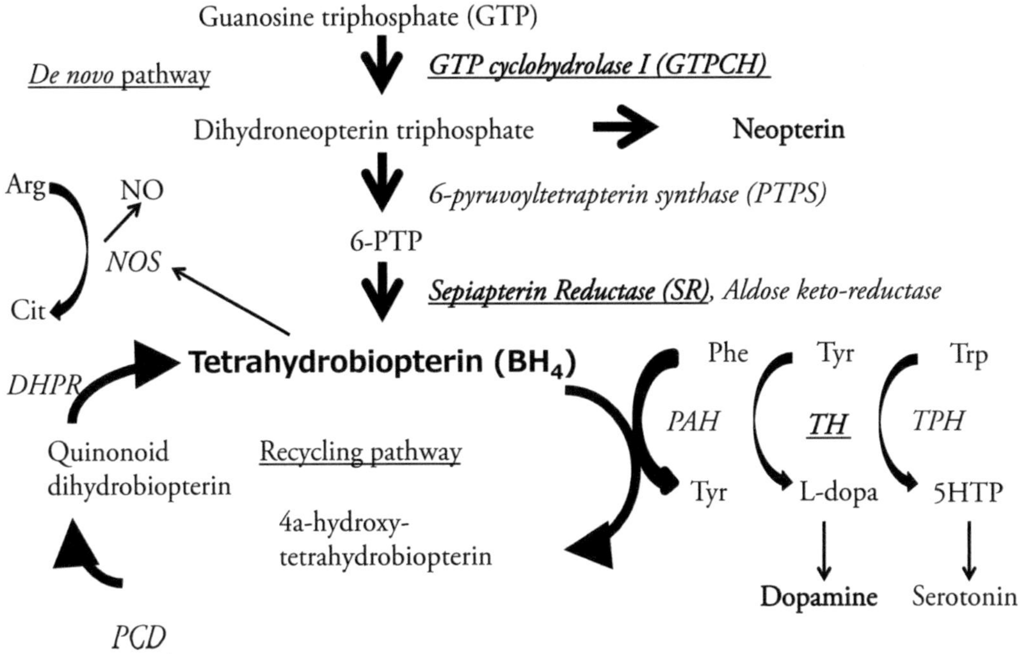

Fig. 2. Scheme of Tetrahydrobiopterin Synthesis and metabolism.

Tetrahydrobiopterin is synthesized from GTP by GTP cyclohydrolase I (GTPCH), Sepiapterin reductase (SR), and other enzymes. BH4 is a co-factor of each aromatic amino acid hydroxylase. Tyrosine hydroxylase (TH) is one of aromatic amino acid hydroxylase, which convert Tyrosine into L-dopa.

As described in original reports, levodopa was effective to many of Segawa disease patients. The maximum dose of levodopa is 20 mg/kg/day. (Segawa et al., 2003; Furusho et al., 1993) Carbidopa is an inhibitor of dopa decarboxylase. To use drugs of the levodopa/carbidopa combination, amount of L-dopa delivering to neurons was increasing, for it prevent to convert L-dopa to dopamine outside the blood-brain barrier. (Nagata et al., 2007; Bernard et al., 2010) In recent report, low dose levodopa and selegiline was helpful. (Yosunkaya et al., 2010) However, in some patients of action type Segawa disease, levodopa was not effective, for it was considered that the dysfunction of D1 receptor of dopaminergic neurons in hypothalamus. (Segawa et al., 2003) In these patients, D1 agonists would be effective. In patients showed shortage of serotonin, 5-hydroxy tryptophan that was the precursor of serotonin would be effective. BH4 is also effective in these patients, for it is known as a co-factor of both tyrosine hydroxylase and tryptophan hydroxylase, which were the rate-limiting enzymes of synthesis of dopamine and serotonin.

As many of Segawa disease are female and their symptoms occur from childhood, a part of them should be pregnant with symptoms and L-dopa replacement therapy. Treatment of Segawa disease during pregnancy has been reported. (Watanabe et al., 2009) A report from Japan, levodopa monotherapy is relatively safe. Six pregnancies with levodopa monotherapy (Levodopa: 250 mg/day) were safe and three pregnancies were fatal loss, two of them were treated with levodopa/carbidopa (100 mg levodopa + 10 mg carbidopa) and the rest one of them was treated without any medication.

2.1.2 Sepiapterin reductase (SR) deficiency

Sepiapterin reductase deficiency has been reported by a patient with progressive psychomotor delay with increase of biopterin and dihydrobyopterin and decrease of 5-hydroxy acetic acid (5-HIAA) and homovanilic acid. (Bonafé et al., 2001) Many of patients were reported around Mediterranean. (Neville et al., 2005) Sepiapterin reductase is one of enzymes to covert sepiapterin into BH4. (See Fig.2)

Patients from Malta showed early motor delay and a significant degree of cognitive impairment. Diurnal variation of the motor impairments and oculogyric crisis occurred from an early stage. Hypotonia was apparent in early stage and later, dystonia was observed. Some of them showed Parkinsonian tremor or chorea. Some of them showed bulbar involvements.

L-dopa dramatically improved motor problems including dystonia, chorea, and oculogyric crisis in those patients. After the treatment, many of them were able to walk. There was no obvious response to cognitive function with learning. In SR deficiency, dysfunction of serotonin was also suspected. It is possible that 5-hydroxy tryptophan is also effective with SR deficiency, for 5-HTP is the precursor of serotonin. Initial dose of L-dopa was 1.5 to 4 mg/kg/day (12.5 to 50 mg/day). (Neville et al., 2005) In these patients, 100 mg L-dopa and 10 mg Carbidopa tablets were used. One case report described incomplete response to treatment during short-term follow-up. (Kusmierska et al., 2009)

Diseases	Segawa Disease	SR deficiency
Cause of Gene	GTPCH I (Heterozygous)	Sepiapterin Reductase (SR)
Inheritance	Autosomal Dominant	Autosomal Recessive
Involuntary Movement	Postural Dystonia, Tremor Action Dystonia	Motor Delay, hypotension Oculogyric crisis, writer's cramp
Convulsion	Very Rare	Rare
Intellectual	Normal	Delay
Hyperphenylalaninemia	-	-
CSF Neopterin Level	Decrease	Normal
CSF Biopterin Level	Decrease	Increase
Dopa Responsibility	+	+
Diagnosis	Gene analysis, decrease of CSF neopterin	Gene analysis
Treatment	L-dopa (or L-dopa with carbidopa)*	L-dopa with carbidopa

*carbidopa is not recommended with pregnant women.

Table 1. Disorders of BH4 metabolism

2.1.3 other tetrahydrobiopterin defects with hyperphenylalaninemia

Tetrahydrobiopterin is a co-factor of aromatic amino acids hydroxylase. There are three aromatic amino acids hydroxylase, which are tyrosine hydroxylase, tryptophan hydroxylase, and phenylalanine hydroxylase. (Fig. 2) Decrease of tetrahydrobiopterin in liver down-regulates the activity of phenylalanine hydroxylase and blood phenylalanine concentration increase. These include autosomal-recessive GTPCH deficiency (Opladen et al., 2011), pterin-carbinolamin dehydratase deficiency, dihydropteridine reductase deficiency, and 6-pyruvoyl tetrahydropterin synthase deficiency. (Shintaku, 2002) All are autosomal recessive inheritance disorders.

Defect of phenylalanine hydroxylase causes phenylketonuria (PKU) and the most common treatment of PKU is restriction of protein. Large neutral amino acid is another treatment, which decrease brain phenylalanine level.

In contrast, oral administration of tetrahydrobiopterin rapidly normalizes hyperphenylalaninemia s with disorders of tetrahydrobiopterin deficiency. Unlike normal PKU, protein restriction is not effective to decrease serum phenylalanine concentration. Treatment of BH4 deficiency is administration of BH4 (10 mg/kg/day). (Shintaku, 2002) Recently, tetrahydrobiopterin responsive PKU was reported and administration of tetrahydrobiopterin is a new treatment of PKU.

Oral supplementation of BH4 improves the activity of liver phenylalanine hydroxylase and normalizes blood phenylalanine concentration. (Shintaku et al., 2004)

However administration of BH4 does not improve movement disorder due to shortage of dopamine and/or serotonin in CNS, for BH4 do not go through blood-brain barrier. To improve their movement disorders due to insufficient dopamine and/or serotonin, administration of precursor of dopamine and/ or serotonin is necessary to go through blood-brain barrier. Clinically, levodopa and 5-HTP are often used to patients with BH4 deficiency. Carbidopa are also used in addition to levodopa.

2.2 Disease of monoamine metabolism

Tyrosine hydroxylase deficiency and Aromatic amino acids decarboxylase deficiency are classified as disorders of monoamine synthesis. In these diseases, symptoms are induced by decrease of amounts of monoamines. Monoamines include dopamine, serotonin, noradrenaline, adrenaline, histamine and other catecholamine. Diseases classified as monoamine breakdown includes monoamine oxidase deficiency and dopamine β-hydroxylase deficiency.

2.2.1 Tyrosine hydroxylase deficiency

Tyrosine Hydroxylase (See Fig. 2 and 3) converts tyrosine into L-dopa, and is a rate-limiting enzyme of dopamine synthesis. (Castaigne et al., 1971; Rondot et al., 1983, 1992) Most of patients with tyrosine hydroxylase deficiency showed progressive encephalopathy. (DE Lonlay et al., 2000; Hoffmann et al., 2003) Some other patients showed typical dopa-effective dystonia. Unlike to Segawa disease, neopterin and biopterin concentration in CSF are normal. (Lüdecke et al., 1996)

The former severe type shows axial hypotonia, hypokinesia, and facial mimicry within a few months after birth. After that, increase of deep tendon reflexes, pyramidal movement disorder, oculogyric crisis, ptosis, miosis, and prolonged diurnal periods of lethargy with increased sweating alternated with irritability are also observed. The progress of those symptoms would be sometimes lethal. No effective treatment has been reported. Recently trial of deep brain stimulation was reported to improve severe involuntary movements with a TH deficiency patient. (Tormenti et al., 2011)

The latter mild type patients show involuntary movements responsible for levodopa however did not show any psychomotor delay or convulsion. Their dystonic symptoms and rigidity occur during infantile period. Many of these patients show lower limb dystonia and then the dystonic symptoms spread to other lesions. Some patients also show tremor. They are treatable by levodopa as Segawa Disease. (Willemsen et al., 2010)

2.2.2 Aromatic amino acid decarboxylase (AADC) deficiency

Aromatic amino acids decarboxylases convert L-dopa into dopamine and 5-HTP into serotonin. (See Fig.3) Patients of AADC deficiency showed intermittent oculogyric crisis and dystonia of four limbs before 6 month-old. (Korenke et al., 1997; Swoboda et al., 1999, 2003) Irritability, ocular convergence spasm, facial dystonia, myoclonus, and dysfunction of voluntary movements were often observed. Hypotonia and increase of deep tendon reflex were observed. Many of patients were lawn down and were not able to speak. However, the symptoms of AADC deficiency were various, for a mild type patient showed only a mild hypotonia and ptosis. The patient could walk and talk. Some of the patients would be misdiagnosed as cerebral palsy. FDG-PET findings indicated decrease of sugar metabolism at striatum. (Sato et al., 2006; Ide et al., 2010) Dysfunction of basal ganglia should be a cause of abnormal movements.

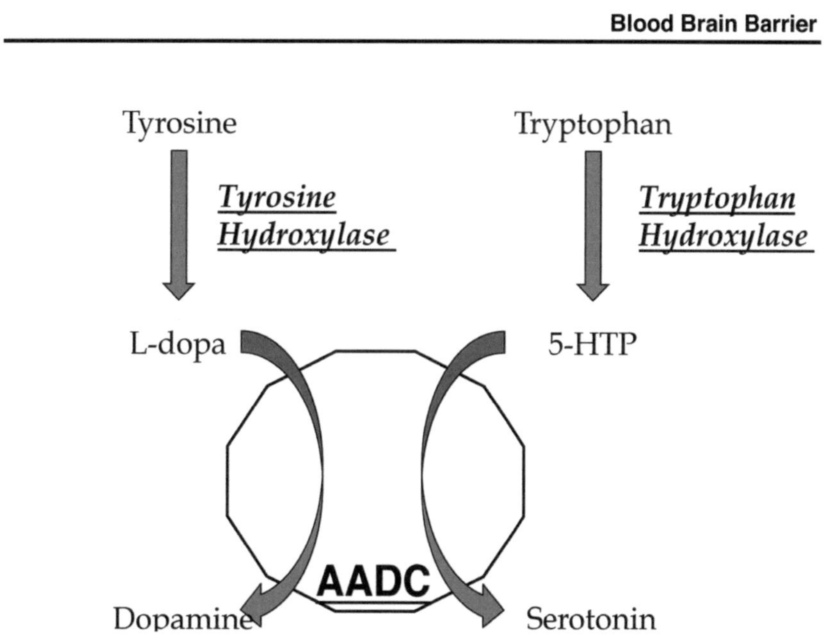

Fig. 3. Structure and Function of Aromatic l-amino acid decarboxylase (AADC).

Due to shortage of catecholamine, sweating, breath holding, diarrhea, and ptosis were observed in most patients with AADC deficiency. In some patients, convulsion due to hypoglycemia was reported. (Korenke et al., 1997; Swoboda et al., 1999, 2003) Sleep disorder was also observed in a part of patients, for amount of melatonin is decreased in patients with AADC deficiency. Melatonin is synthesized from serotonin and amount of serotonin often decrease in patients with AADC deficiency. Some patients have epilepsy or abnormal electroencephalogram. (Pearl et al., 2007; Bräutigam et al., 2002; Ito et al., 2008)

Tyrosine and Tryptophan are converted into L-dopa and 5-HTP by their aromatic acids hydroxylase. The produced L-dopa and 5-HTP are converted into dopamine and serotonin by aromatic l-amino acids decarboxylase (AADC). Increase of L-dopa and decrease of dopamine is observed in CNS when AADC do not work in patients with AADC deficiency, for dopamine is not allowed to go through blood brain barrier

Dopamine agonists, monoamine oxidase inhibitors, and vitamin B6 are used as a medication for AADC deficiency. Vitamin B6 is a co-factor of AADC. (Pons et al., 2004; Brun et al., 2010) However these drugs has not been improved the symptoms of AADC deficiency patients well. Now, gene therapy is expected as a novel therapy for those patients. As the construct of brain in AADC deficiency patients are normal, their symptoms is expected to be improved when AADC enzyme work well in their brain. (Manegold et al., 2009; Allen et al., 2009; Jarraya et al., 2009)

Diseases	TH deficiency	AADC deficiency
Cause of Gene	Tyrosine Hydroxylase	Aromatic L-amino acid Decarboxylase
Inheritance	Autosomal Recessive	Autosomal Recessive
Involuntary Movement	DRD,	Oculogyric crisis,
	Progressive encephalitis	Postural Dystonia of extremities
Convulsion	Rare	Not common
Intellectual	DRD type: normal, encephalitis type: delay	Delay
Diagnosis	Gene analysis, decrease of Homovanilic acid (HVA)	Gene analysis, increase of L-dopa and 5-HTP
Dopa Responsibility	+	-
Treatment	L-dopa (DRD), None (encephalitis)	Dopamine agonist, MAO inhibitor, Vit. B6, Gene therapy

Table 2. Disorders of Dopamine metabolism

2.2.3 Monoamine oxidase deficiency

Monoamine oxidase (MAO) has two isotypes, MAO A and MAO B. Both genes are on the X chromosome. Mutation of MAO A gene was reported in a large family. (Brunner et al., 1993)

All affected males showed mild mental retardation and aggressive behaviour. No MAO B deficiency has been reported.

2.2.4 Dopamine β-hydroxylase deficiency

Dopamine β-hydroxylase is a copper-dependent enzyme and it converts dopamine into noradrenalin. Dopamine β-hydroxylase deficiency (Robertson et al., 1986) is rare autosomal recessive disorder and showed orthostatic hypotension due to deficit in autonomic regulation. Other symptoms of this disease are impaired ejaculation, ptosis, nocturia, hyper flexible joint, high palate, nasal stiffness, and so on. (Robertson et al. 1991) To treat orthostatic hypotension, L-threo-3, 4-dihydroxyphenylserine (DOPS) were reported. (Biagginoni et al., 1986; Freeman et al., 1991)

2.3 Disorders of GABA metabolism

Gamma amino butyric acid is important inhibitory neurotransmitters. Failure of GABA regulation induces various neurologic symptoms. Glutamic acid decarboxylase (GAD) deficiency is disorder of GABA synthesis. GABA transaminase deficiency and succinic semialdehyde dehydrogenase (SSADH) deficiency are disorders of GABA breakdown.

2.3.1 Glutamic acid decarboxylase (GAD) deficiency

Glutamic acid decarboxylase (GAD) synthesizes GABA from glutamate. GAD1 deficiency is autosomal recessive inheritance and it was reported that the disease was a cause of non-progressive form of spastic cerebral palsy. (Lynex et al., 2004) Other report described that animal model of GAD deficiency was related to cleft palate. (Asada et al., 1997) Suppression of GAD by autoantibody was reported to relate Batten disease (Pearce et al., 2001) or epilepsy. (McKnight et al., 2005)

2.3.2 GABA transaminase deficiency

GABA transaminase (See Fig.4) converts GABA into succinate. Deficiency of GABA transaminase is autosomal recessive inheritance. Only three reports have been published about patients with GABA transaminase deficiency. They showed severe psychomotor retardation, hypotonia, hyperreflexia, lethargy, and refractory seizures. (Jaeken et al., 1984; Medina-Kauwe et al., 1999; Tsuji et al., 2010) The patients showed growth acceleration due to elevation of serum growth hormone concentration. Increase of GABA in blood and CSF is important to diagnose GABA transaminase deficiency. The recent study described that increase of intracranial GABA was detected by proton magnetic resonance spectroscopy (^{1}H-MRS). (Tsuji et al., 2010) This report also described that the prenatal exposure of GABA was responsible for the clinical manifestation of this disease, for GABA worked as an excitatory molecule early in life.

2.3.4 Succinic semialdehyde dehydrogenase (SSADH) deficiency

Succinic semialdehyde dehydrogenase (SSADH) converts succinic semialdehyde into succinate. (See Fig.4) In SSADH deficiency patients, dysfunction of SSADH causes increase of 4-hydroxybutylic acids. (Gibson et al., 1983; Rating et al., 1984) However, it is not confirmed that 4-hydroxybutylic acids is the cause of symptoms, for the substance negate the symptoms of SSADH deficiency when it was administrated for patients or model animals. SSADH deficiency is one of disorders of gamma amino butyric acid (GABA) metabolism.

Symptoms of SSADH deficiency are mild to moderate developmental delay, severe hypotonia, sleep disorder, attention deficit, hyperactivity, anxiety, decrease of deep tendon reflex, non-progressive cerebellar ataxia, and convulsions. Most of SSADH patients are non-progressive. However, 10% of SSADH patients are progressive. Cranial T2 weighted MRI indicated high signal in both side of globus pallidus. (Pearl et al. 2011, Yamakawa et al. 2011)

No effective treatment is known. In a part of patients, vigabatrin (gamma vinyl GABA) is reported to improve symptoms of ataxia. Vigabatrin is an inhibitor of GABA transaminase. (Gibson et al., 1989, 1995; Gropman et al., 2003)

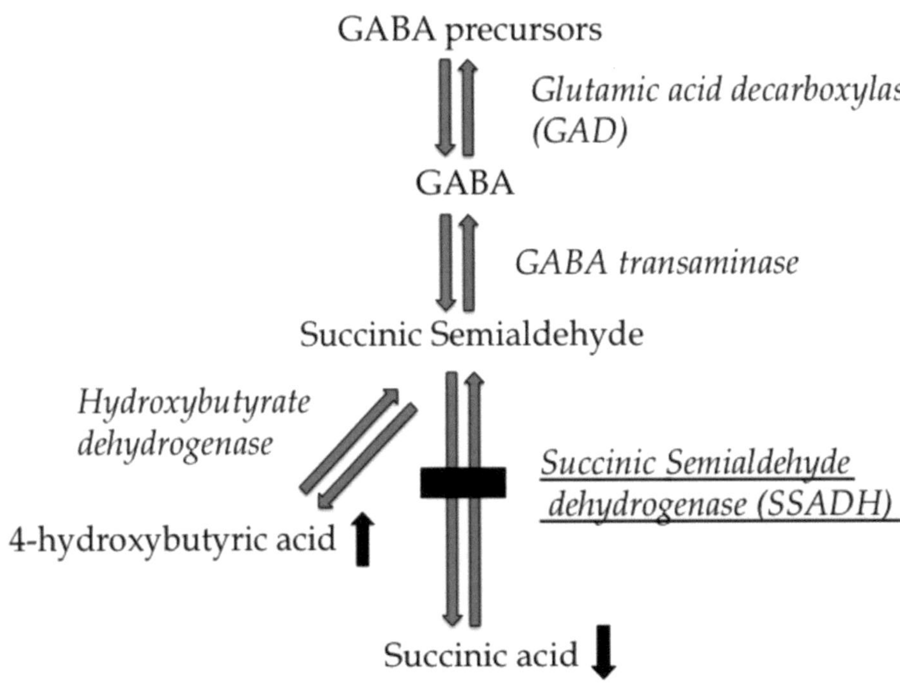

Fig. 4. Metabolism of GABA and SSADH deficiency

GABA is converted into succinic semialdehyde by GABA transaminase. Succinic semialdehyde is catalysed to 4-hydroxybutyric acid and succinic acid. In patients with succinic semialdehyde dehydrogenase (SSADH) deficiency, Succinic acid decrease and 4-hydroxybutyric acid increase.

Diseases	GAD deficiency	GABA transaminase deficiency	SSADH deficiency
Inheritance	Autosomal Recessive	Autosomal Recessive	Autosomal Recessive
Involuntary	Spastic cerebral palsy	Psychomotor delay, hypotonia	Motor delay, hypotonia,
Movement	Cleft palate?	hyperreflexia, lethargy, seizure	convulsion, sleep disorder,
Convulsion	relation to epilepsy?	common	common
Intellectual	Delay	Delay	Delay
Diagnosis	Gene Analysis	Increase of blood and CSF GABA	Gene analysis, increase of
		proton MRS	urine gamma-hydroxy butyrate
Treatment	None	None	Vigabatrin

Table 3. Disorders of GABA metabolism

3. Conclusion

Pediatric neurotransmitter diseases were induced by congenital defects of neurotransmitters. Diseases related to dopamine/serotonin system affected basal ganglia and patients showed dystonia and other involuntary movements. L-dopa was effective to those disorders, for those symptoms were induced by shortage of dopamine in central nervous system. L-dopa is a precursor of dopamine and is able to go through blood-brain barrier. So oral administrated L-dopa is converted into dopamine in brain. Administration of dopamine is no effect because it does not go through blood-brain barrier. In patients with AADC deficiency, L-dopa is not effective. In those patients, dopamine is not synthesized from L-dopa in CNS, for AADC is inactive. (See Fig. 3)

Some of patients of PNDs show decrease of serotonin. Psychiatric symptoms including depression, sleep disorder, obsessive-compulsive disorders, or headache is often observed when serotonin deficiency occurs. In those patients, 5-HTP is useful to supply serotonin, for 5-HTP is a precursor of serotonin and is able to go through blood-brain barrier.

Tetrahydrobiopterin (BH4) is co-factors of dopamine and serotonin synthesis. (Fig. 2) Administration of BH4 is useful to reduce hyperphenylalaninemia in liver. The administration of BH4 could increase the production of innate L-dopa or 5-HTP at outside of CNS, for BH4 do not go thorough blood brain barrier. However, BH4 is insufficient to improve intracranial abnormality of dopamine and serotonin. Administration of L-dopa and 5-HTP to the patients with biopterin deficiency is necessary to prevent appearance of symptoms due to shortage of neurotransmitters.

Carbidopa is an inhibitor of aromatic amino acids decarboxylase. To administrate carbidopa with levodopa increase the amount of levodopa arriving at CNS to reduce degradation of L-dopa before blood-brain barrier. By using carbidopa and levodopa, total dose of levodopa for patients with PNDs could decrease. Other type of PNDs is due to dysfunction of GABA metabolic system. In this manuscript, the author described SSADH deficiency. Previous reports described that an inhibitor of GABA transaminase improved their psychomotor dysfunction al least partially.

AADC deficiency is one of disorders that L-dopa is ineffective. Gene therapy has been expected to improve symptoms of these patients. To replace abnormal enzyme to normal enzyme is enable to convert L-dopa into dopamine in CNS and supplement of dopamine is expected to suppress involuntary movements.

Botulinum toxin therapy (A Pickett and R L Rosales. 2011) and deep brain stimulation (DBS) (K L Collins et al. 2010) have each been shown to be effective mangaement approaches in dystonia. Botulinum toxin is often used in focal dystonia and DBS is usually treated by general dystonia. Both two therapies have not been applied for PNDs because symptoms due to PNDs are often improved by administration of L-dopa. However, in severe patients or patients who are not response to L-dopa, those two therapies will be considered as an alternative therapies.

4. Acknowledgements

The author thanks for Ms. Saori Kusune, Professor Haruo Shintaku, and Professor Masaya Segawa, and other member of PND study group, Ministry of Health, Labor, Welfare, Japan. This work was supported in part by Grants-Aid from Scientific Research from the Ministry of Health, Labor and Welfare of Japan.

5. References

Allen GF, Land JM, Heales SJ. (2009) A new perspective on the treatment of aromatic L-amino acid decarboxylase deficiency. *Mol Genet Metab.* Vol. 97, No. 1, pp. 6-14.

Asada H, Kawamura Y, Obata K. (1997) Cleft palate and decreased brain gamma-aminobutyric acid in mice lacking the 67-kDa isoform of glutamic acid decarboxylase. *Proc Natl Acad Sci* Vol. 94, pp. 6496-6499.

Bandmann O, Nygaard TG, Harding AE. (1996) Dopa-responsive dystonia in British patients: new mutations of the GTP-cyclohydrolase I gene and evidence for genetic heterogeneity. *Hum Mol Genet.* Vol. 5, No. 3, pp. 403-6.

Bandmann O, Goertz M, Oertel W. (2003) The phenylalanine loading test in the differential diagnosis of dystonia. *Neurology.* Vol. 60, No. 4, pp.700-2.

Bernard G, Vanasse M, Chouinard S. (2010) A case of secondary dystonia responding to levodopa. *J Child Neurol.* Vol. 25, No. 6, pp. 780-1.

Biaggioni I and Robertson D. (1987) Endogenous restoration of noradrenaline by precursor therapy in dopamine-beta-hydroxylase deficiency. *Lancet* Vol. 2, pp. 1170-1172.

Bonafé L, Thöny B, Blau N. (2001) Mutations in the sepiapterin reductase gene cause a novel tetrahydrobiopterin-dependent monoamine-neurotransmitter deficiency without hyperphenylalaninemia. *Am J Hum Genet.* Vol. 69, No. 2, pp. 269-77.

Bräutigam C, Hyland K, Sharma R *et al.* (2002) Clinical and laboratory findings in twins with neonatal epileptic encephalopathy mimicking aromatic L-amino acid decarboxylase deficiency. *Neuropediatrics.* Vol. 33, No. 3, pp. 113-7.

Brun L, Ngu LH, Orcesi S. (2010)Clinical and biochemical features of aromatic L-amino acid decarboxylase deficiency. *Neurology* Vol. 75, pp. 64-71.

Brunner HG, Nelen MR, van Oost BA. (1993) X-linked borderline mental retardation with prominent behavioral disturbance: phenotype, genetic localization, and evidence for disturbed monoamine metabolism. *Am. J. Hum. Genet.* Vol. 52, pp. 1032-1039.

Castaigne P, Rondot P, Said G. (1971) Progressive extrapyramidal disorder in 2 young brothers. Remarkable effects of treatment with L-dopa. *Rev Neurol* (Paris) Vol. 124, pp. 162–6.

Chaila EC, McCabe DJ, Murphy RP. (2006) Broadening the phenotype of childhood-onset dopa-responsive dystonia. *Arch Neurol.* Vol. 63, No. 8, pp. 1185-8.

K L Collins, E M Lehmann, P G Patil. (2010) Deep brain stimulation for movement disorders. *Neurobiol Dis.* Vol. 38, pp. 338-345

Freeman R and Landsberg L. (1991) The treatment of orthostatic hypotension with dihydroxyphenylserine. *Clin Neuropharmacol.* Vol. 14, pp. 296-304.

Fujioka H, Shintaku H, Yamano Y. (2009) Plasma phenylalanine level in dopa-responsive dystonia. *Mov Disord.* Vol. 24, No. 15, pp. 2289-2290.

Fujita S and Shintaku H. (1990) Etiology and pteridin metabolism abnormality of hereditary progressive dystonia with marked diurnal fluctuation [in Japanese]. *Med J Kushiro City Hosp* Vol. 2, pp. 64–67.

Furukawa Y, Nishi K, Kondo T, et al. (1993) CSF biopterin levels and clinical features of patients with juvenile parkinsonism. In: Narabayashi H, Nagatsu T, Yanagisawa N, et al. eds. *Advances in Neurology.* Vol 60, pp. 562–567, New York: Raven.

Furukawa Y, Lang AE, Trugman JM, et al. (1998) Gender-related penetrance and de novo GTP-cyclohydrolase I gene mutations in dopa-responsive dystonia. *Neurology.* Vol.50, pp. 1015-1020.

Furukawa Y, Nygaard TG, Gutlich M, et al. (1999) Striatal biopterin and tyrosine hydroxylase protein reduction in dopa-responsive dystonia. *Neurology.* Vol. 53, pp. 1032-1041.

Furukawa Y, Kapatos G, Haycock JW, et al. (2002) Brain biopterin and tyrosine hydroxylase in asymptomatic dopa-responsive dystonia. *Ann Neurol.* Vol. 51, pp. 637-641.

Furusho U, Hirano Y, Hayashi K, et al. (1993) A familial case of juvenile parkinsonism presenting with dystonia with marked diurnal fluctuation at age 5 [in Japanese]. *Tokyo Joshi Ikadaigaku Zasshi (J Tokyo Women's Med Coll)* (Tokyo) Vol. 63, pp. 405–412.

Gibson KM, Nyhan WL, Jakobs C *et al.* (1983) Succinic semialdehyde dehydrogenase deficiency: an inborn error of gamma-aminobutyric acid metabolism. *Clin Chim Acta.* Vol. 133, No. 1, pp. 33-42.

Gibson KM, DeVivo DC, Jakobs C. (1989) Vigabatrin therapy in patient with succinic semialdehyde dehydrogenase deficiency. *Lancet.* Vol. 2, No. 8671, pp. 1105-6.

Gibson KM, Jakobs C, Hagenfeldt L *et al.* (1995) Vigabatrin therapy in six patientswith succinic semialdehyde dehydrogenase deficiency. *J Inherit Metab Dis.* Vol. 18, No. 2, pp. 143-6.

Gropman A. (2003) Vigabatrin and newer interventions in succinic semialdehyde dehydrogenase deficiency. *Ann Neurol.* Vol. 54 Suppl 6: pp. S66-72.

Hoffmann GF, Assmann B, de Klerk JB, et al. (2003) Tyrosine hydroxylase deficiency causes progressive encephalopathy and dopa-nonresponsive dystonia. *Ann Neurol.* Vol. 54 (Suppl 6) pp. S56–65.

Hyland K, Fryburg JS, Trugman JM. (1997) Oral phenylalanine loading in dopa-responsive dystonia: a possible diagnostic test. *Neurology.* Vol. 48, No. 5, pp. 1290-7.

Ichinose H, Ohye T, Takahashi E, et al. (1994) Hereditary progressive dystonia with marked diurnal fluctuation caused by mutations in the GTP cyclohydrolase I gene. *Nat. Gen.* Vol. 8, pp. 236 –242.

Ide S, Kato M, Goto Y. (2010) Abnormal glucose metabolism in aromatic L-amino acid decarboxylase deficiency. *Brain Dev.* Vol. 32, No. 6, pp. 506-10.

Ito S, Ide S, Ito Y *et al.* (2008) Aromatic L-amino acid decarboxylase deficiency associated with epilepsy mimicking non-epileptic involuntary movements. *Dev Med Child Neurol.* Vol. 50, No. 11, pp. 876-8.

Jaeken J, Casaer P, Brucher JM et al. (1984) Gamma-aminobutyric acid-transaminase deficiency: a newly recognized inborn error of neurotransmitter metabolism. *Neuropediatrics* Vol. 15, pp. 165-169.

Jarraya B, Boulet S, Jan C *et al.* (2009) Dopamine gene therapy for Parkinson's disease in a nonhuman primate without associated dyskinesia. *Sci Transl Med.* Vol. 1, No. 2, pp. 2ra4

Korenke GC, Christen HJ, Hyland K. (1997) Aromatic L-amino acid decarboxylase deficiency: an extrapyramidal movement disorder with oculogyric crises. *Eur J Paediatr Neurol.* Vol. 1, No. 2-3, pp. 67-71.

Kusmierska K, Jansen EE, Szymanska *et al.* (2009) Sepiapterin reductase deficiency in a 2-year-old girl with incomplete response to treatment during short-term follow-up. *J Inherit Metab Dis.* Jan 7. [Epub ahead of print]

DE Lonlay P, Nassogne MC, van Cruchten AC *et al.* (2000) Tyrosine hydroxylase deficiency unresponsive to L-dopa treatment with unusual clinical and biochemical presentation. *J Inherit Metab Dis.* Vol. 23, No. 8, pp. 819-25.

Lüdecke B, Knappskog PM, Surtees RA *et al.* (1996) Recessively inherited L-DOPA-responsive parkinsonism in infancy caused by a point mutation (L205P) in the tyrosine hydroxylase gene. *Hum Mol Genet.* Vol. 5, No. 7, pp. 1023-8.

Lynex CN, Carr IM, Markham A F et al. (2004) Homozygosity for a missense mutation in the 67 kDa isoform of glutamate decarboxylase in a family with autosomal recessive spastic cerebral palsy: parallels with stiff-person syndrome and other movement disorders. *BMC Neurol.* Vol. 4, No. 20,.

Manegold C, Hoffmann GF, Ikonomidou H et al. (2009) Aromatic L-amino acid decarboxylase deficiency: clinical features, drug therapy and follow-up. *J Inherit Metab Dis.* Vol. 32, No. 3, pp. 371-80.

McKnight K, Jiang Y, Lang B et al. (2005) Serum antibodies in epilepsy and seizure-associated disorders. *Neurology.* Vol. 65, No. 11, pp. 1730-6.

Medina-Kauwe LK, Tobin AJ, Gibson KM et al. (1999) 4-Aminobutyrate aminotransferase (GABA-transaminase) deficiency. *J. Inherit. Metab. Dis.* Vol. 22, pp. 414-427.

Nagata E, Segawa M, Fujioka H, *et al.* (2007) Dopa-responsive dystonia (Segawa disease) - like disease accompanied by mental retardation: a case report. *Mov Disord.* Vol. 22, No. 8, pp. 1202-3.

Neville BG, Parascandalo R, Felice A. (2005) Sepiapterin reductase deficiency: a congenital dopa-responsive motor and cognitive disorder. *Brain.* Vol. 128, Pt 10, pp. 2291-6.

Nygaard TG, Marsden CD, Duvoisin RC. (1988) Dopa-responsive dystonia. In: Fahn S, Marsden CD, Calne DB, eds. *Advances in Neurology.* Vol. 50, pp. 377–384, New York: Raven.

Opladen T, Okun JG, Blau N. (2010) Phenylalanine loading in pediatric patients with dopa-responsive dystonia: revised test protocol and pediatric cutoff values. *J Inherit Metab Dis*. Vol. 33, No. 6, pp. 697-703.

Opladen T, Hoffmann G, Wolf N. (2011) Clinical and biochemical characterization of patients with early infantile onset of autosomal recessive GTP cyclohydrolase I deficiency without hyperphenylalaninemia. *Mov Disord*. Vol. 26, No. 1, pp. 157-61.

Pearce DA, Atkinson M, Tagle DA. (2004) Glutamic acid decarboxylase autoimmunity in Batten disease and other disorders. *Neurology*. Vol. 63, No. 11, pp. 2001-5.

Pearl PL, Taylor JL, Sokohl A. (2007) The pediatric neurotransmitter disorders. *J Child Neurol*. Vol. 22, No. 5, pp. 606-16.

Pearl PL, Shukla L, Gibson K et al. (2011) Epilepsy in succinic semialdehyde dehydrogenase deficiency, a disorder of GABA metabolism. *Brain Dev*. Jun 9. [Epub ahead of print]

A Pickett and R L Rosales. (2011) New Trends in the Science of Botulinum Toxin-A as applied in Dystonia. *International Journal of Neuroscience* Vol. 121, pp. 22–34

Pons R, Ford B, De Vivo DC. (2004) Aromatic L-amino acid decarboxylase deficiency: clinical features, treatment, and prognosis. *Neurology* Vol. 62, pp. 1058-1065.

Rating D, Hanefeld F, Kneer J *et al.* (1984) 4-Hydroxybutyric aciduria: a new inborn error of metabolism. I. Clinical review. *J Inherit Metab Dis*. Vol. 7 Suppl 1, pp. 90-2.

Robertson D, Haile V, Perry SE. (1991) Dopamine β-hydroxylase deficiency. A genetic disorder of cardiovascular regulation. *Hypertension*. Vol. 18, pp. 1-8.

Robertson D, Goldberg MR, Robertson RM. (1986) Isolated failure of autonomic noradrenergic neurotransmission. Evidence for impaired β-hydroxylation of dopamine. *New Engl J Med*. Vol. 314, pp. 1494-1497.

Rondot P and Ziegler M. (1983) Dystonia–L-dopa responsive or juvenile parkinsonism? *J Neural Transm Suppl*. Vol. 19, pp. 273–81.

Rondot P, Aicardi J, Ziegler M. (1992) Dopa-sensitive dystonia. *Rev Neurol* (Paris) Vol. 148, pp. 680–6.

Sato S, Chiba T, Kakiuchi T et al. (2006) Decline of striatal dopamine release in parkin-deficient mice shown by ex vivo autoradiography. *J Neurosci Res*. Vol. 84, No. 6, pp. 1350-7.

Segawa M, Ohmi K, Itoh S, et al. (1971) Childhood basal ganglia disease with remarkable response to L-dopa: hereditary basal ganglia disease with marked diurnal fluctuation [in Japanese]. *Shinryo* (Tokyo) Vol. 24, pp. 667- 672.

Segawa M, Hosaka A, Miyagawa F, et al. (1976) Hereditary progressive dystonia with marked diurnal fluctuation. In: Eldridge R, Fahn S, eds. *Advances in Neurology*. Vol. 14, pp. 215–233, Raven, New York

Segawa M, Nomura Y, Nishiyama N. (2003) Autosomal dominant guanosine triphosphate cyclohydrolase I deficiency (Segawa disease). *Ann Neurol*. Vol. 54 (Suppl 6), pp. S32-45.

Shintaku H. (2002) Disorders of tetrahydrobiopterin metabolism and their treatment. *Curr Drug Metab* Vol. 3, pp. 123-131.

Shintaku H, Kure S, Ohura T et al. (2004) Long-term treatment and diagnosis of tetrahydrobiopterin-responsive hyperphenylalaninemia with a mutant phenylalanine hydroxylase gene. *Pediatr Res*. Vol. 55, No. 3, pp. 425-30

Swoboda KJ, Hyland K, Levy HL. (1999) Clinical and therapeutic observations in aromatic L-amino acid decarboxylase deficiency. *Neurology*. Vol. 53, No. 6, pp. 1205-11.

Swoboda KJ and Hyland K, (2002) Diagnosis and treatment of neurotransmitter-related disorders. *Neurol Clin*. Vol. 20, pp. 1143-1161

Swoboda KJ, Saul JP, Hyland K. (2003) Aromatic L-amino acid decarboxylase deficiency: overview of clinical features and outcomes. *Ann Neurol*. Vol. 54 Suppl 6, pp. S49-55.

Tarsy D and Simon DK. (2006) Dystonia. *N Engl J Med*. Vol. 355, pp. 818-829.

Tassin J, Dürr A, Brice A et al., (2000) Levodopa-responsive dystonia. GTP cyclohydrolase I or parkin mutations? *Brain*. Vol.123, Pt 6, pp. 1112-21

Tormenti MJ, Tomycz ND, Tyler-Kabara EC. (2011) Bilateral subthalamic nucleus deep brain stimulation for dopa-responsive dystonia in a 6-year-old child. *J Neurosurg Pediatr*. Vol. 7, No. 6, pp. 650-3.

Turjanski N, Bhatia K, Brooks DJ. (1993) Comparison of striatal 18F-dopa uptake in adult-onset dystonia-parkinsonism, Parkinson's disease, and dopa-responsive dystonia. *Neurology*. Vol. 43, No. 8, pp. 1563-8.

Watanabe T, Matsubara S, Suzuki M. (2009) Successful management of pregnancy in a patient with Segawa disease: case report and literature review. *J Obstet Gynaecol Res*. Vol. 35, No. 3, pp. 562-4.

Willemsen MA, Verbeek MM, de Rijk-van Andel JF *et al.* (2010) Tyrosine hydroxylase deficiency: a treatable disorder of brain catecholamine biosynthesis. *Brain*. Vol. 133, Pt 6, pp. 1810-22.

Yamakawa Y, Nakazawa T , Shimizu T. (2011) A boy with a severe phenotype of succinic semialdehyde dehydrogenase deficiency. *Brain Dev*. May 23. [Epub ahead of print]

Yosunkaya E, Karaca E, Yüksel. (2010) A Marked improvement in Segawa syndrome after L-dopa and selegiline treatment. *Pediatr Neurol*. Vol. 42, No. 5, pp. 348-50.

Zirn B, Steinberger D, Müller U. (2008) Frequency of GCH1 deletions in Dopa-responsive dystonia. *J Neurol Neurosurg Psychiatry*. Vol. 79, No. 2, pp. 183-6.

10

Dystonia and Rehabilitation in Children

María Inés Rodríguez S.O.T. and Cynthia Gajardo A.O.T.
Instituto de Rehabilitación Infantil Teletón Santiago
Chile

1. Introduction

Cerebral palsy is defined as a "disorder of movement and posture due to a defect or lesion of the immature brain" (Bax, 1964). The non-progressive brain damage causes a variable impairment of coordination of the muscular action, with the resulting child's inability to maintain proper posture and normal movement. Cerebral palsy (C.P.) is often associated with language, vision and hearing disorders, with different types of alterations of perception and cognition (Fejerman, 2007).

Lesions on the immature brain tend to produce widespread and diffuse damage, with multifocal or generalized dystonia is the third cause of movement disorders, whose most common cause is cerebral palsy (about 15% of them are dystonic dyskinetic). However many of the children with C.P. have spastic dystonia associated (Pascual, 2006).

It is noteworthy that there are dystonias of childhood that are not associated with cerebral palsy and often end up being widespread (Pascual, 2006; Bleton, 2000), so the clinical presentation and treatment lines in the therapeutic management are similar and for purposes of this chapter shall be taken together (Rodriguez-Costelo & Rodríguez- Regal, 2009; Lezcano, 2003).

To evaluate the abnormal movements and patterns of a child with cerebral palsy, we must know what is expected from normal movements. Our central nervous system in relation to motor function gives us the ability to move and perform highly skilled activities, while maintaining posture and balance necessary for proper functional performance. Every movement and postural change causes a variation of the center of gravity over the base of support and this should make a difference and automatic tone fluctuation throughout the body musculature, in order to maintain balance and fluidity of movement. These movements work and / or are learned as dynamic patterns, or chains that involve groups of muscle, determining as a whole, the quality of motion to perform a given task (Rodríguez, 2011).

To ensure that the motor control system is developed and run in harmony, multiple levels of central nervous system (spinal cord, medulla oblongata, pons and midbrain, diencephalon, basal ganglia, cortex and cerebellum) should be involved, since performance of a specific task requires sensory, emotional, and environmental input as well as a context that will determine the motor response needed for a particular task (Afifi, 2006; Gatica, 2005; Machado, 2010; Purves, 2004; Young, 1998).

The functional performance of children with generalized dystonia varies in different stages of development, according to etiology, degree of motor impairment and mental health and socio-cultural context (Machado et. al., 2010; Bleton, 2000). This is why the therapeutic support should be multidisciplinary and continuous throughout the process, to enhance the functional capabilities and prevent complications that may affect occupational performance.

There is some literature available supporting the medical intervention from a pharmacological and surgical approach but there is little to none documents with guidelines or systematization from a rehabilitation team perspective (Bleton, 2000).

The goal of this chapter is to systematize the intervention of children with generalized dystonia from a perspective of their degree of functional difficulties. The systematization is categorized according to the expected performance in different areas according to age of the child, providing a general reference guide for the therapeutic approach in rehabilitation.

Apart from a systematic literature Review on therapy, we incorporated the Clinical experience from a large sample of Children's Rehabilitation Institute of Santiago, Chile. This center, called Teletón, has a patient population base of 30,000 children having musculoskeletal disorders. Cerebral palsy constitutes the majority and serves 20% of the population nationally.

This chapter describes the clinical characteristics of children with cerebral palsy and generalized dystonic. It also provides neuro-rehabilitation plans with emphasis on describing evaluation and treatment processes at different stages of development.

2. Clinical characteristics of children with dystonic cerebral palsy

In order to better understand the movement development of a child with dystonic cerebral palsy it is important to remember that the basal ganglia receives information from the context in which they perform a task. The role of the basal ganglia is to regulate the automatic postural adjustment, facilitating the execution of movements required and block the ones which do not support an action, providing quality depending on the required movement to a given goal (Afifi, 2006; Gatica, 2005; Purves, 2004; Young, 1998).

When basal ganglia circuitry is altered, the control over the axial and proximal muscles is affected as a result of a fluctuating tone. This eventually will affect the fixation and stability of these muscle group (especially shoulder girdle and pelvis), decreasing the chances of dynamics co-contraction and encouraging abnormal patterns or strings that do not allow control of this mechanism through automatic postural reflex (Afifi, 2006; Bleton, 2000; Bobath, 2000; Gatica, 2005; Purves, 2004; Young, 1998). These phenomena ultimately alter the fluidity of movement, and the child in this distorted way, may have difficulties perceiving the sensory input from internal and external sources.

Also the sensory integration as an adaptive precursor response will be affected which in effect, will determine the interaction with the physical and social environment. Much of the exploration is done through vision and hearing as the possibilities to explore through the body and later on of hands as to reach, touch and manipulate objects is limited or distorted by volatile movements especially in the ability to grasp. Thus, the child can not perceive shapes, textures, weights and therefore cannot perceive the relationship of objects with the space (Rodríguez, 2011; Machado et. al., 2010).

The clinic of a child with dystonia is varied and complex given to the cognitive, emotional and motor elements involved. There is literature that relates the basal ganglia with the cognitive functions of the child. Therefore in a clinical observation it is necessary to assess if there is some cognitive impairment. However this is not always the case and there are a large number of children without cognitive difficulties even with a comprehensive level close to normal, being able to understand instructions, be alert, and expressive (Purves, 2004; Young, 1998).

It has also been described that many may have difficulty in controlling impulsivity and low frustration tolerance, which is expressed in behavioral changes such as irritability and emotional liability. The latter varies in each child, according to etiology, age and context, but often in the clinic one can find that this is reinforced by the consistent failure of their relationship with the environment, undermining their self-esteem and motivation to engage with more complex purpose, which results in greater difficulty in controlling voluntary movement, exercise tolerance and maintain the activities.

It is important to understand some key concepts about the mechanism of the generation of normal movement like the automatic postural reflex in order to understand children with generalized dystonia. This can help you identify and point out possible alterations.

The mechanism of generation of normal movement contempls; normal postural-tone, which refers to the adjustments necessary to maintain a muscular stance and anti-gravity balance, reciprocal innervations, that refers to the simultaneous contraction of opposing muscle groups around the waist and proximal parts denominating co-contraction. This dynamic fixation of the proximal parts allows us to perform distal activity with the skills necessary for a task. We can say that reciprocal innervation is of great importance for the regulation of postural tone in maintaining balance and performing normal movements. It exerts a remarkable stabilizing influence and guiding the developing movement. Finally, it considers the variety of patterns of posture and movement, which refers to the increased complexity and evolutionary patterns of movement as a result of maturation and development. (Bobath, 2000; Bobath 1992).

In generalized dystonia this aspects are alterate and they can be found on clinical examination (Bobath, 2000). In relation to the tone, it's observe hypertonia recognizing the lack of changes in the strength of a muscle group in the entire range of motion, in both cases as to flexion and extension. However, this feature is not maintained consistently, the fluctuation of the tone depends on the severity of symptoms and also on emotional and environmental factors, as well as if you are resting or in motion. Therefore, one can observe that different types of tone in the same child may change over time as the brain matures.

In relation to the reciprocal innervations, the child with dystonia seems to have, on the one hand, a disturbance of reciprocal innervations given to an excess of co-contraction, where hypertonic muscles oppose equally or more hypertonic muscles (especially in the hip and scapular girdle). On the other hand, when the case is associated with involuntary movements or ataxia it may have an excess of reciprocal inhibition with marked instability of the shoulder and pelvic girdle, varying degrees of commitment to each child. The lack of co-contraction is also responsible for the lack of action in support of synergists, which explains the excessive mobility, lack of fixation and lack of postural control of this group of children. Movements are characterized by lack of control, extreme ranges and poor coordination.

In relation to abnormal patterns, the child learns knows through exploration and play. The success of these activities sets a learning process of the motor patterns. In children with dystonia occurring movement patterns and erroneous chains are learned by positive feedback, which is provided by the ultimate success of the activity. This positive feedback is recorded even if it means that this child had to stabilize the position from proximal fixation and sometimes distal. This is required in order to compensate for the lack of postural adjustments and synergies that provide proximal stability required to run dissociated and precise movements distally.

Finally what is observed in the clinic of a child with dystonia is the consequence of the three elements above described, in which unstable postural tone, and movements are jerky, uncontrolled and of extreme ranges, with poor control of the middle ranks. As a result, the child cannot maintain a stable position against gravity to fixed posture, in addition to a mobile zone, interfering in the overall functional performance. Therefore, it is important to identify items that are altered and how these interfere with the development of normal movement patterns and functional performance.

Muscle tone, reciprocal innervations and movement patterns are crucial when planning an intervention treatment. Each child will have different clinical characteristic, so the therapist must propose alternatives treatment, considering the child's abilities and motivations, family characteristics, and social context to maximize the autonomy and independence (Crepeac, 2005).

3. Neuro rehabilitation of the child with dystonic cerebral palsy

The therapeutic approach of children with generalized dystonia should be multidisciplinary, since each discipline makes a contribution to improving functional performance.

For purposes of this chapter there will be an overview of the therapeutic management under the foundations of Occupational Therapy, differentiated by degree of commitment and age groups in order to guide treatment and to provide guidelines.

It is important to understand that the occupation is the essence of "doing" in the human being, which determines and identifies the person in a context, set in a social and cultural environment. There must be a promotion of balance in the different areas of performance (basic and instrumental activities of daily living, productive activities as well as leisure and entertainment), maximizing components (cognitive perceptual, sensory, motor, psychological and social) that enable the development and the achievement of each life cycle stage (Crepeac, 2005; Kielhofner, 2004).Occupational therapy approach considers the child as an interacting system and a whole, considering also the environment in which the child develops. This appreciation facilitates a better understanding of the child's problems and contributes to a better approach.

The intrinsic and extrinsic motivation of the child in combination with a properly selected therapeutic activity, close related to the child's abilities, should raise an interesting challenge as a key to successful therapy. The right challenge promotes the child's learning or relearning of the conscious and successful voluntary motor program. Whit repetition, this successful movement becomes finally as an automatic motor pattern (Csikszentmihayi, 1997).

Children with generalized dystonia are permanently seeking body stability. Therefore the work position must provide axial support to lessen the need to seek stability through postural fixation or abnormal patterns. An unstable position can in the future cause permanent alterations of the posture, inefficient chains of movements, and not functional movement. As for the activity, this should ensure success and avoid frustration; creating an atmosphere that encourages repetition of the voluntary action, encouraging people to learn more stable motor schemes, more functional and appropriate movements (Bleton, 2000; Rodríguez, 2011).

The aim of the therapeutic approach is to achieve a better occupational performance whit the remaining capacity, development potential, according to the age and context of the child (Mulligan, 2006; Rodríguez, 2011).

There is a large literature referring to drug therapies available for children with dystonic cerebral palsy. Regarding intervention approaches performed by non-medical disciplines (Kinesiology, Occupational Therapy, Speech Therapy, etc.) the literature is scars. There are only short articles about overall management and very specific to certain rehabilitation centers. These studies are in general not validated nor statistically significant or representative (Blanco, 2006; Bleton, 2000; Pascual, 2006).

Below are areas and evaluation criteria, methodology of intervention based on characteristics of children in an age group, level of motor impairment and level of understanding. The therapeutic management is discussed according to the criteria of postural control, hand function, movement, activities of daily living and school management. In each of these points is considered the orthotic management, adaptations and furniture recommended (Mulligan, 2006; Rodríguez, 2011).

3.1 Assessment

The generalized dystonia often interfere whit the functional and occupational performance of children. Therefore assessment process must consider a broad range of tools to assess the multiple elements involved in child development.

Regarding the evaluation tools there is a wide range of standardized guidelines, however, most seek to measure the intensity of dystonia in a segmental way and only a few refer to a functional evaluation of performance (Bleton, 2000; Rodríguez, et.al. 2006).

Observing the motor control from the neurodevelopment model (Bobath, 2000; Bobath, 1992), helps to have a reference of the degree of assistance in the activities of daily living using for example the Wee-FIM (Uniform Data System for Médical Rehabilitation, 2005) of International classification of functioning assessment scale (CIF) (Herrera, 2008). These assessments allow us to classify and guide the treatment. Also the Scales evaluating functional compromise and involuntary upper extremity movements in children with extra pyramidal disorders (Rodríguez, et.al., 2006) scale categorizes clinically the level of functional compromise from normal to severe in the areas of sitting posture, basic activities daily living and manual functionality. It is also a good resource to use the Gross Motor (Russel, 2002) assessment to evaluate gross motor control associated with walking. There are psychomotor development test and games, which could be useful in milder cases and in young children. Incorporating quality of life test as KIDSCREEN (Urzúa, et.al., 2009) allows us to know the perception of child welfare and family.

All these tests are feasible to use with children with involuntary movements, or with those who have no oral language difficulties and can communicate through oral language. Tests assessing manual functionality are not always useful, because these tests are very specific and strict about the times and methods of implementation, so it could be used in milder cases in terms of difficulties of upper extremities.

Below you will find a comprehensive way to evaluate the child and family more holistically, using direct observation methods. Some of the items listed above may be evaluated based on standardized tests, leaving to the discretion of the evaluator their implementation (Bleton, 2000; Mulligan, 2006; Rodríguez, 2011).

Direct observation

It is suggested that the initial assessment is done with the mother or primary caregiver, to learn their attitudes, what elements are positively reinforced and what are not, how the caregiver holds the child and moves the child and what are the voice commands used. Following the interview with the caregiver, observe the child in a free and spontaneous play session to see rhythms, patterns, compensation, fixings and surfaces in which the child feels more comfortable and successful for performing the tasks.

Assessment should include an interview to the parents along with an observation of free play of the child. The mother or caregiver can provide information regarding daily routine as well as context in which the activities are performed. It is also important to record the child's interest and participation within and outside the home.

Following the interview, a structure evaluation is recommended, where the environment is prearranged to guide the child's activity to record all aspects needed to detect difficulties in skills and functional performance.

3.1.1 Cognitive aspects

Frequently, children with dystonic cerebral palsy have a comprehensive level enough to follow simple commands and even have a comprehensive level close to normal. Measuring the cognitive ability of children with generalized dystonia is very challenging, given that standardized psychometric tests include verbal and motor tests to assess a score. Generally these children have many difficulties to successfully complete such tests which often results in scores that do not reflect the actual learning abilities of children with dystonic cerebral palsy (Ramirez, 2005).

3.1.2 Sensory aspects

It is important to know that the basal ganglia participate as environmental regulators. Therefore it is important to assess how the child is receiving the internal and external sensory information, which is observed through the adaptive response against a variety of sensory input (Ayres, 2006).

Consider that these children have insufficient or altered vestibular and propioceptive experiences generated by difficulties presented to move against gravity in different planes. This alters the sensory processing and reduces the possibility for organizing the body in relation to self and the space, affecting the proximal stability, righting reactions, balance and accuracy of movements.

3.1.3 Neurological aspects

It is important to determine the different types of tones that the child presents. Determine which tone is the one present when the child is resting and not moving and which one is the tone during action. It is also important to determine the intensity and form of presentation when the dystonic pattern appears and how this pattern interferes with the function. Observe if the child has a primitive reflex present and if these reflexes begin to be used as a functional resource to be able to move.

3.1.4 Postural development

The assessment of the postural development has to follow the neurodevelopmental approach which observes and assesses (sagittal, frontal and transverse). Assessing postural development from a normal developmental sequence would allow you the early identification of disorders that could hinder the acquisition of normal patterns (Bobath, 2000; Bobath, 1992).

To facilitate the process, it is recommended to evaluate the child in different positions according to what is expected to be normal motor development (prone, supine, traction to sitting, sitting, transition points and four intermediate positions, crawling, transition to bipedal, bipedal, and assisted start up independent). After this, the evaluator should identify how the child is gradually moving against gravity as well as which are the normal or abnormal patterns used to successfully move against gravity. It is also important to identify what postural fixation and involuntary movements appear when the child is activating the movement. Note the range, speed and rhythm presented during the movement in order to identify the way and how much these patterns interfere in the achievement of postural control and functional performance.

3.1.5 Active mobility of upper extremities

It is important to observe the mobility of upper extremities at different levels. It is suggested to observe the quality of the child active movement that can be performed in space or in relation to their own bodies and what strategy is being used to compensate for the lack of axial stability. One must distinguish the pattern and rhythm of movements used in relation to speed and amplitude and whether this is appropriate for the target in order to determine the functional level in relation to energy consumption and execution time (Rodríguez, 2011).

3.1.6 Manual function

It is frequently observed in children with dystonia movement patterns of total flexion-extension of the wrist and fingers. This pattern is due to the lack of reciprocal innervations caused by the excessive co-contraction. Wrist extension with fingers in fist and wrist in flexion with fingers extended prevents the flow of movement in intermediate ranges which makes more difficult to perform a voluntary control of the grasp. It is rare to observe dissociation of fingers and fine grasps and usually the children tend to use the grip type of rake.

Assessment is made with single-handed and bimanual activities going from the simple to the complex. It is necessary evaluate the active mobility of the wrist and fingers, digital dissociation and the ability to perform gross and fine grips on functional activities. Consider the pace or chain movement used to perform a successful grasp. This information is crucial when choosing the necessary aids and orthotics for the child (Rodríguez, 2011). When assessing the manual function it is important to register if the observation was done using orthotic or any accommodations. In case some external accommodations were used, register what type of external elements and what is the indication of use they had as well as the functional benefit that these elements are offering to the child.

3.1.7 Play

It is important to provide different types of play activities, challenging both cognitive and motor abilities to demonstrate skills, abilities and interests, in addition to handling emotional and social response to success and failure. All these aspects will establish the level of autonomy and ultimately determine the quality of occupational performance of the child.

The frustration tolerance in children with dystonia is usually very low which often promotes caregivers and parents to supply children with toys that are easier to handle to avoid frustration. This particular situation diminishes the challenge to explore more complex type of toys and most of the times these "easier toys" end up not being adequate for the child's cognitive or emotional age.

The context in which the child is developing and the toys and elements that the child uses frequently to play can provide important information to determine if adequate stimulation is being provided to promote the potential development.

3.1.8 Routine and daily life activities

The evaluation includes a direct interview with the mother or caregiver about the child's daily routine to check if it is balanced and healthy. Also evaluate the basic and instrumental activities of daily living considering the level of independence, autonomy and degree of assistance. The way how they are performing the tasks and how much power this implies for the caregiver are also important to be considered (Rodríguez, 2011).

3.1.9 Orthotics, furniture, technical aids, adaptations and architectural barriers

In general, they have a low postural control and low function and will require assistance from third parties and adaptations to facilitate the tasks. It is important to register the type of furniture, adaptations and orthotics used in terms of functional goals, frequency and tolerance. It is also important to assess whether the use of these elements are creating a postural or functional benefit to the child. These elements must be permanently checked because of the possible occurrence of postural compensations.

In the case of children who use wheelchairs it is important to assess whether the posture is appropriate, if it provides stability, head and trunk alignment, position and symmetry of the pelvis, lower extremities posture and alignment, restraint or postural support (Fife, et. al., 1991). In appropriate cases it is required to evaluate the potential self-propelled option with either rings or electrical control.

In relation to architectural barriers, it should be evaluated whether or not there are barriers present in the environment where they are and how the family deals with these situations.

3.1.10 Family and school context

It is necessary to assess the family and school context in terms of integration, monitoring the therapeutic indications and how to facilitate the independence, autonomy and socialization.

In relation to the familiar context, it is important to assess who are the primary and secondary caregiver of the child, the type of link they have and if they are facilitating integration, independence and autonomy of the child in the family or in the community contexts.

In relation to the school, it is important to highlight the type of link with the authority and with peers, level of attendance and participation. In addition to registering if you have some kind of specialist support from other professionals or rating systems adapted to a formal integration plan.

It is essential to know what furniture you use and the ease or difficulty about this in relation to the sitting posture and upper extremity function, considering always recording the specific adaptations necessary for the implementation of homework. It is very important to consider the level of accessibility offered by the educational establishment as well.

3.2 Treatment

The treatment of children diagnosed with generalized dystonia is based on terms of greater functionality by a better voluntary control of movement (Blanco, 2006). For this it is necessary to work with different sensory and motor skills that promote learning, relearning and improving motor patterns, achieving a better postural adjustment, a more appropriate speed, better directionality and fluidity of movement in relation to the body and different levels in space (Bobath, 2000; Gracies, 1997; Rannie, 2000; Rodríguez, 2011; Rodríguez, et.al., 2006).

The lines of treatment can be projected after having clarity about the degree of functional compromise and also knowing the family and social context, which is achieved after a comprehensive evaluation and in conjunction and together with the child and family.

This treatment information is projected mainly through frameworks that include sensory stimulation (tactile, propioceptive and vestibular) (Ayres, 2006), neuro-developmental (Bobath, 2000) framework (facilitation based on sequences and normal movement patterns) and rehabilitation framework (to facilitate posture, functionality and independence through activities and elements such as therapeutic aids, orthotics and adjustments) (Creapeac, 2005).

Below you can find a description of the therapeutic management used according to the age of the children, the degree of motor impairment and comprehensive level. These descriptions include some suggestions and considerations.

Children with severe generalized dystonia present difficulties in establishing contact with the environment and/or have cognitive impairments obstruct the understanding of simple instructions. These children will be addressed as multi deficit where the emphasis of the therapeutic management will be placed in relation to family child care.

The cases of dystonia that have mild intellectual disability will have a major alteration of their functional performance primarily from cognitive impairment, so it will not be described under the guidelines of this chapter since these areas are generally handled properly in special schools.

Children with generalized dystonia with moderate motor impairment present a comprehensive level enough to follow simple instructions; this group of children will be described by two distinct age groups, involving them as active participants in the rehabilitation process, with emphasis on motor control and overall functional performance. The more detailed description will be in this group, as we understand that is requiring more therapeutic intervention, highlighting the potential gains to obtain from the functional performance.

Children with mild motor impairment and a high level of understanding will be addressed in two separate age groups. This is because the therapeutic action contemplates an intervention plan focused on facilitating normal development and functional performance appropriate to the age and context of the child.

Children with a severe motor impairment with a good understanding will also be addressed in two age groups. There are no major changes expected in terms of functional capacity and postural control in short periods of time for this group of children, being important for these cases to enhance the function and prevent complications.

It should be considered across the board that in children with a good understanding, the treatment should emphasize the identification of aspects that contribute to optimize the function of the child. It is also important to suggest to the family the self management of aspects that can facilitate the improvement of the child's performance, such as furniture, or adaptations that optimizes the child's performance.

3.2.1 Children with mild motor impairment level and good understanding. Ages 0 to 6 year

This group of children will benefit from models such as neurodevelopmental and sensory integration, cognitive and behavioral rehabilitation.

The intervention aims to normalize psychomotor development facilitating movement sequences and patterns in a more organized, automatic, economical way with a better voluntary control. In this range of age, gross and fine motor demands become more complex and therefore require more postural control to prevent and reduce functional bindings and decrease involuntary movements.

Along with this, the sensory aspect is reinforced to provide better input to these stimuli, facilitating the integration and maturation of the systems involved, promoting a favorable adaptive response. Activities are conducted using vestibular and propioceptive sensations and promoting the development of righting and equilibrium reactions, with synergies to promote the organization of movement in relation to body and space (Ayres, 2006).

It is also important to generate patterns of controlled and rhythmic breathing, as this has great impact on the voluntary control of movements and spoken language. Initially, it is suggested putting the child to work on the mother's breast, to feel the respiratory patterns to later do so voluntarily.

At this stage, play is the main occupation of the child, which develops through social, emotional, cognitive, sensory, and motor functions. From this, it is essential that play is constantly referred to within the therapeutic activity and according to the therapy goals. Games should also be selected according to the abilities and interests of children, looking to present interesting challenges in order to promote the interest necessary to generate action. The relevance is focused in one punctual aspect: learning will occur to the extent that the activity has both significance and success for the child (Maturana, 2007).

Some children will require external support such as furniture, orthotic or adaptation, but these are mostly transitory.

In relation to postural control: The child that has interest and contact with the environment initiates movements to go out against gravity spontaneously, developing near-normal patterns. Progressively the child should be dominating higher positions and perform activities according to age. The therapist must accompany this process based on the sequences of normal development, safeguarding that the child does not use fixed resources by setting in abnormal postural patterns learned as functional. Treatment should be focused on correct and facilitate normal motor chain repetition reinforced by activities that bring success in a functional way. From a sensory point of view, treatment should include propioceptive and vestibular elements in order to stimulate the harmonious development of the movements.

It is important to address the sitting posture as this is often used for play and influence the stability of hand function. If the child is seated early you may have the need for proximal postural fixation to stabilize the pelvis and trunk, making the transfer of weight and the degrees of freedom more difficult, limiting the possibility of developing movements in different planes which establish harmonic synergy for space exploration.

In relation to the role of hands: The function of the hands is largely determined by a stable axial and proximal control, reason why it should be offered a work setting that provide adequate support for the position and sensory registration.

In relation to the development of grips you can see a greater mastery of the gross grips, making it difficult or delayed acquisition of fine grips and digital dissociation. To promote the sound development, the child should experience tactile and propioceptive sensation in different games in two motor ways, globally and manipulative. This provides information on weight, texture, shape and size, which determines the progressive development of manual skills necessary for a variety of grasps, dissociated intermediate ranges and movements that will facilitate the execution of increasingly complex tasks according to age of development.

The need of proximal fixation to reach stability and distal control needs to be avoided. This fixation reduces the degree of freedom of movement in space of upper extremities. Therefore, it is recommended that activities involving the use of hands are performed in a sitting position. The sitting position should include a stable chair with a rigid seat base and a table with cutout appropriate to the child's size in order to provide stability to the forearms.

For this age group and level it is suggested to postpone the use of orthotics in order to facilitate normal development.

In relation to the movement: This group of children often succeeds crawling, but with a pattern of increased pelvic instability as in jumping rabbit, being useful assisted systems for crawling or walking. Be mindful not to encourage postural proximal fixation, but provide stability and assistance with some element of temporary external support.

In most cases walking is acquired close to six years old. Therapeutic support should be cautious and towards a proper gait pattern. In some cases it will require a transitional element of external support. It is not uncommon to use a gait trainer or wheelchair for long transfers.

In relation to the activities of daily living: To carry out these tasks it should be considered to place the child in a stable position that allows him to have better resources to perform these activities.

It is important that the family favors the development of activities as self-feeding, hygiene and clothing according to their age and thereafter provide environmental support with elements or adaptations to facilitate appropriate and successful implementation. Do not lose of sight that the difficulties in proximal stability and involuntary movements require to modify the pattern and sequence of execution to accomplish the task, since most of the movements' performed to do these tasks require to go out against gravity which increases involuntary movements.

It is suggested that during feeding, forearms are flat on a surface permanently; preventing that the elbow loses contact with the surface, thereby decreasing the involuntary movements. Along with this, if necessary, provide a thickened spoon and always give an indication of moving the head toward the spoon. In these activities the child may need adult assistance or elements that give stability to the plate like an antiskid or an adapted tray.

As for hygiene and clothing the child must be an active participant in this routine, to internalize and reinforce appropriate sequences and energy efficiency. It is important to remember the age appropriate tasks watching runtimes to support achievement in the everyday as functional. Also you need to consider the necessary changes in terms of access, items available in the space, utensils and/or some element of temporary or permanent support or adaptation to facilitate the task.

In this age self-care activities take on greater relevance with the gain of progressive independence in regards to the activities of basic daily life (Mulligan, 2006).

In relation to school activities: It is recommended that this group of children start their schooling in regular school system of selection. Sometimes you need professional support to adapt specific elements related to specific subjects and tasks that require more accuracy or quality of execution. It may also be useful to assess if the furniture provides suitable positions favoring a proper execution of tasks, offering suggestions when necessary.

3.2.2 Children with mild motor impairment level and good understanding. Ages 6 and older

Treatment in this group has a profile of progressively making a difference in the development of autonomy, independence and community involvement. After 12 years of age, the self-management of elements of support that foster a better occupational performance are well established.

In relation to the position: At this point it is important to constantly reassess all aspects of the postural adjustment because as growth implies a reorganization of motor schemes, were compensations or patterns may appear abnormal but, in most cases these are temporary. It must be safeguarded that these are not made permanent, damaging in a long-term the postural control and functional performance.

In relation to hand function: Insofar as the child progresses through the school system, increasing demands will require greater demands on the quality and speed of execution, which could lead to a decrease in occupational performance, "both given" by the more demanding task and the stress.

Assess and define strategies to optimize performance and in some cases it might be required the use of accommodations, furniture and technical assistance.

In children over twelve years old, manual abilities are largely developed. The possible difficulties that might occur should be evaluated and corrected to avoid a significant detriment to the functional performance that has already being achieved.

In relation to movement: At this stage, most will walk independently. In periods of high growth they may become unstable, so it is recommended to reevaluate constants gait pattern to intervene therapeutically if the case requires so. Some children retain the use of a wheelchair for long transfers.

In relation to activities of daily living: A child this age should increase the autonomy and independence according to age levels in activities of basic daily life, expanding progressively toward the instrumental activities. It must be constantly evaluated to decrease the third-party assistance, providing accommodations or modifications conducive to the attainment of independence.

In the instrumental activities daily living it is suggested to increase tasks and responsibilities of intra domiciliary in addition to provide spaces for an active community participation, including documents management, money use, transportation and occupational activities, all age appropriate. In some cases these activities require therapeutic support and training to habituation, as well as to provide strategies, social skills and safety for a satisfactory performance.

In relation to school activities: At this point they may demonstrate difficulties in relation to the time of execution, specifically in terms of writing. It is suggested to check if the furniture and tools are providing stability to optimize performance. In many cases, it is required to use support systems or alternative technologies that facilitate the execution of the task.

Children older than twelve years should be identifying skills and interests to focus on alternative vocational and employment preferences that must be consistent with the real possibilities of the young.

3.2.3 Children with moderate motor impairment level and good understanding. Ages 0 to 6 year

This group of children presents clinical signs that can be seen early by a professional in the area. Treatment should be approached from models such as neurodevelopmental, sensory integration, behavioral and cognitive rehabilitation.

The intervention must accompany psychomotor development facilitating movement sequences and patterns in a more organized way and with a better voluntary control. From early stages when the child tries out against gravity, compensation and abnormal patterns emerge in response to the lack of control and axial synergies. In some cases we observe prolonged primitive reflexes that can be used as a functional resource, transforming it into a learned pattern that is pathological.

It becomes important that the development of low postures should take special care and attention as it is on this stage when they begin to strengthen postural and proximal fixation.

Managing the child that is less than one year old provides a postural control with elements or implements that help the organization in space, is important to achieve synergies and midline line which are precursors of visual monitoring and of the use of hands.

In children over one year, in addition to the above, it begins to favor the functional activity of higher positions such as sitting and bipedal. Parallel to this, it is important to provide vestibular and propioceptive sensory input to enhance and promote afferential information to organize properly a functional motor and adaptive response.

Efforts must be placed on patterns of controlled and rhythmic breathing to organize movements to facilitate and promote oral language. In the early stages this work is suggested by the mother who provides rhythmic breathing patterns, after this, the child should work this voluntarily or therapy could help to increase the quality of movement.

In children older than three years, gross and fine motor demands become more complex, so the chances of feeling frustration or anxiety increases, making even more difficult the control of movement. This requires special attention when treating and choosing the activity and postural control support which needs to be both static and dynamic.

Play and school activities are the main occupation of the child, which develops through social, emotional, cognitive, sensory and motor functions. It becomes relevant the child preferences and interests. The therapist must reconcile this with the selected therapeutic activity, not to mention that an activity generates significant and successful learning. Also at this stage the child enters a school system, which sometimes requires guidance or counseling in handling furniture and specific elements of technical assistance.

In relation to postural control: In the early stages environmental elements must be conducive to proper posture and the ability to explore spontaneously.

Supine flexion should be favored, using elements of containment that provide slight bend of the head and pelvis in order to provide a midline upper extremities, visual and abdominal activity.

In prone, use a wedge to allow the right use of forearms or arm support on the surface to weight bearing and allow synergies of shoulder girdle, neck and head. Avoid a pattern of abnormal extension or hyperextension of the neck to be a precursor to every action.

Often when turning there is a tendency to one side only and initiated from the head in hyperextension. In this case it will be necessary to facilitate synergies and dissociation in lateral planes.

In managing the sitting posture observe if the overall patterns are initiated from the head and/or pelvis, as this will be a critical control point to consider for the functional use of this position.

In the case that the movement originates at the head, descending tactile and propioceptive information must be submitted in the sterna, to stimulate flexor muscles. In the event of involuntary movement generated in the pelvis, hip flexion facilitated greater than 90 degrees is required, in order to shift the weight to this area and reduce the chances of making an involuntary extensor pattern.

In children less than one year sitting posture will be fully assisted given that the head and trunk control are still developing. The righting reactions and support do not offer enough control.

Until the extent that the child is about three years old the control of head and trunk stability improves, but still continues to require assistance. There is instability due to weak righting reactions, slow or nonexistent, in addition to the predominance of the sagital plane flexion and extension patterns in total ranges. This makes more difficult the postural automatic control and intermediate ranges needed to maintain a stable sitting posture.

It is important to consider providing a strong support level to promote sciatic propioceptive information at various levels to facilitate the automatic postural control. The use of postural seating made for each child ensures good posture avoiding that the child resort to fixation to stabilize posture against gravity. Along with this, the feet should also be in contact with a surface to provide support and control.

On the other hand, although sometimes the child can sit independently at times on a bench, the child will lose stability when needed to go out and try different planes of motion or when using upper extremities for functional activity. This happened because these items require more automatic adjustments of posture. However as a therapeutic target it will be beneficial to consider, because it is related to the axial control and it can provide lower assistance in postural and lower demand from the upper extremities function, or conversely if the goal is to increase functionality, further assist hands posture will be required.

As for four points' posture, crawling and transition to bipedal, the child will require great assistance as these positions involve transitions and intermediate ranges which should be assisted or facilitated by the therapist. For this, you can use external support elements to organize the space both physically and visually. Subsequently, the bipedal posture becomes important and can make an assisted start with some gait trainer with brachial support adaptation.

In upper body it is recommended the support in the forearm on a surface as a tray or table with cutout in order to provide information at the proximal and shoulder girdle to stimulate axial and head control. This provides visual information regarding body position in space and promotes greater organization and global control. At the level of the pelvis it is helpful to use a cushion of sand to provide weight and more stability information to the seat bones, reducing the involuntary movements at this level.

The use of compressive clothing must be evaluated for treatment and in some children may be useful regulating the tone and decreasing the degrees of freedom giving stability to the pelvic girdle, providing axial and proximal control (Rannie, 2005; Allen, 1997).

In relation to the role of hands: As for the function of hands, the tasks become more complex progressively looking for a greater coordination, dissociation and accuracy, which require proximal stability and motion control to distal for a successful performance. It must be anticipated and address early the proximal fixations made by the child when looking for proximal stability and distal control. Surge the dichotomy between stabilize the trunk or use their hands to play. Subsequently this generates that the child will choose the upper extremity with less difficulties to perform the tasks, and the other extremity will be used as a postural fixation, which in the long term, will reduce the function and generate an asymmetry in the trunk and shoulder girdle producing postural scoliosis as a result of maintaining this position.

Given the above, to facilitate the manual functionality it should be considered to provide axial stability to the pelvic girdle as a basis for proximal control. The greater functional requirement involving upper extremities movements in space at a proximal level and distal level as well as manual dexterity will require more support or postural control. This is why, efforts should consider pelvic and trunk stability by providing a stable sitting posture as a basis to support the role of hands in different planes in space. The use of tray or table with cutout helps control the movement of upper limbs when supporting the forearm.

The upper extremity presents a pattern to the action of co-contraction with internal rotation of shoulder, elbow in extension, forearm in pronation and wrist in flexion or extension, thumb included, with difficulty in opening and closing the hand on a voluntary way. Therefore they prefer to work in extension, distal to the body, having trouble with proximal tasks. Gross grasps are performed using a functional tenodesis to facilitate grasp, using mechanically a maximum flexion and maximum extension of the wrist as a resource, not being able to perform intermediate ranges. This abnormal pattern allows the opening and closing of the hand but significantly limits the ability to grasp.

To facilitate the manual function it is suggested to use games and therapeutic activities adequate for the comprehensive level but easy to handle, considering the challenge versus the child's ability to ensure the success of the activity. There are alternative therapies such as compression bandaging and abduction bandage that provides tactile and propioceptive information to agonist and antagonist groups helping the tone regulation, providing a mechanical effect of a reverse pattern favoring the dominant one. This element must be used therapeutically as training for re learning a normal pattern.

To facilitate the grasp use a wrist stabilizing orthotic and thumb positioning, considering that the wrist should be neutral or in slight flexion to ensure the start of the string or pattern learned. To this orthotics, adaptations can be attached such as pencil, to expand activities in order to increase significance. It is not recommended the use of weight in the upper extremities.

Often these children prefer to use the extremity with less difficulties of movement, assigning the contra lateral fixing element in either extension or flexion, for which an adequate remedies to position the extremity, is a stick attached to the table or tray to provide symmetry and closed string promoting the role of the dominant limb.

To encourage the voluntary control of movement, improving the quality in terms of amplitude and speed, and decreasing the involuntary movements, it is recommended to provide verbal cue to regulate these aspects, so that the child displays improved performance and energy economic movement. The therapist or caregiver must establish a climate of trust, giving timeouts and pauses to self-regulate using breathing as a relaxation tool.

In relation to the activities of daily living: At this stage, it is important that the caregiver engages in the activities in a stable posture, encouraging the collaboration of the child in parts of the activity, facilitating normal movement sequences. At this age and level of commitment of basic activities daily living, in most tasks assistance should be given by a third party.

Self-care activities provide progressive independence in regards to the activities of basic daily life, but the low postural control hinders the attainment of independence and also the functional result in terms of execution time and physical effort. Do not forget the required holding for seated posture for these activities.

The family must provide the space and time to develop or encourage participation in activities of feeding, hygiene and clothing, according to functional conditions of the child, bearing in mind that in most cases they will be able to implement some part of the tasks and will require specific adaptations and training.

In relation to self-feeding, proper posture should consider supporting the pelvis and a table with cutout to provide support to avoid leaving forearms permanently against gravity. Also consider adjustments in the spoon to ensure a good grip, the plate which must not be too high to have to raise your arm, should be fixed to the table with an anti slip. Indication remains ideally to lead head to the spoon.

As for the dressing, facilitate the child performance during the initiation or by the end of the activity providing a proper posture. Usually this activity will not be functional in daily life.

In hygiene, if it can grant the appropriate posture and environmental conditions this may help the child to participate in parts of the activity like washing hands and face, but brushing teeth will be difficult by the possibility of self injury. Regardless, it will require assistance from a third party to complete the task.

In relation to the movement: This group of children usually does not achieve the transition to crawling or bipedal, being useful assisted systems for standing or running. Keep in mind not to encourage postural proximal fixation, when providing stability and assistance with some element of external support.

The walking will not be functional; it will require a gait trainer with forearm support and adaptations with pelvis support, separating lower extremities, and trunk and head support to prevent the extension discharge, to diminish to the maximum fixation resources and abnormal patterns. Thus, the child may make an intra domiciliary assisted walk to start favoring independence and sense of accomplishment. This activity must be accompanied by stretching to maintain flexibility and range of motion and bipedal to protect bone development and provide propioceptive information.

Regarding the movement it is recommended if possible a wheelchair with 5 degrees of reclining, watching the same premises described in sitting posture, which means, support the postural control with accessories and fastening systems that provide alignment and stability to the pelvis and trunk. At least it should be encouraged intra domiciliary self-propulsion.

In relation to school activities: Regarding the school system it is suggested to evaluate whether the child has conditions to enter a regular school with integration program. There will be a need for professional support to bring environmental elements related to the furniture and access. It will also be required the support in making various adjustments to facilitate implementation of the tasks, the implementation of mechanisms or alternative technology that facilitates learning and communication. Differentiated evaluation is suggested in relation to the methodology used, to ensure that children have the opportunity to express their knowledge.

3.2.4 Children with moderate motor impairment level and good understanding. Ages 6 and more

This group maintains the treatment scheme of the previous section in all areas. In children older than twelve it becomes important the development of autonomy and community involvement. Self-management must be a condition that favors the young to reach a better occupational performance according to their age and abilities.

In relation to the position: The reassessment will be dominant because of the possibility of generating postural scoliosis due to rapid growth typical of this stage. The child cannot adapt quickly enough and being against gravity will be a difficult effort to maintain over time, especially increasing the residence time of the sitting posture. It is recommended medical evaluation of the spine and hip to prevent complications, and thereby provide early support to external elements of containment and alignment and stimulate within your daily routine the changes in posture as well as passive and active mobilization to maintain a proper balance in this area.

The child will require supportive care, and in some cases external aid elements of temporary or permanent use to provide axial support and postural alignment.

In relation to hand function: The role of hands should not be affected in relation to that achieved in previous stages. It is necessary to assess whether the support elements and adaptations are sufficient and whether they are facilitating the function according to the requirements for the type of activities typical of the age.

According to the assessment and skills it is suggested to facilitate necessary resources that support performance based on abilities and interests. It can be incorporated for example, pointers, adapted scissors, pencils and thickening brushes; orthotics (with the same considerations of the previous group), among others.

In relation to the movement: As the child grows taller, they have greater possibility of muscle imbalance, so it should be permanently reassessed if the walker offers stability and sufficient alignment and what musculoskeletal functional benefits and which function are promoted.

In relation to the movement in a wheelchair, which may be electrical or mechanical, should be supported with postural control accessories and restraint systems to provide alignment and stability to the pelvis and trunk. Self-propulsion should be considered only when the position is adequate and does not involve excessive energy expenditure; it is important new elements of postural restraint if necessary.

In relation to activities of daily living: At this age it should be important encourage the child to achieve greater autonomy in their daily activities, understanding that they must be progressively making the right decisions about how to choose and which tasks to be performed considering the help of others, and custody that the activities are executed properly.

Children over twelve years that are independent or partially independent should continue to be independent, with the exception of architectural barriers that restrict their access. As for activities where the patient is dependent, it will be leading the autonomy as a fundamental self-management and social integration.

In relation to school activities: We suggest adding elements of assistive technology that promotes communication and access to search information, global literacy and learning, providing speed and efficiency.

In the age of twelve skills and interests of the young can be assessed more clearly. It is important to provide guidance that considers the pre vocational skills, motivations and social context that allow objectify professional development options.

3.2.5 Children with severe motor serious commitment and a good level understanding. Ages 0 to 6 year

This group presented a severe motor or serious condition will have no major changes from the postural and functional over time. The emphasis will be given in preventing deformities and finding activities that provide purpose and a sense of accomplishment with a healthy routine.

In relation to the position: In children younger than 2 years old, it will be vital to perform therapeutic activities that tend to decrease the extensor pattern and normalize the tone, promoting voluntary movements. For this we suggest considering working with neurodevelopmental framework, learning normal patterns at different levels. This should be complemented with activities and age-appropriate games that are possible to implement in order to ensure success in the task and thus achieve the repetition and learning. Accessories and furniture will be required to provide symmetrical positions conducive to reducing overall patterns of flexion and extension.

The position should include the head avoiding abnormal extension; the arms tending to the midline, and the pelvis in flexion and abduction. It is suggested the use of straps or cushion of sand to facilitate posture. It is intended to perform the movements not in a total and repetitive pattern, but rather try to dissociate and promote variability.

Special attention should be placed to the management with the family. The family should keep the child posture, avoiding abnormal postures to play in order to avoid give a positive feedback to these patterns.

In regards to furniture is suggested that the sitting posture contains adapted seating surface or shaped to give alignment of head and trunk flexion and hip abduction at least 90 degrees to move the center of gravity backwards, favoring the reduction of extensor discharges. The inclination in this position depends on the condition of each child and must always make sure that the hips remain in the position described above. The weight pad on the pelvis favors stability. The use of trays with cut will be a great support for the position, manual function and cephalic control from the visual record.

Regarding the lateral position it should maintain the alignment conditions mentioned in the sitting posture considering the use of furniture and adapted cushions for this purpose.

In regards to the prone position be aware that the child does NOT make a total extensor reaction and facilitate conditions for the arms forward with support in the forearm, the trunk should be neutral and have a half bent pelvis. For this, use a roll and therapeutic wedge as elements to position while the child is on the lap of a caregiver.

As for the biped this position will have greater relevance starting at the age of one as a therapeutic action for development and joints nutrition.

In relation to hand function: The mobility of upper extremities and hands is severely affected by the presence of dystonic discharges. Often permanence of primitive reflexes exists and becomes pathological functional resource, limiting the proper development of movement in space and manual functionality.

Considering adequate postural support, the child should develop the full potential for the use of the hands. Central to the therapeutic approach is to provide sufficient postural support to provide stability and reduce the intensity of the shock, facilitating the movement of upper extremities. But this movement is not functional and it will be very difficult to address accurately enough to achieve the reach and grasping capacity.

Orthotics primarily target to correct or maintain healthy joints and muscles to prevent deformities and improve capabilities that support remaining function, even if it is assisted (Gajardo & Rodríguez).

The tray or table with cutout and the use of stick fixed to the table provides stability and symmetry.

In relation to movement: The movements are dependent on a third party, usually the child moves with an adapted gait trainer or wheelchair without the possibility of self-propelled. It is advisable to consider for sitting the described above options, using seats made for the child or adapted that can be considered as an accessory to the chair or gait trainer. The trunk usually requires a four point vest to maintain alignment and facilitate bending.

In relation to activities of daily living: This area is totally dependent; the intervention plan should look to fully develop the child's autonomy as managing his routine of self care. The therapist must evaluate, guide and train the family in healthy strategies to accomplish these tasks, in order not to further enhance abnormal patterns in the child and not harm the health of the primary caregiver.

In relation to school activities: These children should be educated with therapeutic care in terms of permanent aids and adaptations, both in general management, and assessment systems. This favors a level appropriate to support general motor and postural control to facilitate autonomy, the level of access to information, communication and integration.

3.2.6 Children with severe motor serious commitment and a good level understanding. Ages 6 and more

In relation to the position: These children have severe dystonic discharges affecting global posture and therefore severely interferes the function and communication. Treatment should include the management of postural control by promoting normal patterns in order to keep the remaining capacity favoring achievements and possible to develop. While the daily postural change should be maintained, the sitting posture becomes important, as it is the one that offers greater functionality, so you have to pay special attention on supporting the axial and proximal body to decrease abnormal patterns and encourage the functionality. The use of soft corset with rigid frame or bivalve type can be helpful for activities in chair. The considerations for proper sitting posture and furnishings are similar to those described in the previous age group. Added to this it should be considered the choice of activities possible to be performed by them with purpose and according to their interests, as part of treatment and considering the adjustments necessary for a successful outcome.

Some of the suggested furniture to maintain postural changes at home can be a side table, wedges, standing tables and custom made seats.

In relation to hand function: The hands could or is severely affected by dystonic discharges observed globally both distal and axial, which increases with the intention to move and execution of some task or activity. Postural support is still relevant; adjustments and orthotics provide control and function, which should also be considered as preventive of any deformities. Activities that generate excessive emotional involvement and energetic cost should be restricted.

In relation to movements: Like the previous group, the child will be dependent on a third party. In most cases the movement will be in wheelchairs with no possibility of self-propelled. It is important to use brackets and fasteners at the pelvis and trunk level and other accessories and modifications needed to maintain symmetry such as, for example, wedges and molded side bumpers and seats.

In relation to activities of daily living: As for these activities they should further enhance the child's autonomy, but being mindful that the child will remain dependent. The therapist must include the training of the family in terms of everyday activities, using healthy strategies for both the child and the caregiver. The child must have the space to express needs and preferences.

In relation to school activities: It is important to integrate these children into the school system, where supportive and therapeutic care is essential in order to attend the requirements specific to this area. Assistive technology can be a great facilitator of learning and integration. In young people with possibilities for higher education it is required orienting with respect to interests that are commensurate with their abilities and career possibilities.

3.2.7 Children with severe motor impairment and low serious understanding

Although these groups of patients have a profound dystonia, the cognitive impairment makes the therapeutic management be addressed as a child with multi deficit, this means that the emphasis on treatment will be given in the area of postural management described above, also focusing on strategies and routines and health care of the caregiver.

3.2.8 Children with mild motor impairment and low understanding

Like the previous group we will not describe the management of these patients from the perspective of dystonia. In these cases the most affected area is their occupational performance and social integration given the mental commitment and therefore it must be addressed primarily through management guidelines specific to this area.

3.2.9 General information about orthotics and adjustments used in children with generalized dystonia

As mentioned in the description of each age group, there are some orthotics and adjustments frequently used in children with generalized dystonia, however it will depend on the condition of each child which model will be use and the material indicated. This must be previously being assessed by the therapist.

Below are described some general considerations.

3.2.9.1 Orthotics

Orthotics in children with dystonia meets the objective of correcting the position of the hand in order to facilitate the function and prevent deformity. The model chosen will depend upon the pattern used, the dystonic discharge and the muscle tone manifested when performing an active movement.

Because the movement is generated for a functional objective based on a pattern or muscle string, when manufacturing the orthotic the therapist should consider the position and angulations of the wrist in order to facilitate the initiation of the chain movement (neutral or minimal flexion). It is important to mention that in many cases this does not correspond to established biomechanically functional positions. For material it is suggested to use thin thermoplastic (1.6-2.0) and allow a minimum degree of freedom of motion, while the thicker provides rigidity but blocks the function, which prevents the beginning of the chain created as a functional pattern. As for soft materials and combined materials, it depends on muscle tone when performing a movement and the extent of the maximum ranges of flexion and wrist extension. If muscle tone is too high it is not recommended soft brace or semi-rigid thermoplastic neoprene with thermoplastic. If the pitch is lower the soft brace helps the functional position during movement, containing the joint and giving propioceptive information.

In some cases, long orthotics as long resting hand orthotic (figure 1) for use during the night and sometimes during the day is the best option, in order to position and stretch the muscles in children with increased muscle tone. To position the thumb a soft or rigid abductor splint made of thin material (figure 1) is a good option. In case to also need to align wrist, a semi-rigid cock- up or a long abductor of thin material (figure 1and 1) is a good option. It can facilitate the direction of the movement the use of a derotation bandage for therapeutic purposes (Fig. 1).

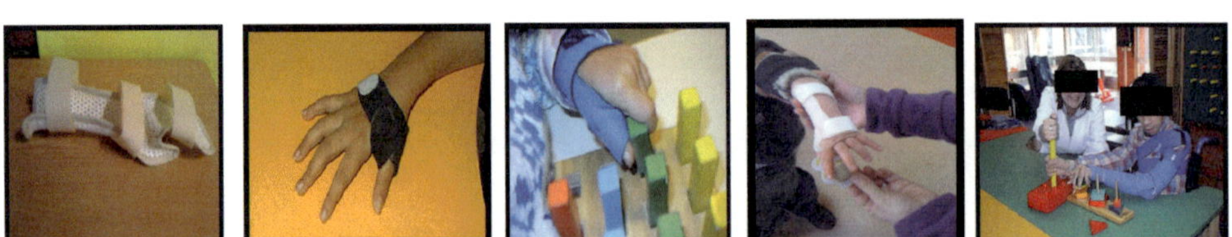

Fig. 1. From left to right: Resting splint, Soft thumb abduction, soft orthotics to stabilize the thumb and the wrist, thumb abductor long version, derotating band with shoulder strap.

3.2.9.2 Furniture and accessories

Chairs should provide sufficient stability and symmetry in the pelvis. The seat model depends on how much axial support needed, in moderate to severe cases we recommend the use of adapted or shaped sitting (figure 2, 3, 4) as they provide containment of the pelvis and trunk, facilitating the use of upper extremities in different planes, without the need for proximal fixation in the extremities (Alvarez, et. al., 2003; Fife, 1991; Rodríguez, 2011).

For wheelchair and sitting it is a priority to give abduction and flexion at an angle less than 90 degrees to the pelvis to make sure the center of gravity is back and avoid the extensor pattern. It also recommended increasing the lateral restraint of the trunk to help the symmetry and stability. These can be supplemented with different types of pelvis and torso straps whose design depends on the needs of each child (Rodríguez, 2011).

The table or tray with cutout with or without containment caps (figure 2) is an important addition as it provides support to stabilize the upper girdle, the trunk alignment from the visual and manual functionality point of view and to allow more fluidity and freedom of movement. The use of a stem fixed to the table (figure 3) is a good contribution to the less functional extremity, and also to promote symmetry and closed chains.

As for adapted gait (figure 5), it is important the alignment and containment of the pelvis as well as the back support to prevent extensor discharges and forearm support with or without stem to facilitate the alignment of upper body.

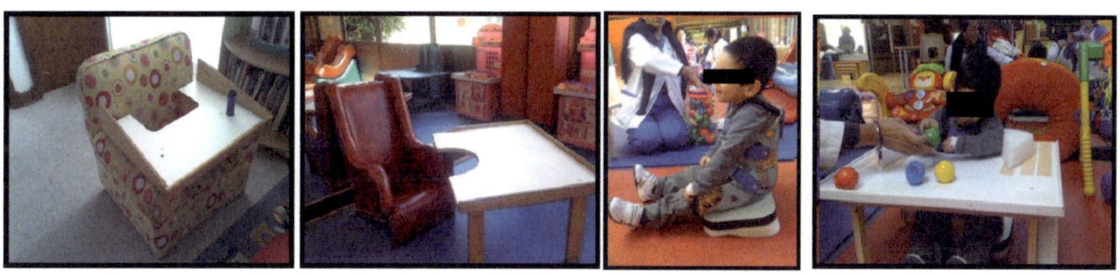

Fig. 2. Table with cutout and lateral borders; table with cutout and chair whit inclination, molded sitting, sitting and dining table with cutout molding and rear bumpers forearm

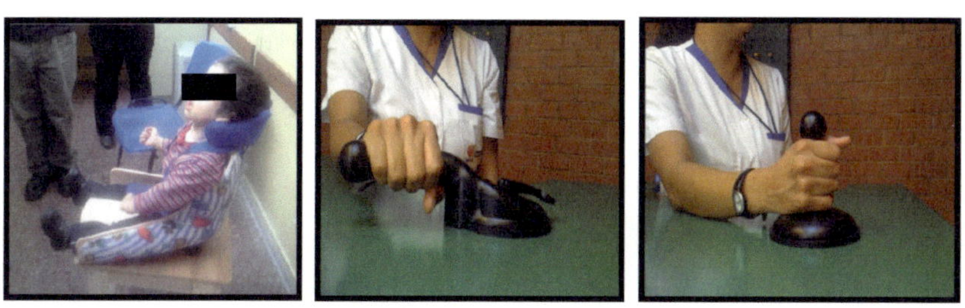

Fig. 3. Molded sitting with leg extension; Stems in prone and neutral

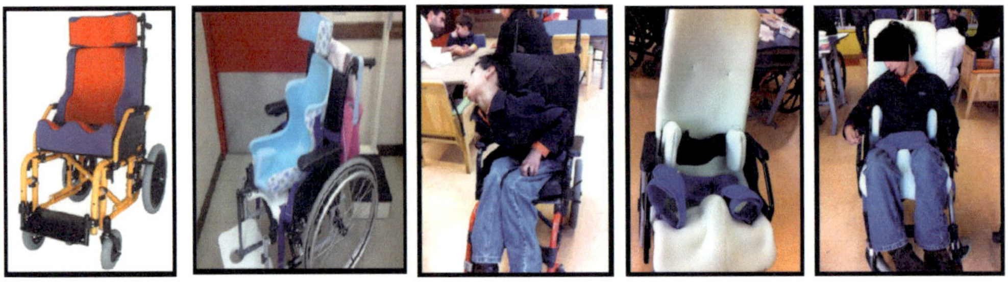

Fig. 4. Wheelchair with adapted set of cushions; wheelchair with molded sitting, wheelchair without molded sitting, molded sitting, wheelchair with molded sitting

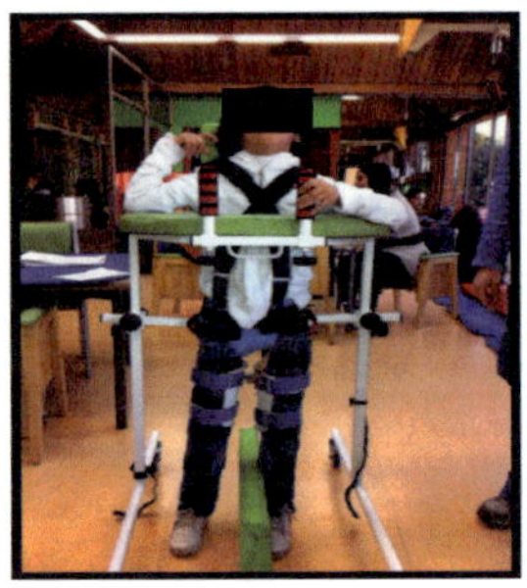

Fig. 5. Walking gait with forearm support and adaptations

4. Conclusion

Children with cerebral palsy who have generalized dystonia require therapeutic management throughout their development process. Due to the varied clinical presentation and evolution, it is difficult to find significant documentation regarding treatment lines to guide the rehabilitation team to address these.

This chapter describes some aspects of assessment and treatment based on bibliographic information and the experience of the program for children with dystonic cerebral palsy of the Occupational Therapy Unit from the Child Rehabilitation Institute of Chile Teletón.

The purpose is to systematize and provide baseline information that will provide general guidelines regarding treatment options, differentiated by degree of functional compromise and age groups, addressing both elements of assessment and intervention on postural control, hand function, activities of daily living, movements and school activities.

External elements mentioned, complement the therapeutic action such as furniture, adaptations, orthotics and accessories that facilitate the positioning, function and occupational performance, enhancing the development, wellbeing and preventing complications.

5. References

Afifi A., Bergman R. (2001). *Neuroanatomía Funcional Texto y Atlas* (2ª edición), Ed. Interamericana. ISBN 9789701022481. México.

Allen H. (1997). The development and use of SPIO Lycra Compression Bracing in Children with Neuromotor Deficits. *Pediatric Rehabilitation*, vol 1. nº2, (109-116). (Febrero 1997)ISSN

Alvarez et.al., (2003), III Congreso Internacional ORITEL, *Guía metodológica de ayudas y adaptaciones*, Unidad de Terapia Ocupacional, Santiago, Chile. (Agosto, 2003)

Ayres J. (2006). *La Integración Sensorial y el Niño.* Ed. Mad. ISBN 9788466546232. España

Bax MCO. (1964). Terminology of Cerebral Palcy Developmental Medicine and Child. *Neurology* 6: 295-307.

Blair E, Ballantyne J, Horsman S, Chauvel P. (1995). A study of a dynamic proximal stability splint in the management of children with cerebral palsy. *Dev Med Child Neurol* 1995;37:544-54.

Bobath K. (1992). *Base neurofisiológica para el Tratamiento de la Parálisis Cerebral* (2°edición), Ed. Panamericana. Buenos Aires, Argentina.

Bobath B., Bobath K. (2000). *Desarrollo Motor en Distintos tipos de Parálisis Cerebral* (1° edición), Ed. Panamericana. Buenos Aires, Argentina

Blanco A., et. al. (2006). *Enfermedades Invalidantes de la Infancia.* (2° edición). Instituto de Rehabilitación Teletón Santiago, Chile. ISBN 978-956-7484-03-4.

Bleton J-P. (2000) Papel de la Rehabilitación en el Tratamiento de las Distonías. *Encyclopédie Médico Chirurgicale.* (1-14)

Csikszentmihalyi M. (1997), *Finding Flow The Psychology of Engagement with everyday Life.* Basic Books. A Division of HarperCollins Publishers, Inc.pp. 181. NY. USA.

Crepeac B, (2005). *Willard and Spackman: Terapia Ocupacional.* (10ª edición). Panamericana, Madrid.

Fejerman N. (2007). *Neurología Pediátrica* (3° Edición), Panamericana, Madrid.

Fife S., Roxborough L., Armstrong R., Harris S., Gregson J., Field D. (1991) Development of a Clinical of Postural Control for Assessment of Adaptive Seating in Children with Neuromotor Disabilities. *Physical Therapy Journal.* Vol. 71, Nº 12. Ed. PTG Editorial, ISSN 1538-6724 (diciembre 1991)(113-125)

Gajardo C., Rodríguez M. (2003): *Efecto de la aplicación de ayudas técnicas en niños con movimientos involuntarios, en Terapia ocupacional, Teletón Santiago.* Instituto de rehabilitación Teletón Santiago, Chile.

Gatica V. (2005). Segunda Jornada Teórica Instituto de rehabilitación Infantil, *Sistemas Corticales que organizan el Movimiento.*, Santiago Chile.

Gracies J-M. (1997). Lycra Garments Designed for Patients with upper limb spasticity: mechanical Effects in normal subjects, *Arch. Phys. Med. Rehabilitation,* vol. 78, October 1997.

Hermosilla M, (1982). Mnual WAIS-R, *Estandarización para adolecentes chilenos 16 y más.* Ediciones Universidad de Chile. Santiago (1-66)

Herrera S, Vazquez J, Gaite L. (2008). International Classification of Functioning, Disability and Health (ICF), *Rehabilitación (Mad).* Vol.42 Nº6; (269-75). Ed. Elsevier. España.

Kielhofner G. (2004). *Modelo de Ocupación Humana. Teoría y Aplicación.* 3ª edición, Ed. Panamericana. ISSN 9788479038366. Bs. Aires, Argentina.

Lezcano- Garcia E. (2003). Distintos Tipos de Temblores y otros Movimientos Anormales, *Gaceta Medica Bilbao.* Ed. Elsevier, Bilbao España.

Merello M, Cerquetti D. (2004) Actividad neuronal del Globo pálido en pacientes con Distonía Generalizada. Instituto de Investigaciones Neurológicas FLENI. *Archivos de neurología, Neurocirugía y Neuropsiquiatría.* Vol 9, N° 1. ISSN 1669-709x, Buenos Aires, Argentina.

Machado S, Cunha M, Velasques B. (2010). Integración Sensitivomotora: Conceptos básicos, anomalías relacionadas con trastornos del movimiento y reorganización cortical inducida por el entrenamiento sensitivomotor, *Revista de Neurología,* Ed. Elsevier. vol. 51, (Abril 2010),(427-436) España.

Maturana H, (2007). *Amor y Juego. Fundamentos olvidados de lo humano.* Ed. J.C. Sáez, EAN: 9789567802524, Chile.

Mulligan S. (2006). *Terapia Ocupacional en Pediatría, proceso de Evaluación* (1ª edición), Panamericana, ISBN 9788479039813. Madrid, España.

Pascual-Pascual S.I. (2006) *Estudio y Tratamiento de las Distonías en la infancia.* Revista de neurología, 43. (Septiembre 2006), (161-168). España.

Purves D. (2004). *Invitación a la Neurociencia (3° Edición),* Ed. Panamericana, ISBN 8479039892, Argentina.

Ramírez V. (2005) *Estandarización del Wisc para niños Chilenos de 6 anos a 16 años.* (3 edición) Ediciones Universidad Católica, Santiago, Chile. (1-74)

Rennie D. (2000) Attfield, S., Morton, R., Polak, F., & Nicholson, J.. An Evaluation of Lycra Garments in the Lower Limb Using 3D Gait Analysis and Functional Assessment (PEDI). *Gait and Posture,* Ed. Elsevier, vol. 12 (1). (Enero 2000), (1-6). ISSN 0966-6362.

Rodríguez M. (2011). Curso Rehabilitación del Paciente Pediátrico con Parálisis Distónica. *Visión de Terapia Ocupacional en el fundamento y manejo del niño con movimientos involunatarios,* Instituto de Investigación Príncipe Felipe, Valencia, España, Marzo 2011.

Rodríguez- Costelo I., Rodríguez-Regal A. (2009). Distonía, Epidemiología, Diagnóstico y Tratamiento, *Revista de Naurología*, vol. 48, Ed. Elsevier, España.

Rodríguez M., Gajardo C., Solis F. (2010). Escalas de compromiso funcional y de movimientos involuntarios en extremidades superiores, en niños con trastornos del movimiento de tipo extrapiramidal. Instituto de Rehabilitación Teletón Chile. *Rehabilitación (Mad),* vol. 44, n° 4, octubre, 2010, (336-44), ISSN 0048-7120, Ed. Elsevier, España.

Russel D, Rosenbaum P, Avery L, Lane M. *Gross Motor Function Measure* (GMFM-66 & GMFM- 88). User's manual. Ontario, Canada. Cambridge University, 2002. 234p.

Trombly C, (1995). *Occupational therapy for physical dysfunction.* (4ª edición). Williams & Wilkins, ISBN 9780781724616. Boston, USA.

Uniform data system for medical rehabilitation: (2005). *The Wee-fim II Sistem Clinical Guide,* Buffalo, Ed. Uniform data system for medical rehabilitation, a division of UB Foundation Activities, inc. 2005. (41-116)

Urzúa A, Cortés E, Vega S, Prieto L, Tapia K.(2009). *Propiedades Psicometricas del cuestionario de auto reporte de la calidad de vida Kidscreen-27 en adolecentes chilenos.* Terapia Psicológica 2009.27 (1):83-p2.

Young P. (1998). *Neuroanatomía Clínica Funcional,* Masson-Williams y Wilkings, España. http://www.distonia.org/revistas/alde23/1719.pdf. Tratamiento de la distonía apoyado en la evidencia.

11

Dystonia and DBS: The Jury Arrives

Han-Joon Kim and Beom S. Jeon
Seoul National University
Korea

1. Introduction

Even before the deep brain stimulation (DBS) era, stereotactic functional neurosurgery such as thalamotomy and pallidotomy had been used for control of medically intractable dystonia (Cooper, 1976; Lozano et al., 1997). However, unreliability and variability in the results and furthermore, needs for bilateral surgery in most patients with generalized dystonia and the occurrence of unacceptable adverse effects including dysarthria and cognitive impairment have greatly limited their use. In this regard, DBS, which provides a more stable response with fewer side effects, has revolutionized the treatment of dystonia. The first report of DBS for dystonia was by Mundinger in 1977 (Mundinger, 1997). Since then, over the past few decades, bilateral globus pallidus internus (GPi) DBS has emerged as the best therapeutic option for medication-refractory dystonia (Lang, 2011).

Generally, bilateral GPi DBS is effective and safe for primary dystonias whether it is generalized or segmental (Bronte-Stewart et al., 2011). However, its effects on secondary dystonias are variable and generally less favorable (Eltahawy et al., 2004).

This Chapter will focus on factors that should be considered before and after DBS in patients with dystonia and the outcome of GPi DBS for the different forms of dystonia.

2. Mechanism of GPi DBS in dystonia

Since the pathophysiological mechanism of dystonia is not clearly understood, the mechanism by which GPi DBS improves dystonia remains elusive. The proposed mechanism of GPi DBS involves (1) silencing of stimulated neurons, which results in blocking of the pathological outflow from the target structure (i.e. GPi), and (2) introduction of new activity in the network (Hammond et al., 2008). Neuronal activity is altered in the GPi, thalamic ventral oral posterior nucleus (Vop), and subthalamic nucleus (STN) in dystonia (Zhuang et al., 2004); thus, it is suggested that GPi DBS modulates the activity of GABAergic GPi efferent exons, which inhibits Vop neurons through one or both of the above mentioned mechanisms (Hammond et al., 2008).

3. General consideration: Presurgical

3.1 Patient selection

When facing a surgical decision, several factors should be taken into account (Volkmann & Benecke, 2002). First and most important, the diagnosis of dystonia should be correct. It is especially true for patients with phasic hyperkinetic movement or patients with dystonic tremor because sometimes very careful evaluation is needed to differentiate these conditions from chorea and tremor disorders, respectively. Second, DBS should be considered only when medical treatment has proven to be ineffective. Third, it should be determined whether the target symptom is the predominant source of the disability and severe enough to do surgery despite its cost and the risk of adverse events. Finally, the patient should have the realistic goals and expectations because not all the dystonic symptoms that the patient has had before surgery will disappear or improve after DBS.

3.2 Target selection

GPi is an established and the most commonly used target for DBS in the treatment of dystonia. Many studies have shown that GPi DBS improves motor symptoms and quality of life in patients with medically intractable dystonia.

Recently, several reports showed that STN DBS also improved dystonia and suggested that it may be an alternative target. Bilateral STN DBS improved primary cervical dystonia with an efficacy comparable to that of GPi DBS (Ostrem et al., 2011). Improvements in secondary dystonia such as neurodegeneration with brain iron accumulation (NBIA) also have been reported (Ge et al., 2011; Zhang et al., 2006). Moreover, it has been claimed that STN is a better target than GPi for segmental dystonia because stimulation-related adverse effects such as bradykinesia, which has been repeatedly reported in GPi DBS, does not occur with STN DBS (Ostrem et al., 2011). However, STN is still a novel target for dystonia and further studies are needed to see whether STN DBS is an effective and safe therapy for dystonia. Successful treatment of writer's cramp with thalamic DBS has been reported (Fukaya et al., 2007), but generally, it is not considered as a therapeutic option for dystonia (Andrews et al., 2010).

4. Primary dystonia

4.1 Primary generalized dystonia

Primary generalized dystonia responds well to GPi DBS. Actually, it is the only form of dystonia, in which, the effect of GPi DBS was confirmed by randomized controlled trials. The mean improvement in the Burke-Fahn-Marsden Dystonia Rating Scale (BFMDRS) movement score was 46% at 6 months in one study (Kupsch et al., 2006) and 51% at 1 year and 58% at 3 year in another study without permanent adverse effects (Vidailhet et al., 2005, 2007). A recent long-term follow-up study showed that improvement by GPi DBS was sustained for up to 8 years (Isaias et al., 2009). Although results from early studies suggested that patients positive for DYT1 mutation have a greater benefit (Coubes et al., 2000; Krauss et al., 2003), it is now widely accepted that there is no difference in the outcome between DYT1-posivie and DYT1-negative patients (Isaias et al., 2008, 2011; Kupsch et al., 2006; Vidailhet et al., 2005). Results from a small group of DYT6-positive patients were less favorable, with 16-55% of motor improvement (Groen et al., 2010).

The magnitude of response to GPi DBS varies considerably among patients, and factors possibly associated with poor or good outcomes have been suggested. Patients with diffuse phasic hyperkinetic movements tend to improve more rapidly and better than patients with severe tonic posturing (Kupsch et al., 2006; Vidailhet et al., 2005; Wang et al., 2006). Fixed skeletal deformity, longer disease duration at surgery, older age at surgery, and more severe motor symptoms at surgery have been associated with a poor outcome (Andrews et al., 2010; Isaias et al., 2008, 2011). Speech and swallowing symptoms are less responsive than axial or limb dystonia (Isaias et al., 2009; Vidailhet et al., 2007), even within an individual patient.

4.2 Cervical dystonia (spasmodic torticollis)

Many case reports and several studies indicate that bilateral GPi DBS is an effective treatment for cervical dystonia (Jeong et al., 2009; Kiss et al., 2007; Kupsch et al., 2006; Pretto et al., 2008). Two long-term follow-up studies showed 67% and 55% improvement in Toronto Western Spasmodic Torticollis Rating Scale (TWSTRS) severity scores at 38 and 32 months after surgery, respectively (Cacciola et al., 2010; Hung et al., 2007). TWSTRS pain scores were also reduced by more than 50% and TWSTRS disability score improved by 81% and 59%.

Usually the age of the patient at surgery is greater in cervical dystonia than in generalized dystonia and DBS in older subjects in their 60s and 70s appears to be safe. Until now, there has been not enough data to prove that the age or duration of disease at surgery affects the outcome in cervical dystonia. However, since a longer duration of disease may run a risk of fixed skeletal deformities, DBS should be considered before these problems occur (Bronte-Stewart et al., 2011).

As described above, a recently study reported that STN DBS improved cervical dystonia with an efficacy comparable to that of GPi DBS (Ostrem et al., 2011).

4.3 Craniofacial and craniocervical dystonia (Meige syndrome)

Data from the literature suggest that GPi DBS is an effective and safe treatment for Meige syndrome. Recent case reports with long-term follow-up (1 to 4 years) show sustained improvement in cranio-facio-cervical dystonia by GPi DBS. Improvement in terms of the BFMDRS movement score was 53% in one report and 82 - 86% in the other reports (Ghang et al., 2010; Lyons et al., 2010; Reese et al., 2011; Sako et al., 2011). However, in a recent case series, the effect of GPi DBS on Meige syndrome was variable with some patients having less than 20% improvement (Limotai et al., 2011). Speech and swallowing did not improve. The authors pointed out that a careful re-examination of the selection criteria for surgery for Meige syndrome is needed.

5. Secondary dystonia

5.1 Myoclonus-dystonia (ε-Sarcoglycan mutation, DYT11)

Several case reports showed that bilateral GPi DBS improves motor symptoms in patients with myoclonus-dystonia with an overall improvement of 60% to 90% (Cif et al., 2004; Foncke et al., 2007; Jog & Kumar, 2009; Kurtis et al., 2010). A recent case series of 5 patients with myoclonus-dystonia reported that both myoclonus and dystonia improved with GPi DBS more than 80% and this improvement was sustained after 15-18 months of follow-up (Azoulay-Zyss et al., 2011). Improvement in myoclonus but not in dystonia by thalamic DBS was reported in 2 cases of myoclonus-dystonia (Kuncel et al., 2009; Trottenberg et al., 2001).

5.2 X-linked dystonia parkinsonism (DYT3, 'Lubag')

In the literature, 5 case reports of GPi DBS on X-linked dystonia parkinsonism are available (Aguilar et al., 2011; Evidente et al., 2007; Martinez-Torres et al., 2009; Oyama et al., 2010; Wadia et al., 2010). All cases showed improvement in dystonia. Of note, dysarthria, oromandibular dystonia, and stridor, which usually show poor response to GPi DBS in primary generalized dystonia, also improved. Interestingly, improvements in dystonia were immediate in all cases. However, the effect on parkinsonism was variable: parkinsonism improved in 3 patients but not in the other 2 patients.

5.3 Rapid-onset dystonia parkinsonism (ATA1A3 mutation, DYT12)

Only 2 case reports of bilateral GPi DBS in this rare disease are available. One patient did not receive any benefit from the surgery (Deutschländer et al., 2005) and the other patient had only mild (30%) improvement in dystonia, mainly in the craniocervical and truncal area. Limb dystonia and parkinsonism did not improve (Kamm et al., 2008).

5.4 Tardive dystonia

DBS is a very effective treatment for tardive dyskinesia. Recent studies showed that GPi DBS improves tardive dystonia motor symptoms for more than 80% and this benefit was sustained during long-term follow-up up to 80 months (Capelle et al., 2010; Gruber et al., 2009; Trottenberg et al., 2005). In contrast to primary generalized dystonia, patients experienced distinct improvement within days or even hours after stimulation. Improvements of tardive dystonia with STN DBS also have been reported (Sun et al., 2007; Zhang et al., 2006).

5.5 NBIA

Responses to GPi DBS are variable in NBIA. There are reports of favorable (65-91%) responses (Castelnau et al., 2005; Clement et al., 2007; Krause et al., 2006; Mikati et al., 2009; Umemura et al., 2004), but others reported only 20-30% improvement (Isaac et al., 2007; Shields et al., 2007). A single case report of STN DBS on a NBIA patient showed 84% improvement at 3 years after surgery (Ge et al., 2011). It is surprising that motor symptoms in NBIA can improve with DBS, given that structural abnormalities in the brain MRI usually meet the exclusion criteria for DBS in primary dystonia (Kupsch et al., 2006; Vidailhet et al., 2005).

5.6 Cerebral palsy

A wide range of responses has been reported on the effect of GPi DBS in cerebral palsy. Some patients had favorable outcomes but others experienced no or only minimal improvement (Alterman and Tagliati, 2007; Pretto et al., 2008; Zorzi et al., 2005). This variability in response is most likely due to the heterogeneity of this condition. Recently, a multicenter prospective study investigating the effect of bilateral GPi DBS on dystonia-choreoathetosis cerebral palsy showed 24% improvement in the BFMDRS movement score at 1 year after surgery (Vidailhet et al., 2009). However, as the authors mentioned, cerebral palsy patients who meet the criteria of this study (i.e. prominent dystonia-choreoathetosis, little or no spasticity, unimpaired intellectual function, and only slight abnormalities of the basal ganglia on MRI) was only about 10% of the cerebral palsy population.

5.7 Other secondary dystonias

There are many causes of secondary dystonias and the number of patients with each secondary dystonia who underwent DBS is small. There are reports of DBS in postanoxic dystonia, postencephalitic dystonia, and posttraumatic dystonia (Eltahawy et al., 2004; Pretto et al., 2008; Katsakiori et al., 2009; Zhang et al., 2006; Krause et al., 2004; Ghika et al., 2002). Improvements in dystonia in Lesch-Nyhan syndrome (Cif et al., 2007; Pralong et al., 2005) and GM1 gangliosidosis (Roze et al., 2006) also have been reported. Generally, the effects of DBS on secondary dystonias are variable and less favorable.

6. Task-specific dystonias

For writer's cramp, contralateral unilateral thalamic DBS has been tried with favorable results (Cho et al., 2009; Fukaya et al., 2007). Improvements were immediate in all cases. It appears that thalamic DBS is more effective than GPi DBS for writer's cramp (Fukaya et al., 2007).

7. Complications

There is no compelling evidence that DBS surgery- or device-related adverse effects are more common in dystonia than in Parkinson disease (PD). However, it has been suggested that lead migration and lead fracture is more common in dystonia than in parkinsonian patients (Yianni et al., 2003). Stimulation-related adverse effects specific for GPi DBS in dystonia include the development of reversible bradykinesia and parkinsonian gait problems in previously nondystonic body regions (Berman et al., 2009; Ostrem et al., 2007; Zauber et al., 2009).

8. Postsurgical management

Several points should be kept in mind when managing dystonic patients after DBS surgery (Kupsch et al., 2011).

In contrast to PD where maximal clinical effect of DBS occurs within hours of switching on of the device, the beneficial effects of DBS in dystonia are not immediate and slowly progress over weeks to months, possibly beyond 1 year after surgery. This protracted improvement is more prominent in older patients (Isaias et al., 2011). There is no evidence that tolerance develops with long-term stimulation (Tagliati et al., 2011).

Battery lifetime in GPi DBS for dystonia is usually shorter compared to that in DBS for PD because of higher voltages and greater pulse widths. Thus, a more frequent battery change is required. In a recent study, the mean battery life in patients with GPi DBS for dystonia was 25 months (Blahak et al., 2011). Regarding inadvertent depletion of the battery or discontinuation of stimulation during procedures for battery replacement, it should be noted that sudden bilateral cessation of stimulation can lead to acute and possibly life threatening rebound dystonia or respiratory difficulty (Grabli et al., 2009; Tagliati et al., 2011).

9. Conclusion

So, has the jury arrived at a verdict as to the usefulness of DBS in treatment of dystonia? The answer appears to be yes for primary dystonias. However, for secondary dystonias, more evidences are needed.

Literatures show that bilateral GPi DBS is an effective and safe therapy for medically intractable primary dystonia and it provides a sustained benefit. Not only good surgical technique, but also appropriate selection of patients and individualized postsurgical management are crucial for optimized patient care.

In secondary dystonias, its effects are heterogeneous, and at this stage, data are not enough to determine whether it can be considered as an effective therapy for each form of the disease. Further studies are needed for re-examination of the inclusion criteria and selection of targets other than GPi.

10. References

Aguilar JA, Vesagas TS, Jamora RD et al. (2011). The promise of deep brain stimulation in X-linked dystonia parkinsonism. *Int J Neurosci.* Vol.121, pp.57-63, ISSN 0020-7454

Alterman RL & Tagliati M. (2007). Deep brain stimulation for torsion dystonia in children. *Child's Nervous System.* Vol.23, pp.1033-1040, ISSN 0256-7040

Andrews C, Aviles-Olmos I, Hariz M et al. (2010). Which patients with dystonia benefit from deep brain stimulation? A metaregression of individual patient outcomes. *Journal of Neurology, Neurosurgery & Psychiatry.* Vol.81, pp.1383-1389, ISSN 0022-3050

Azoulay-Zyss J, Roze E, Welter ML et al. (2011). Bilateral Deep Brain Stimulation of the Pallidum for Myoclonus-Dystonia Due to -Sarcoglycan Mutations: A Pilot Study. *Archives of neurology.* Vol.68, pp.94-98, ISSN 0003-9942

Berman BD, Starr PA, Marks Jr WJ et al. (2009). Induction of bradykinesia with pallidal deep brain stimulation in patients with cranial-cervical dystonia. *Stereotact Funct Neurosurg.* Vol.87, pp.37-44, ISSN 1011-6125

Blahak C, Capelle HH, Baezner H et al. (2011). Battery lifetime in pallidal deep brain stimulation for dystonia. *European Journal of Neurology.* Vol.18, pp.872-875, ISSN 1468-1331

Bronte-Stewart H, Taira T, Valldeoriola F et al. (2011). Inclusion and exclusion criteria for DBS in dystonia. *Movement disorders.* Vol. 26, pp.S5-S16, ISSN 0885-3185

Cacciola F, Farah JO, Eldridge PR et al. (2010). Bilateral Deep Brain Stimulation for Cervical Dystonia: Long-term Outcome in a Series of 10 Patients. *Neurosurgery.* Vol.67, pp.957-963, ISSN 0148-396X

Capelle HH, Blahak C, Schrader C et al. (2010). Chronic deep brain stimulation in patients with tardive dystonia without a history of major psychosis. *Movement disorders.* Vol.25, pp.1477-1481, ISSN 0885-3185

Castelnau P, Cif L, Valente EM et al. (2005). Pallidal stimulation improves pantothenate kinase-associated neurodegeneration. *Annals of neurology.* Vol.57, pp738-741, ISSN 0364-5134

Cho CB, Park HK, Lee KJ et al. (2009). Thalamic deep brain stimulation for writer's cramp. *Journal of Korean Neurosurgical Society.* Vol.46, pp52-55, ISSN 2005-3711

Cif L, Biolsi B, Gavarini S et al. (2007). Antero ventral internal pallidum stimulation improves behavioral disorders in Lesch–Nyhan disease. *Movement disorders.* Vol.22, pp.2126-2129, ISSN 0885-3185

Cif L, Valente EM, Hemm S et al. (2004). Deep brain stimulation in myoclonus–dystonia syndrome. *Movement disorders.* Vol.19, pp.724-727, ISSN 0885-3185

Clement F, Devos D, Moreau C et al. (2007). Neurodegeneration with brain iron accumulation: clinical, radiographic and genetic heterogeneity and corresponding therapeutic options. *Acta neurologica belgica.* Vol.107, pp.26-31, ISSN 0300-9009

Cooper IS. (1976). 20-year followup study of the neurosurgical treatment of dystonia musculorum deformans. *Advances in neurology.* Vol.14, pp.423-452, ISSN 0091-3952

Coubes P, Roubertie A, Vayssiere N et al. (2000). Treatment of DYT1-generalised dystonia by stimulation of the internal globus pallidus. *The Lancet.* Vol.355, pp.2220-2221, ISSN 0140-6736

Deutschländer A, Asmus F, Gasser T et al. (2005). Sporadic rapid onset dystonia–parkinsonism syndrome: Failure of bilateral pallidal stimulation. *Movement disorders.* Vol.20, pp.254-257, ISSN 0885-3185

Eltahawy HA, Saint-Cyr J, Giladi N et al. (2004). Primary dystonia is more responsive than secondary dystonia to pallidal interventions: outcome after pallidotomy or pallidal deep brain stimulation. *Neurosurgery.* Vol.54, pp613-619, ISSN 0148-396X

Evidente VGH, Lyons MK, Wheeler M et al. (2007). First case of X linked dystonia parkinsonism ("Lubag") to demonstrate a response to bilateral pallidal stimulation. *Movement disorders.* Vol.22, pp1790-1793, ISSN 0885-3185

Foncke EMJ, Bour LJ, Speelman JD et al. (2007). Local field potentials and oscillatory activity of the internal globus pallidus in myoclonus–dystonia. *Movement disorders.* Vol.22, pp369-376, ISSN 0885-3185

Fukaya C, Katayama Y, Kano T et al. (2007). Thalamic deep brain stimulation for writer's cramp. *Journal of Neurosurgery: Pediatrics.* Vol.107, pp.977-982, ISSN 1933-0707

Ge M, Zhang K, Ma Y et al. (2011). Bilateral Subthalamic Nucleus Stimulation in the Treatment of Neurodegeneration with Brain Iron Accumulation Type 1. *Stereotactic and Functional Neurosurgery.* Vol.89, pp.162-166, ISSN 1011-6125

Ghang JY, Lee MK, Jun SM, Ghang CG. (2010). Outcome of pallidal deep brain stimulation in meige syndrome. *Journal of Korean Neurosurgical Society.* Vol.48, pp.134-138, ISSN 2005-3711

Ghika J, Villemure J, Miklossy J et al. (2002). Postanoxic generalized dystonia improved by bilateral Voa thalamic deep brain stimulation. *Neurology.* Vol.58, pp311-313, ISSN 0028-3878

Grabli D, Ewenczyk C, Coelho Braga MC et al. (2009). Interruption of deep brain stimulation of the globus pallidus in primary generalized dystonia. *Movement disorders.* Vol.24, pp2363-2369, ISSN 0885-3185

Groen JL, Ritz K, Contarino MF et al. (2010). DYT6 dystonia: Mutation screening, phenotype, and response to deep brain stimulation. *Movement disorders.* Vol.25, pp.2420-2427, ISSN 0885-3185

Gruber D, Trottenberg T, Kivi A et al. (2009). Long-term effects of pallidal deep brain stimulation in tardive dystonia. *Neurology.* Vol.73, pp.53-58, ISSN 0028-3878

Hammond C, Ammari R, Bioulac B et al. (2008). Latest view on the mechanism of action of deep brain stimulation. *Movement disorders.* Vol.23, pp.2111-2121, ISSN 0885-3185

Hung S, Hamani C, Lozano A et al. (2007). Long-term outcome of bilateral pallidal deep brain stimulation for primary cervical dystonia. *Neurology.* Vol.68, pp.457-459, ISSN 0028-3878

Isaac C, Wright I, Bhattacharyya D et al. (2008). Pallidal stimulation for pantothenate kinase-associated neurodegeneration dystonia. *Archives of disease in childhood.* Vol.93, pp.239-240, ISSN 0003-9888

Isaias IU, Alterman RL, Tagliati M. (2008). Outcome predictors of pallidal stimulation in patients with primary dystonia: the role of disease duration. *Brain.* Vol.131, pp.1895-1902, ISSN 0006-8950

Isaias IU, Alterman RL, Tagliati M. (2009). Deep brain stimulation for primary generalized dystonia: long-term outcomes. *Archives of neurology.* Vol.66, pp.465-470, 0003-9942

Isaias IU, Volkmann J, Kupsch A et al. Factors predicting protracted improvement after pallidal DBS for primary dystonia: the role of age and disease duration. *Journal of Neurology.* DOI 10.1007/s00415-011-5961-9, ISSN 0340-5354

Jeong SG, Lee MK, Kang JY et al. (2009). Pallidal deep brain stimulation in primary cervical dystonia with phasic type: clinical outcome and postoperative course. *Journal of Korean Neurosurgical Society.* Vol.46, pp346-350, ISSN 2005-3711

Jog M & Kumar H. (2009). Bilateral pallidal deep brain stimulation in a case of myoclonus dystonia syndrome. *Movement disorders.* Vol.24, pp1547-1549, ISSN 0885-3185

Kamm C, Fogel W, Wachter T et al. (2008). Novel ATP1A3 mutation in a sporadic RDP patient with minimal benefit from deep brain stimulation. *Neurology.* Vol.70, pp1501-1503, ISSN 0028-3878

Katsakiori P, Kefalopoulou Z, Markaki E et al. (2009). Deep brain stimulation for secondary dystonia: results in 8 patients. *Acta Neurochirurgica.* Vol.151, pp473-478, ISSN 0001-6268

Kiss ZHT, Doig-Beyaert K, Eliasziw M et al. (2007). The Canadian multicentre study of deep brain stimulation for cervical dystonia. *Brain.* Vol.130, pp2879-2886, ISSN 0006-8950

Krause M, Fogel W, Kloss M et al. (2004). Pallidal stimulation for dystonia. *Neurosurgery.* Vol.55, pp.1361-1370, ISSN 0148-396X

Krause M, Fogel W, Tronnier V et al. (2006). Long term benefit to pallidal deep brain stimulation in a case of dystonia secondary to pantothenate kinase associated neurodegeneration. *Movement disorders.* Vol.21, pp2255-2257, ISSN 0885-3185

Krauss JK, Loher TJ, Weigel R et al. (2003). Chronic stimulation of the globus pallidus internus for treatment of non-dYT1 generalized dystonia and choreoathetosis: 2-year follow up. *Journal of neurosurgery.* Vol.98, pp785-792, ISSN 0022-3085

Kuncel AM, Turner DA, Ozelius LJ et al. (2009). Myoclonus and tremor response to thalamic deep brain stimulation parameters in a patient with inherited myoclonus-dystonia syndrome. *Clinical neurology and neurosurgery.* Vol.111, pp.303-306, ISSN 0303-8467

Kupsch A, Benecke R, Müller J et al. (2006). Pallidal Deep-Brain Stimulation in Primary Generalized or Segmental Dystonia. *New England Journal of Medicine.* Vol.355, pp1978-1990, ISSN 0028-4793

Kupsch A, Tagliati M, Vidailhet M et al. (2011). Early postoperative management of DBS in dystonia: programming, response to stimulation, adverse events, medication changes, evaluations, and troubleshooting. *Movement disorders.* Vol. 26, pp.S41-S57, ISSN 0885-3185

Kurtis MM, San Luciano M, Yu Q et al. (2010). Clinical and neurophysiological improvement of SGCE myoclonus-dystonia with GPi deep brain stimulation. *Clinical neurology and neurosurgery.* Vol.112, pp149-152, ISSN 0303-8467

Lang AE. (2011). Deep brain stimulation for dystonia. *Movement disorders.* Vol. 26, pp.S43-S4, ISSN 0885-3185

Limotai N, Go C, Oyama G et al. Mixed results for GPi-DBS in the treatment of cranio-facial and cranio-cervical dystonia symptoms. *Journal of Neurology.* DOI: 10.1007/s00415-011-6075-0, ISSN 0340-5354

Lozano AM, Kumar R, Gross R et al. (1997). Globus pallidus internus pallidotomy for generalized dystonia. *Movement disorders.* Vol.12, pp865-870, ISSN 0885-3185

Lyons MK, Birch BD, Hillman RA et al. (2010). Long-term follow-up of deep brain stimulation for Meige syndrome. *Neurosurgical focus.* Vol.29, p.E5, ISSN 1092-0684

Martinez Torres I, Limousin P, Tisch S et al. (2009). Early and marked benefit with GPi DBS for Lubag syndrome presenting with rapidly progressive life threatening dystonia. *Movement disorders.* Vol.24, pp.1710-1712, ISSN 0885-3185

Mikati MA, Yehya A, Darwish H et al. (2009). Deep brain stimulation as a mode of treatment of early onset pantothenate kinase-associated neurodegeneration. *European Journal of Paediatric Neurology.* Vol.13, pp.61-64, ISSN 1090-3798

Mundinger F. (1977). Neue stereotaktisch-functionelle Behandlungsmethode des Torticollis spasmodicus mit Hirn-stimulatoren. *Medizinische Klinik.* Vol.72, pp.1982-1987, ISSN 0025-8458

Ostrem JL, Marks Jr WJ, Volz MM et al. (2007). Pallidal deep brain stimulation in patients with cranial–cervical dystonia (Meige syndrome). *Movement disorders.* Vol.22, pp.1885-1891, ISSN 0885-3185

Ostrem JL, Racine CA, Glass GA et al. (2011). Subthalamic nucleus deep brain stimulation in primary cervical dystonia. *Neurology.* Vol.76, pp.870-878, ISSN 0028-3878

Oyama G, Fernandez HH, Foote KD et al. (2010). Differential Response of Dystonia and Parkinsonism following Globus Pallidus Internus Deep Brain Stimulation in X-Linked Dystonia-Parkinsonism (Lubag). *Stereotactic and Functional Neurosurgery.* Vol.88, pp329-333, ISSN 1011-6125

Pralong E, Pollo C, Coubes P et al. (2005). Electrophysiological characteristics of limbic and motor globus pallidus internus (GPI) neurons in two cases of Lesch–Nyhan syndrome. *Clinical Neurophysiology.* Vol.35, pp.168-173, ISSN 1388-2457

Pretto TE, Dalvi A, Kang UJ, Penn RD. (2008). A prospective blinded evaluation of deep brain stimulation for the treatment of secondary dystonia and primary torticollis syndromes. *Journal of Neurosurgery: Pediatrics.* Vol.109, pp.405-409, ISSN 1933-0707

Reese R, Gruber D, Schoenecker T et al. (2011). Long term clinical outcome in Meige syndrome treated with internal pallidum deep brain stimulation. *Movement disorders.* Vol.26, pp.691-698, ISSN 0885-3185

Roze E, Navarro S, Cornu P et al. (2006). Deep brain stimulation of the globus pallidus for generalized dystonia in GM1 Type 3 gangliosidosis: technical case report. *Neurosurgery.* Vol.59, p.E1340, ISSN 0148-396X

Sako W, Morigaki R, Mizobuchi Y et al. (2011). Bilateral pallidal deep brain stimulation in primary Meige syndrome. *Parkinsonism & Related Disorders.* Vol.17, pp.123-125, ISSN 1353-8020

Shields DC, Sharma N, Gale JT, Eskandar EN. (2007). Pallidal stimulation for dystonia in pantothenate kinase-associated neurodegeneration. *Pediatric neurology.* Vol. 37, pp.442-445, ISSN 0887-8994

Sun B, Chen S, Zhan S et al. (2007). Subthalamic nucleus stimulation for primary dystonia and tardive dystonia. *Acta Neurochirurgica Supplementum.* Vol.97 pp.207-214, ISSN 0065-1419

Tagliati M, Krack P, Volkmann J et al. (2011). Long Term management of DBS in dystonia: Response to stimulation, adverse events, battery changes, and special considerations. *Movement disorders.* Vol.26, pp.S54-S62, ISSN 0885-3185

Trottenberg T, Meissner W, Arnold G et al. (2001). Neurostimulation of the ventral intermediate thalamic nucleus in inherited myoclonus dystonia Syndrome. *Movement disorders.* Vol.16, pp769-771, ISSN 0885-3185

Trottenberg T, Volkmann J, Deuschl G et al. (2005). Treatment of severe tardive dystonia with pallidal deep brain stimulation. *Neurology.* Vol.64, pp.344-346, ISSN 0028-3878

Umemura A, Jaggi JL, Dolinskas CA et al. (2004). Pallidal deep brain stimulation for longstanding severe generalized dystonia in Hallervorden-Spatz syndrome. *Journal of neurosurgery.* Vol.100, p706-709, ISSN 0022-3085

Vidailhet M, Vercueil L, Houeto J et al. Bilateral deep-brain stimulation of the globus pallidus in primary generalized dystonia. *N Engl J Med.* 2005;352:459-467, ISSN 0028-4793

Vidailhet M, Vercueil L, Houeto JL et al. (2007). Bilateral, pallidal, deep-brain stimulation in primary generalised dystonia: a prospective 3 year follow-up study. *The Lancet Neurology.* Vol.6, pp.223-229, ISSN 1474-4422

Vidailhet M, Yelnik J, Lagrange C et al. (2009). Bilateral pallidal deep brain stimulation for the treatment of patients with dystonia-choreoathetosis cerebral palsy: a prospective pilot study. *The Lancet Neurology.* Vol.8, pp.709-717, ISSN 1474-4422

Volkmann J and Benecke R. (2002). Deep brain stimulation for dystonia: patient selection and evaluation. *Movement disorders.* Vol.17, pp.S112-S115, ISSN 0885-3185

Wadia PM, Lim SY, Lozano AM et al. (2010). Bilateral pallidal stimulation for x-linked dystonia parkinsonism. *Archives of neurology.* Vol.67, pp.1012-1015, ISSN 0003-9942

Wang S, Liu X, Yianni J et al. (2006). Use of surface electromyography to assess and select patients with idiopathic dystonia for bilateral pallidal stimulation. *Journal of neurosurgery.* Vol.105, pp.21-25, ISSN 0022-3085

Yianni J, Nandi D, Shad A et al. (2004). Increased risk of lead fracture and migration in dystonia compared with other movement disorders following deep brain stimulation. *Journal of Clinical Neuroscience.* Vol.11, pp.243-245, ISSN 0967-5868

Zauber SE, Watson N, Comella CL et al. (2009). Stimulation-induced parkinsonism after posteroventral deep brain stimulation of the globus pallidus internus for craniocervical dystonia. *Journal of neurosurgery.* Vol.110, pp.229-233, ISSN 0022-3085

Zhang J, Zhang K, Wang Z et al. (2006). Deep brain stimulation in the treatment of secondary dystonia. *Chinese medical journal.* Vol.119, pp.2069-2074, ISSN 0366-6999

Zhuang P, Li Y, Hallett M. (2004). Neuronal activity in the basal ganglia and thalamus in patients with dystonia. *Clinical Neurophysiology.* Vol.115, pp.2542-2557, ISSN 1388-2457

Zorzi G, Marras C, Nardocci N et al. (2005). Stimulation of the globus pallidus internus for childhood onset dystonia. *Movement disorders.* Vol.20, pp.1194-1200, ISSN 0885-3185

12

Dystonia and Peripheral Nerve Surgery in the Cervical Area

Bunpot Sitthinamsuwan and Sarun Nunta-Aree
Division of Neurosurgery, Department of Surgery, Faculty of Medicine Siriraj Hospital, Mahidol University, Bangkok Thailand

1. Introduction

Cervical dystonia is the most common form of focal dystonia (Dashtipour et al., 2007). It is characterized by involuntary movement of the neck resulting in abnormal neck posture (Brin & Benabou, 1999; Dent, 2002). Cervicalgia and headache sometimes occur in patients suffering from the disease (Albanese, 2005; Brashear, 2004, Schim, 2006). A critical long-term sequelae of this kind of movement disorder is premature cervical spinal degenerative disease (Chawda et al., 2000) which possibly progresses to cervical spondylotic myelopathy (Hagenah et al., 2001; Jameson et al., 2010; Konrad et al., 2004; Krauss et al., 2002; Spitz et al., 2006; Tonomura et al., 2007; Waterston et al., 1989).

Fundamentally, cervical dystonia is categorized into several patterns, including torticollis (head rotation), anterocollis (head forward flexion), retrocollis (head backward extension), laterocollis (lateral head bending), and combined pattern (Brin & Benabou, 1999; Feely, 2003; Sitthinamsuwan & Nunta-aree, 2010; Sitthinamsuwan et al., 2010a). The last mentioned pattern is comprised of two or more dystonic patterns. Dystonic muscles in each pattern are quite unique. For instance, involved muscles in torticollis include the posterior cervical muscles (mainly splenius capitis, semispinalis capitis and semispinalis cervicis) on the same side of turning head and the contralateral sternocleidomastoid. The various dystonic patterns and corresponding neck muscles are summarized in Fig.1 (Brashear, 2004; Brin & Benabou, 1999; Dashtipour et al., 2007; Dent, 2002; Feely, 2003; Huh et al., 2005; Sitthinamsuwan & Nunta-aree, 2010; Sitthinamsuwan et al., 2010a). An example of the combined pattern is presented in Fig.2.

Conventional treatment of cervical dystonia consists of oral medication, botulinum toxin injection, and physical therapy. For patients who do not respond to such therapies or are refractory cases, surgical treatment is an appropriate option (Nunta-aree & Sitthinamsuwan, 2009; Nunta-aree et al. 2010a, 2010b). Surgical therapy for cervical dystonia has been continuously developed for a significant period to improve outcome and diminish complication. Some operations have been abandoned because of their potential complications while some of them have been used increasingly and are currently popular on account of their effectiveness and safe (Albanese, 2005; Albanese et al., 2006; Brin & Benabou, 1999; Feely, 2003). Overview of surgical treatment for cervical dystonia is described in the following.

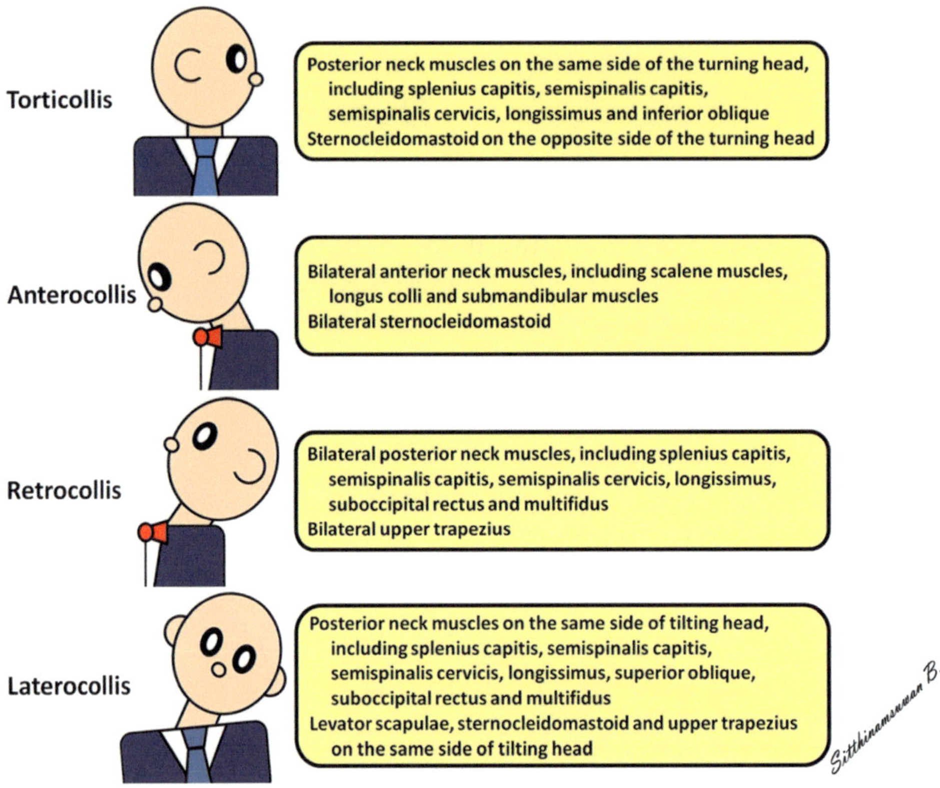

Fig. 1. Various patterns of cervical dystonia. The involved cervical muscles are shown in the yellow boxes.

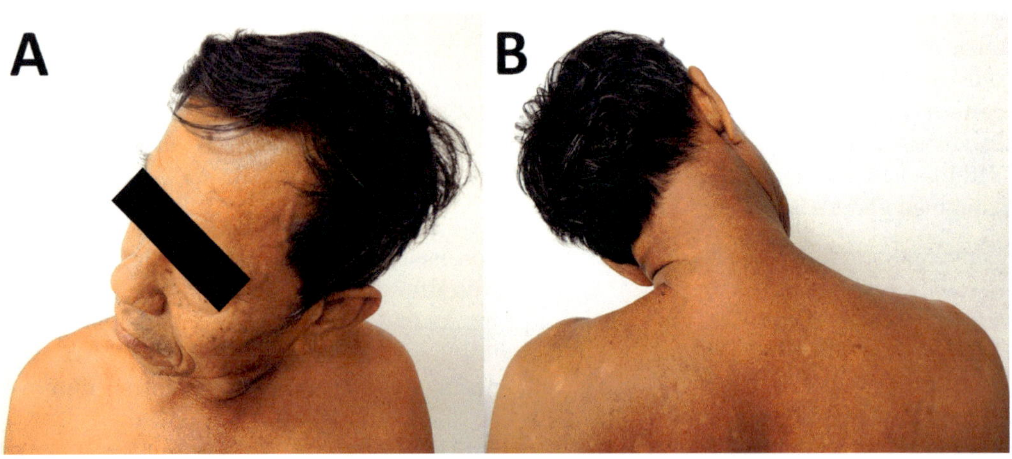

Fig. 2. A combined pattern of cervical dystonia in the same patient. A, The anterior view shows right torticollis with left laterocollis. B, Left laterocollis can be clearly seen in the posterior view.

a) Intradural anterior cervical rhizotomy

Originally, bilateral C1-C3 anterior spinal nerve roots were resected intradurally in this operation (Münchau et al., 2001a; Taira, 2009). A significant numbers of patient developed swallowing dysfunction following the surgery while improvement of cervical dystonia was not appreciable. Consequently, there is no use of bilateral C1-C3 anterior rhizotomy in the present (Brin & Benabou, 1999; Bronte-Stewart, 2003; Taira, 2009). However, recently, intradural C1-C2 anterior rhizotomy has been successfully combined with selective denervation of C3-C6 posterior rami successfully without serious adverse effect (Taira et al.; 2002; Taira & Hori, 2003; Taira, 2009).

b) Intradural posterior cervical rhizotomy

The formerly common procedure was bilateral C1-C4 posterior rhizotomy (Vogel et al., 2010) which was ultimately proved ineffective in the treatment of cervical dystonia. It sometimes caused respiratory insufficiency as a result of diaphragmatic dysfunction (Fraioli et al., 1977). Nowadays, posterior rhizotomy in the cervical level are performed only on C5 to T1 posterior nerve spinal roots and it aims to treat bilateral upper limb spasticity (Benedetti et al, 1977; Bertelli et al., 2000, 2003; Heimburger 1973; Hsin et al., 2004, Laitinen et al., 1983).

c) Intradural accessory nerve denervation

This abandoned method was resection of the accessory nerve situated in the posterior cranial fossa (Adams, 1984; Hernesniemi & Keränen, 1990). It affected not only motor fibers to the sternocleidomastoid but also those to the trapezius. Postoperative trapezius atrophy and shoulder instability inevitably occurred (Bronte-Stewart, 2003; Sorensen & Hamby 1965).

d) Stereotactic brain lesioning

Bilateral thalamotomy used to be an effective stereotactic ablative surgery for cervical dystonia (Bronte-Stewart, 2003; Dashtipour et al., 2007). Bilateral procedures, however, commonly resulted in speech disturbance (Bronte-Stewart, 2003; Imer et al., 2005; Krauss, 2010). Presently, it is completely replaced by pallidal deep brain stimulation.

e) Microvascular decompression of the accessory nerve

This rarely used operation primarily aims to rectify dystonia of the sternocleidomastoid and trapezius in patients with torticollis (Sun et al, 2009). Nevertheless, the hypothesis of accessory nerve decompression cannot explain improvement of cervical dystonia in the individuals who have no dystonia of both the muscles (Albanese et al., 2006; Brin & Benabou, 1999; Bronte-Stewart, 2003; Taira, 2009).

f) Selective peripheral denervation

This relatively safe and popularly used procedure is an ablative surgery specific on peripheral motor nerves innervating dystonic neck muscles whereas motor branches supplying normal muscles and sensory nerves will be entirely preserved (Bertrand, 1987, 1993; Braun & Richter, 1994). Good to excellent outcome is often achieved by the operation, so it has become a common surgical treatment for cervical dystonia (Albanese, 2005; Albanese et al., 2006; Krauss, 2010). This type of surgery is the central idea of the present chapter and its content will be stated in detail.

g) Myotomy or myectomy

Resection of dystonic muscles is occasionally combined with selective peripheral denervation (Albanese et al., 2006; Bronte-Stewart, 2003; Chen et al., 2000; Huh et al., 2005; Krauss, 2010; Münchau et al., 2001a; Xingkang, 1981). In the authors view, muscle section is an adjunctive procedure for cervical dystonia and should be considered in cases with long-standing dystonia which exhibit evidence of soft tissue stiffness or muscle shortening. Furthermore, it may be performed on muscles which are difficult to denervate (Ondo & Krauss, 2004), such as the scalene muscles.

h) Pallidal deep brain stimulation

High-frequency stimulation of the globus pallidus internus often yields outstanding result in dystonic individuals, including patients with cervical dystonia (Albanese et al., 2006; Bittar et al., 2005; Cacciola et al., 2010; Hung et al., 2007; Krauss et al., 1999, 2004; Krauss, 2007; Parkins et al., 2001; Vercueil, 2003; Volkmann & Benecke, 2002; Yianni et al., 2003). However, among our patients with uncomplicated or simple cervical dystonia, we did not encounter substantial difference of outcome between the patients who underwent pallidal deep brain stimulation and those who underwent peripheral denervation. Therefore, we always chose peripheral nerve resection as the primary surgical therapy in the uncomplicated cases. On the other hand, we consider the deep brain stimulation as the prerequisite treatment of complex cervical dystonia, such as mobile cervical dystonia, segmental dystonia, head tremor, anterocollis, severe retrocollis, in the patients who have significant extracervical symptoms, or who have never been improved by botulinum toxin injection (primary botulinum toxin non-responder). Such complicated cases are always difficult to deal with through selective peripheral denervation (Albanese et al., 2006; Krauss, 2010; Nunta-aree & Sitthinamsuwan, 2009; Nunta-aree et al., 2010a, 2010b).

i) Intrathecal baclofen therapy

Implantation of this kind of intraspinal drug delivery system is more suitable for generalized dystonia or multifocal dystonia than focal dystonia at the neck (Albright et al., 2001; Dykstra et al., 2005).

j) Spinal cord stimulation

Dorsal column stimulation of the spinal cord gave inconstant outcome and there was no continuous study in dystonic patients since 1990s (Fahn, 1985; Taira & Hori, 2007; Taira, 2009). However, currently, it appears to be a good surgical option in various pain disorders, particularly in neuropathic pain and pain of ischemic origin (Forouzanfar et al., 2004; Kunnumpurath et al., 2009).

This chapter focuses on peripheral nerve surgery in the cervical region for cervical dystonia which refers to selective peripheral denervation in terms of patient selection, preoperative evaluation, operative procedures with relevant surgical anatomy, and surgical outcome.

2. Patient selection

Selective peripheral denervation is chiefly indicated in patients with failed botulinum toxin injection, including those who have never responded to the injection (primary botulinum toxin non-responder) or who have a change from significant previous response to poor recent response (secondary botulinum toxin non-responder) (Albanese et al., 2006; Brin & Benabou,

1999; Bronte-Stewart, 2003; Feely, 2003; Taira, 2009;). Good surgical candidates for the operation include those who meet the following parameters (Braun et al., 1995; Brin & Benabou, 1999; Chen et al., 2000; Dashtipour et al., 2007; Feely, 2003, Nunta-aree et al., 2010b).

a. Patients who are botulinum toxin responder or even secondary non-responder
b. Dystonic symptoms have been stable or not progressed at least 1 year
c. Dystonic disorder mainly confines in the neck region
d. Pure torticollis with slight laterocollis or retrocollis
e. Preoperative electromyography and imaging of the cervical muscles are concordant with clinical manifestation

Furthermore, selective peripheral denervation is sometimes considered as a major alternative to botulinum toxin injection in the treatment of cervical dystonia. For example, for patients who do not require multiple repeated injections or who cannot afford the cost of the toxin, the operation is meaningful for them (Taira, 2009). Nevertheless, some kinds of cervical dystonia are not suitable for the procedure, including head tremors, anterocollis, complex cervical dystonia or cervical dystonia with marked phasic movement. In such kinds of dystonia, pallidal deep brain stimulation should be considered first (Albanese et al, 2006; Nunta-aree et al., 2010b).

3. Preoperative evaluation

In the surgical point of view, consideration before decision of the denervating procedure should cover the following.

3.1 Identification of dystonic muscles

Basically, dystonic muscles must be always defined by using clinical observation and physical examination. Visualization of abnormal posture of the neck, palpable deviant muscle tone and tension usually give valuable preliminary information about the group of involved muscles. Electromyography or video-electromyography is an important tool to define the specific group of dystonic muscles (Brin & Benabou, 1999; Dressler, 2000; Feely, 2003; Krauss et al., 1997; Münchau et al., 2001a; Ostergaard et al., 1996), for which it is very helpful in operative planning. Recently, FDG PET-CT was introduced in localization of dystonic muscles in the neck region (Sung et al., 2007).

3.2 Prior response to botulinum toxin injection

As mentioned above, patients with good prior response to the toxin have tendency to achieve good outcome following the operation, whereas the primary non-responders may not (Braun et al., 1995). The information about injected muscles which accomplish good outcomes is very critical for operative planning.

3.3 Fixed bony deformity

This secondary change should be investigated, especially in patients who have long-lasting cervical dystonia. It can be simply revealed by noting passive range of motion of the neck and plain radiographic studies of the cervical spine. Limitation of passive neck motion implies probable fixed deformity which often impairs surgical outcome, particularly in terms of postoperative neck posture.

3.4 Measure of cervical dystonia

The commonly used measures of cervical dystonia severity and its impacts are The Toronto Western Spasmodic Torticollis Rating Scale (TWSTRS) and Tsui score (Cano et al., 2004; Ceballos-Baumann, 2001; Comella et al., 2003; Taira, 2009; Tsui et al., 1986). The TWSTRS (Comella et al., 1997) (Table 1) is comprised of three main sections, including torticollis severity scale, disability scale, and pain scale. The Tsui score (Moore & Blumhardt, 1991; Tsui et al., 1986) (Table 2) is a composite score calculated by a formula. By both the methods, a higher level of score indicates increased severity of cervical dystonia (Comella et al., 1997; Moore & Blumhardt, 1991). The score can be used for comparison between before and after a treatment or between among various alternatives of treatment.

1. Torticollis severity scale (maximum = 35)			
A. Maximal excursion			
Rotation *(turn: right or left)*		0	None (0°)
		1	Slight (< 1/4 range, 1° - 22°)
		2	Mild (1/4 - 1/2 range, 23° - 45°)
		3	Moderate [1/2 - 3/4 range, 46° - 67°)
		4	Severe (>3/4 range, 68° - 90°)
Laterocollis *(tilt: right or left, exclude shoulder elevation)*		0	None (0°)
		1	Mild (1° - 15°)
		2	Moderate (16° - 35°)
		3	Severe (> 35°)
Anterocollis or retrocollis (a or b)	a. Anterocollis	0	None
		1	Mild downward deviation of chin
		2	Moderate downward deviation (approximates 1/2 possible range)
		3	Severe (chin approximates chest)
	b. Retrocollis	0	None
		1	Mild backward deviation of vertex with upward deviation of chin
		2	Moderate backward deviation (approximates 1/2 possible range)
		3	Severe (approximates full range)
Lateral shift *(right or left)*		0	Absent
		1	Present
Sagittal shift *(forward or backward)*		0	Absent
		1	Present
B. Duration factor *(weighted x 2)*			
Duration factor *(weighted x 2)*		0	None
		1	Occasional deviation (< 25% of the time, most often submaximal)
		2	Occasional deviation (< 25% of the time, often maximal) or Intermittent deviation (25 - 50% of the time, most often submaximal)
		3	Intermittent deviation (25 - 50% of the time, often maximal) or Frequent deviation (50 - 75% of the time, most often submaximal)
		4	Frequent deviation (50 - 75% of the time, often maximal) or Constant deviation (>75% of the time, most often submaximal)
		5	Constant deviation (>75% of the time, often maximal)

C. Effect of sensory tricks		
Effect of sensory tricks	0	Complete relief by one or more tricks
	1	Partial or only limited relief by tricks
	2	Little or no benefit from tricks
D. Shoulder elevation/ Anterior displacement		
Shoulder elevation/ Anterior displacement	0	Absent
	1	Mild (< 1/3 possible range, intermittent or constant)
	2	Moderate (1/3 - 2/3 possible range and constant, > 75% of the time) or Severe (> 2/3 possible range and intermittent)
	3	Severe and constant
E. Range of motion *(without aid of sensory tricks)*		
Range of motion *(without aid of sensory tricks)*	0	Able to move to extreme opposite position
	1	Able to move head well past midline but not to extreme opposite position
	2	Able to move head barely past midline
	3	Able to move head toward but not past midline
	4	Barely able to move head beyond abnormal posture
F. Time *(up to 60 seconds) for which patient is able to maintain head within 10° of neutral position without using sensory tricks (mean of two attempts)*		
Time	0	> 60 seconds
	1	46 - 60 seconds
	2	31 - 45 seconds
	3	16 - 30 seconds
	4	< 15 seconds
2. Disability scale (maximum = 20)		
A. Work *(occupation or housework/home management)*	0	No difficulty
	1	Normal work expectations with satisfactory performance at usual level of occupation but some interference by torticollis
	2	Most activities unlimited, selected activities very difficult and hampered but still possible with satisfactory performance
	3	Working at lower than usual occupation level; most activities hampered, but all possible with less than satisfactory performance in some activities
	4	Unable to engage in voluntary or gainful employment; still able to perform some domestic responsibilities satisfactorily
	5	Marginal or no ability to perform domestic responsibilities
B. Activities of daily living *(e.g., feeding, dressing, or hygiene, including washing, shaving, makeup, etc.)*	0	No difficulty with any activity
	1	Activities unlimited but some interference by torticollis
	2	Most activities unlimited, selected activities very difficult and hampered but still possible using simple tricks
	3	Most activities hampered or laborious but still possible; may use extreme tricks
	4	All activities impaired; some impossible or require assistance
	5	Dependent on others in most self-care tasks

C. Driving	0	No difficulty (or has never driven a car)
	1	Unlimited ability to drive but bothered by torticollis
	2	Unlimited ability to drive but requires tricks (including touching or holding face, holding head against head rest) to control torticollis
	3 4 5	Can drive only short distances Usually cannot drive because of torticollis Unable to drive and cannot ride in a car for long stretches as a passenger because of torticollis
D. Reading	1	Unlimited ability to read in normal seated position but bothered by torticollis
	2	Unlimited ability to read in normal seated position but requires use of tricks to control torticollis
	3	Unlimited ability to read but requires extensive measures to control torticollis or is able to read only in nonseated position (e.g., lying down)
	4	Limited ability to read because of torticollis despite tricks
	5	Unable to read more than a few sentences because of torticollis
E. Television	0	No difficulty
	1	Unlimited ability to watch television in normal seated position but bothered by torticollis
	2	Unlimited ability to watch television in normal seated position but requires use of tricks to control torticollis
	3	Unlimited ability to watch television but requires extensive measures to control torticollis or is able to view only in nonseated position (e.g., lying down)
	4 5	Limited ability to watch television because of torticollis Unable to watch television more than a few minutes because of torticollis
F. Activities outside the home *(e.g., shopping, walking about, movies, dining, and other recreational activities)*	0	No difficulty
	1	Unlimited activities but bothered by torticollis
	2	Unlimited activities but requires simple tricks to accomplish
	3	Accomplishes activities only when accompanied by others because of torticollis
	4	Limited activities outside the home; certain activities impossible or given up because of torticollis
	5	Rarely if ever engages in activities outside the home
3. Pain scale (maximum = 20)		
A. Severity of pain		Rate the severity of neck pain due to spasmodic torticollis during the last week on a scale of 0 - 10 where a score of 0 represents no pain and 10 represents the most excruciating pain imaginable. Score calculated as: [worst + best + (2 x usual)]/4 Best ____ Worst ____ Usual ____ Score____
B. Duration of Pain	0	None
	1	Present < 10% of the time
	2	Present 10 - 25% of the time
	3	Present 26 - 50% of the time
	4	Present 51 - 75% of the time
	5	Present > 75% of the time

C. Disability due to pain	0	No limitation or interference from pain
	1	Pain is quite bothersome but not a source of disability
	2	Pain definitely interferes with some tasks but is not a major contributor to disability
	3	Pain accounts for some (less than half) but not all of disability
	4	Pain is a major source of difficulty with activities; separate from this, head pulling is also a source of some (less than half) disability
	5	Pain is the major source of disability; without it most impaired activities could be performed quite satisfactorily despite the head pulling

Table 1. The Toronto Western Spasmodic Torticollis Rating Scale (TWSTRS) (Comella et al., 1997)

A. Amplitude of head deviation A = A1 + A2 +A3	A1. Rotation	0	Absent
		1	< 15°
		2	15 - 30°
		3	> 30°
	A2. Lateral head tilt	0	Absent
		1	< 15°
		2	15 - 30°
		3	> 30°
	A3. Antero/retrocollis	0	Absent
		1	< 15°
		2	15 - 30°
		3	> 30°
B. Duration of sustained movements		1	Intermittent
		2	Constant
C. Shoulder elevation		0	Absent
		1	Mild, intermittent
		2	Mild constant or severe intermittent
		3	Severe constant
D. Unsustained head movements *(head tremor/jerk)* D = D1 x D2	D1. Severity	1	Mild
		2	Severe
	D2. Duration	1	Occasional
		2	Continuous
Total score = (A x B) + C + D			

Table 2. The Tsui score (Tsui et al., 1986)

4. Operative procedures and relevant surgical anatomy

Selective peripheral denervation consists of several surgical procedures. One well-known operation is the Bertrand procedure which originally included section of peripheral branches of the cervical spinal nerve and selective denervation of the sternocleidomastoid nerve. Taira's method is a modification of the classic procedure of Bertrand aiming to overcome some drawbacks of the original method. Cutting of peripheral branches supplying the sternocleidomastoid or levator scapulae endeavors to reduce their dystonia resulting in improved neck posture and function. The authors simply divide the denervating procedures into three main themes, including denervation of the posterior cervical paraspinal, sternocleidomastoid, and levator scapulae muscles. In order to understand these operations, each of them will be preceded by exposition of its relevant surgical anatomy. In addition, identification of nerves by using intraoperative electrical nerve stimulator, conclusion of nerve supply to the neck muscles, options in selective denervation, and combined operations will be discussed consecutively.

4.1 Surgical anatomy of the posterior cervical paraspinal muscles and related nerve supply

In all patterns of cervical dystonia except for anterocollis, the posterior cervical paraspinal muscles have the key role in occurrence of dystonic postures. They are abnormal on the same side of rotating or tilting head in torticollis or laterocollis, respectively (Anderson et al., 2008; Krauss et al., 1997). This group of muscles are found to be dystonic bilaterally in retrocollis (Taira, 2009). The commonly involved muscles include the splenius capitis, semispinalis capitis, semispinalis cervicis, multifidus, suboccipital muscles (rectus capitis posterior major and minor, obliquus capitis superior and inferior), and upper trapezius (Taira, 2009) (Fig.3).

Aside from the trapezius, all of them are innervated by the posterior rami of the C1 to C8 spinal nerves while the upper twig of the accessory nerve directly supplies the trapezius. The most influent muscles are controlled by the C1 to C6 posterior rami. Consequently, a common procedure of posterior neck muscle denervation is C1-C6 posterior ramisectomy (Krauss et al., 1997).

The C1 dorsal root and its ganglion are usually absent (Tubbs et al., 2007), so the C1 spinal nerve mostly originates from the C1 ventral nerve root which contains pure motor fibers. The C1 segmental nerve emerges from the atlanto-occipital space located superior to the atlas, then it abruptly branches into the anterior and posterior rami. Unlike the C2 to C6 posterior rami, the C1 posterior ramus does not ramify into medial and lateral branches (Fig.4A) while those of the C2-C6 spinal nerves do (Clemente, 1985; Kahle & Frotscher, 2003; Kayalioglu, 2009; Roman, 1981). The posterior ramus of the C2 spinal nerve always bifurcates into medial and lateral branches. The medial branch mainly contains sensory fibers which it terminates as the greater occipital nerve supplying the posterior scalp up to the vertex (the C2 dermatome). The lateral branch is composed of motor fibers supplying the upper portion of the posterior cervical group (Fig.4B). The C3-C6 posterior rami often divide into medial and lateral branches innervating the corresponding skin as well as paraspinal muscles of the neck (Clemente, 1985; Kayalioglu, 2009; Roman, 1981) (Fig.4C).

4.2 Denervation of the posterior cervical paraspinal muscles

The two main strategic options in selective denervation of the posterior neck muscles are posterior cervical ramisectomy in the Bertrand procedure and Taira's modified method. The details of both alternatives are described as the follows.

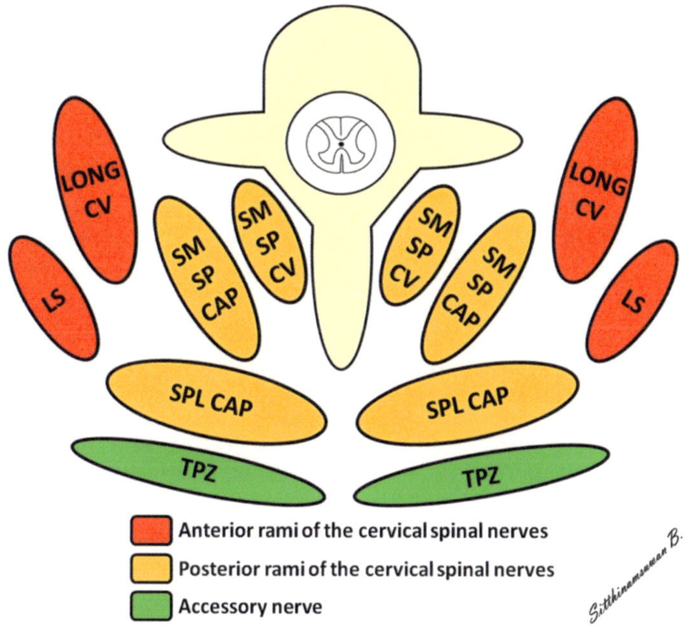

Fig. 3. Major cervical paraspinal muscles involved in cervical dystonia and their nerve supply. LONG CV, longissimus cervicis; LS, levator scapulae; SM SP CAP, semispinalis capitis; SM SP CV, semispinalis cervicis; SPL CAP, splenius capitis; TPZ, trapezius.

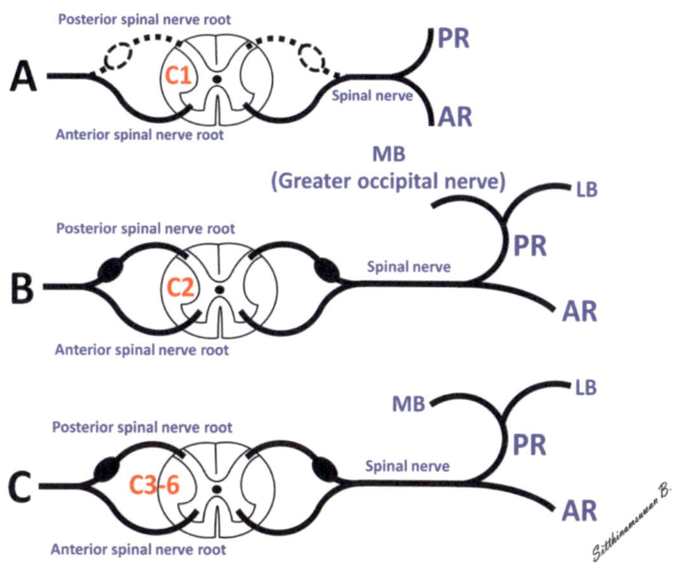

Fig. 4. The C1 - C6 spinal nerves and their branches. A, The C1 posterior root and ganglion are usually absent (dashed lines). The C1 spinal nerve directly arises from the C1 anterior spinal nerve root. The C1 spinal nerve branches into anterior ramus (AR) and posterior ramus (PR). The latter has no further ramification. For B and C, The posterior rami of C2 - C6 spinal nerves branch into medial branch (MB) and lateral branch (LB). The former, originating from the C2 level, terminates as the greater occipital nerve.

4.2.1 Posterior cervical ramisectomy in Bertrand procedure

Classically, peripheral denervation for torticollis in the Bertrand procedure is comprised of selective peripheral denervation of the posterior cervical muscles ipsilateral to the rotating head and selective denervation of the contralateral sternocleidomastoid muscle (Anderson et al., 2008; Bertrand, 1993; Braun & Richter, 1994; Feely, 2003; Krauss, 2010; Sitthinamsuwan et al., 2010b; Taira, 2009). This genuine extraspinal procedure provides good surgical outcome and is currently a widely used operation for cervical dystonia (Bronte-Stewart, 2003; Krauss, 2010; Sitthinamsuwan & Nunta-aree, 2010; Taira, 2009). Denervating procedure on peripheral nerves supplying the posterior cervical group is typically performed on those arising from the C1 to C6 spinal cord segment (Brin & Benabou, 1999; Dashtipour et al., 2007; Krauss, 2010; Sitthinamsuwan & Nunta-aree, 2010) through a midline posterior cervical incision (Fig.5). Original Bertrand's denervation of the posterior cervical muscles is comprised of extraspinal resection of C1-C2 spinal nerve roots (extraspinal C1-C2 rhizotomy) with section of C3-C6 posterior rami (C3-C6 posterior ramisectomy) (Bertrand, 1993; Huh et al., 2005, 2010). Alternatively, C1-C2 posterior ramisectomy can be used instead of C1-C2 extradural rhizotomy (Brin & Benabou, 1999; Münchau et al., 2001a; Ondo & Krauss, 2004). In the authors' practice deriving from C1-C2 operation, we preferred posterior ramisectomy rather than extraspinal rhizotomy. Therefore, C1-C6 posterior ramisectomy was always performed in our denervation. During dissection, muscular branches emerging from the C1-C6 posterior rami are identified by using an electrical stimulator and prepared for ramisectomy. The ablation is done just before the peripheral nerves penetrating the targeted muscles (Fig.6).

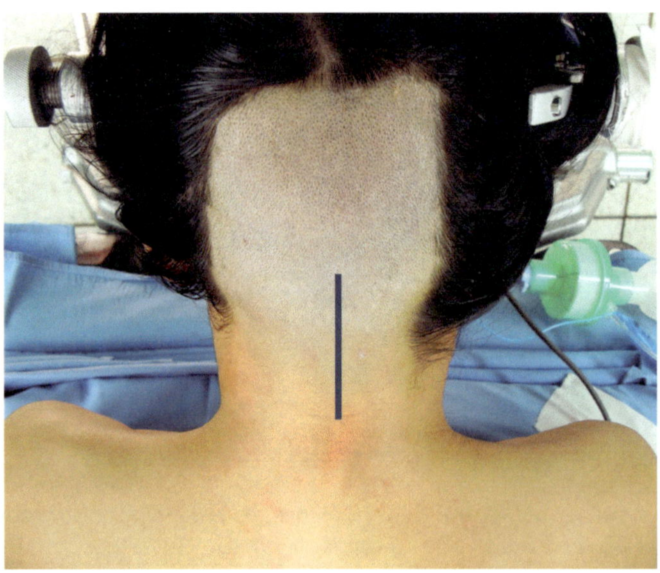

Fig. 5. A midline surgical incision on the back of the neck in posterior cervical ramisectomy

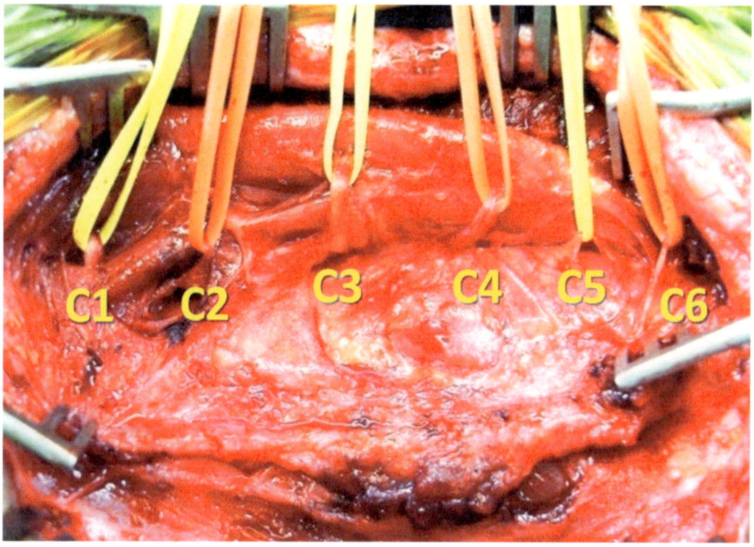

Fig. 6. Operative exposure of selective denervation in the posterior neck region. The muscular branches of the C1-C6 nerves supplying dystonic muscles on the affected side are identified and subsequently sectioned.

A common pitfall of posterior cervical ramisectomy is inadequate denervation of the semispinalis capitis resulting in residual or recurrent cervical dystonia. The pitfall may occur as a result of complex innervation of this muscle comprised of two entities. The first one is motor branches originating from the medial branches of the posterior cervical rami. They intervene in the plain between the semispinalis capitis and semispinalis cervicis and then enter into the deep surface of the semispinalis capitis (Fig.7A). In the same manner, the other entity is muscular branches coming from the lateral branches of the posterior cervical rami which they are situated in the plain between the semispinalis capitis and splenius capitis, then supply the semispinalis capitis through its superficial aspect (Taira, 2009) (Fig.7B). Hence, to accomplish complete denervation of the semispinalis capitis, exploration and resection of the motor nerves in both the plains are mandatory.

In patients suffering from retrocollis, bilateral posterior cervical muscle denervation is required. With caution, bilateral section of the C6 posterior rami should be avoided, particularly in elderly females who have thin neck muscles. Following bilateral C6 posterior ramisectomy, such patients probably develop difficulty in their neck extension and swallowing (Bertrand, 1988; Taira 2009). In our experience of bilateral posterior cervical denervation for intractable retrocollis, we always performed C1-C6 posterior cervical ramisectomy on a more severe side and cut from the C1 posterior ramus caudally to the C4 or C5 posterior ramus with total preservation of the C6 one on the contralateral side.

A major sequelae of Bertrand procedure is dysesthesia over the skin innervated by the C2 spinal nerve. The sensory disturbance of the C2 dermatome is inevitable in almost all cases who undergo this procedure. It always occurs in the early postoperative period as a result of resection of the proximal C2 dorsal ramus containing both motor and sensory nerve fibers (Albanese et al., 2006; Braun & Richter, 1994; Feely, 2003; Münchau et al., 2001a;

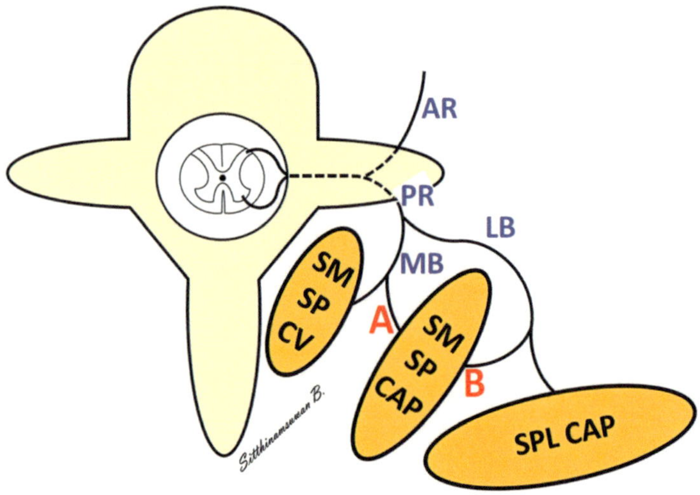

Fig. 7. Innervation of the semispinalis capitis muscle (SM SP CAP). A and B are the muscular branches arising from the medial branch (MB) and lateral branch (LB) of the posterior cervical rami (PR), respectively. They supply the semispinalis capitis through its opposite surfaces. AR, anterior cervical rami; SM SP CV, semispinalis cervicis; SPL CAP, splenius capitis.

Sitthinamsuwan & Nunta-aree, 2010; Taira, 2003, 2009). Additionally, considerable bleeding from the paravertebral venous plexuses adjacent to the C1 and C2 posterior rami sometimes happens intraoperatively (Braun & Richter, 2002; Taira, 2009). Other potential complications include transient occipital neuralgia which usually disappears within 3 months (Braun & Richter, 2002; Huh et al., 2005), weakness of non-dystonic muscles (Taira, 2009) caused by excessive denervation (Feely, 2003), surgical site infection (Huh et al., 2005; Münchau et al., 2001a), swallowing dysfunction (Braun & Richter, 2002; Münchau et al., 2001a, 2001b; Taira, 2009), and injury of the extradural vertebral artery located close to the C1 dorsal ramus (Braun & Richter, 2002; Taira, 2009).

4.2.2 Taira's modified method

Because of some critical disadvantages of Bertrand operation, especially C2 dysesthesia and bleeding around the C1 and C2 posterior branches, the C1-C2 procedure was modified to minimize these drawbacks (Taira & Hori, 2002; Taira et al., 2006). In Taira's method, the operation on C1 and C2 spinal nerves was adapted from extraspinal C1-C2 rhizotomy (or C1-C2 dorsal ramisectomy) in Bertrand procedure (Fig.8A) to intradural C1-C2 anterior rhizotomy (Fig.8B), while the C3 to C6 procedure is identical to that of Bertrand (Fig.8C). Therefore, the modified method is a combination of intradural C1-C2 anterior rhizotomy performed through the C1 hemilaminectomy and conventional C3-C6 posterior ramisectomy (Sitthinamsuwan & Nunta-aree, 2010; Taira, 2009).

Resection of the C1 and C2 anterior spinal nerve roots (C1-C2 anterior rhizotomy) can entirely preserve sensory function of the C2 posterior spinal nerve root, so C2 dysesthesia does not occur. Furthermore, the unilateral C1-C2 procedure does not bring about swallowing trouble. Although the efficacy of Taira's modified method in the treatment of cervical dystonia was not significantly different from that of the Bertrand procedure, the C2 sensory disturbance, operative time, and intraoperative blood loss were appreciably minimized by Taira's operation (Taira & Hori, 2001; Taira et al., 2002; Taira & Hori, 2003). Potential complications of intradural C1-C2 operation may have occurred, such as cerebrospinal fluid leak, meningitis, spinal cord injury, and spinal cord ischemia. However, all of them are preventable and avoidable.

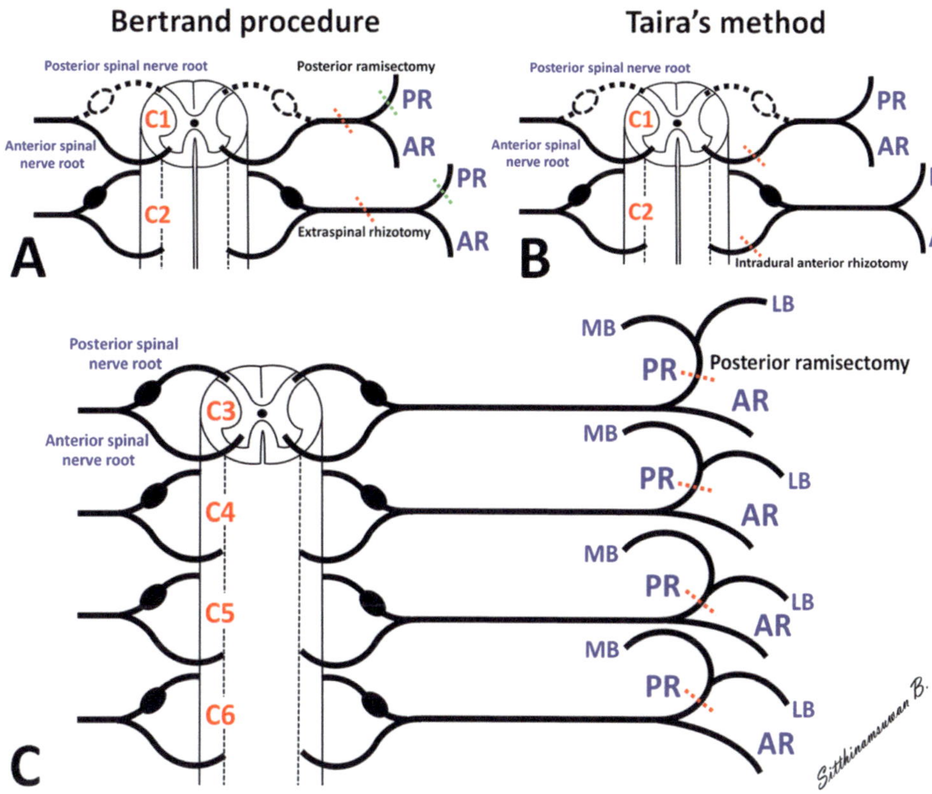

Fig. 8. A, B and C, A comparison between Bertrand procedure and Taira's method. A, C1-C2 denervation in Bertrand procedure. The C1-C2 nerves can be cut on either the spinal roots (extraspinal rhizotomy) presented by red dashed lines or posterior rami (PR) displayed by green dashed lines. B, Intradural C1-C2 anterior rhizotomy in Taira's method. The resection will be performed on the C1 and C2 anterior spinal nerve roots (red dash lines), while the C2 posterior spinal nerve root will be entirely preserved. For A and B, The C1 posterior spinal nerve root and its dorsal root ganglion are usually absent in the majority of humans. Therefore, they are presented in a dashed appearance. C, C3-C6 posterior ramisectomy is identical in both the operations.

4.3 Surgical anatomy of the accessory nerve and its peripheral branches

The accessory nerve originates from its cranial and spinal roots. After the nerve exits the posterior cranial fossa through the jugular foramen, it runs underneath the sternocleidomastoid muscle where it gives motor branches to the muscle and appears in the posterior triangle of the neck after that (Aramrattana et al., 2005; Clemente, 1985; Frank 1997; Roman 1981). In the triangle, it emerges from the posterior border of the sternocleidomastoid at the punctum nervosum (Erb's point) (Anderson et al., 2008; Aramrattana et al., 2005). There are several nerves arising from this point, including the great auricular, lesser occipital, transverse cervical, and supraclavicular nerves (Anderson et al., 2008; Aramrattana et al., 2005; Dailiana et al., 2001). From the punctum nervosum, the accessory nerve courses inferolaterally, then ramifies into numerous branches supplying the trapezius (Aramrattana et al., 2005; Clemente, 1985; Dailiana et al., 2001; Kierner et al., 2000; Roman 1981; Shiozaki et al., 2000) (Fig.9).

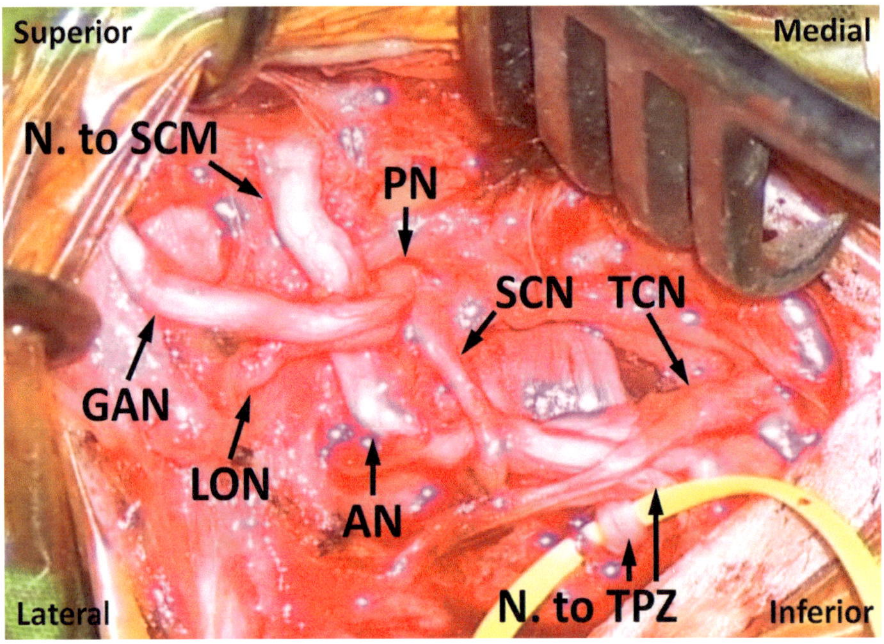

Fig. 9. The posterior cervical triangle, right side. Several nerves, including the great auricular nerve (GAN), lesser occipital nerve (LON), accessory nerve (AN), supraclavicular nerve (SCN), and transverse cervical nerve (TCN) emerge from the punctum nervosum (PN). After the accessory nerve gives nerve(s) to the sternocleidomastoid (N. to SCM), it runs inferolaterally and then terminates as nerve(s) to the trapezius (N. to TPZ).

In addition to the accessory nerve, motor branches of the cervical plexus derived from the C2-C3 anterior rami participate in innervation of the sternocleidomastoid and trapezius muscles (Aramrattana et al., 2005; Bertrand, 2004; Clemente, 1985; Dailiana et al., 2001; Pu et al., 2008; Roman 1981; Stacey et al., 1995; Zhao et al., 2006). Among the entire phalanx of nerves to both the muscles, multiple variations can be encountered during surgical exploration (Brennan et al., 2002; Brown et al., 1988; Caliot et al., 1984, 1989; Latarjet, 1948; Stacey et al., 1995; Taira, 2009) (Fig.10 and Fig.11). Knowledge of the variations is essential in accessory nerve denervation. Incomplete denervation of the sternocleidomastoid usually occurs in individuals who have hidden extra nerve supply from the cervical plexus. Failure of improvement or recurrent dystonia is occasionally due to this aberration. Furthermore, ignorance of diversity of trapezius innervation perhaps gives rise to injured trapezius nerves resulting in shoulder dysfunction.

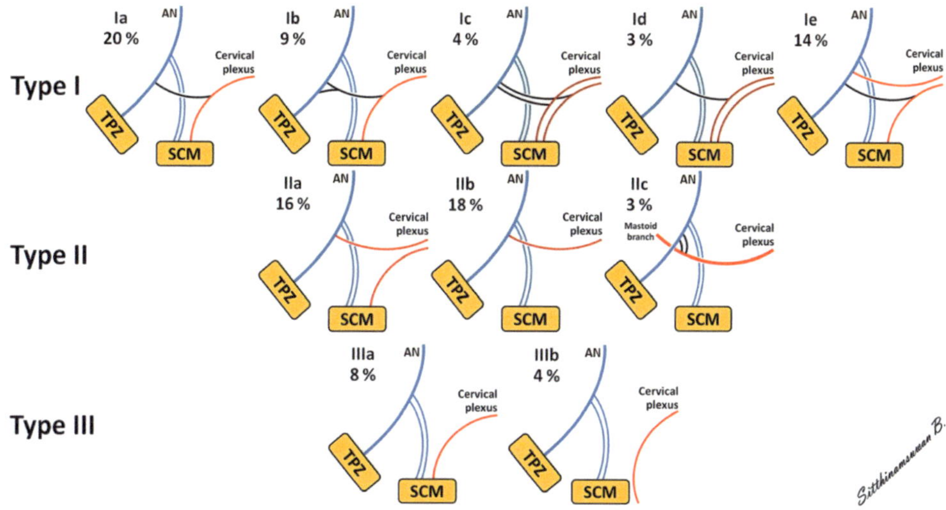

Fig. 10. Variations of the sternocleidomastoid (SCM) innervation and their frequencies in percentage. Type I, Presence of a connecting branch between the accessory nerve (AN) and cervical plexus. Type II, The accessory nerve directly connects to the cervical plexus. Type III, no connection between either of them. TPZ, trapezius. [Modified from Caliot et al., 1984].

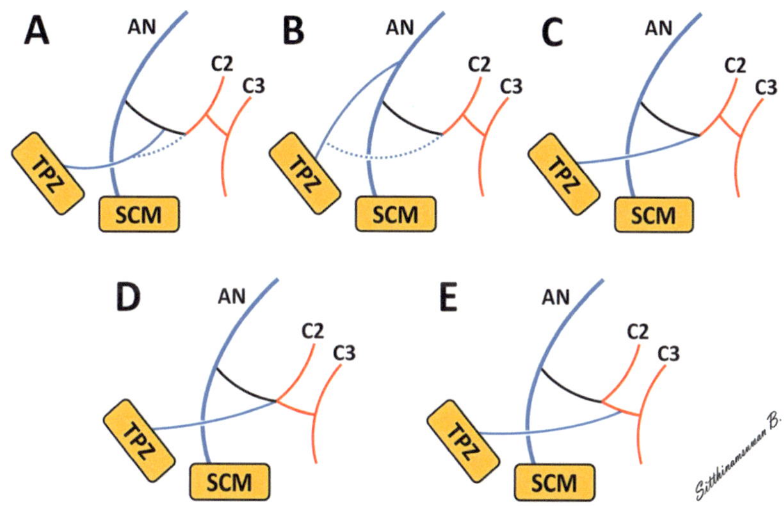

Fig. 11. Variation of the nerve to the trapezius (TPZ). A, The nerve originates from a connecting branch between the accessory nerve (AN) and anterior ramus of the C2 spinal nerve (C2). A direct branch from the C2 anterior rami (dotted line) may participate in the supply. B, The accessory nerve gives a direct branch to supply the trapezius. An additional twig perhaps comes from the C2 anterior ramus to join the main supply (dotted line). C, The trapezius is innervated by the nerve arising from the junction between the C2 anterior ramus and a connecting branch from the accessory nerve. D, The nerve emerges from the union of the connecting branches of the accessory nerve, C2, and C3 anterior rami (C3). E, A connection between C2 and C3 anterior rami gives the nerve supplying the trapezius muscle. SCM, sternocleidomastoid. [Modified from Latarjet, 1948].

4.4 Selective denervation of the sternocleidomastoid muscle

Selective resection of nerve to the sternocleidomastoid with sparing of the trapezius nerve is commonly used in the treatment of torticollis and laterocollis. It is one of two main parts of Bertrand procedure. In our viewpoint, we considered sternocleidomastoid denervation on the contralateral side of posterior cervical muscle denervation in all patients with torticollis. In addition, we used the ipsilateral procedure in some laterocollic cases, particularly in patients with absence of shoulder elevation, which probably indicated hyperactivity of the sternocleidomastoid rather than that of the levator scapulae. The denervation can be done through a small incision along the posterior boundary of the sternocleidomastoid muscle (Fig.12A). Medial retraction of the sternocleidomastoid is helpful in visualization of the nerve. The nerve is often seen underneath the retracted muscle (Fig.12B).

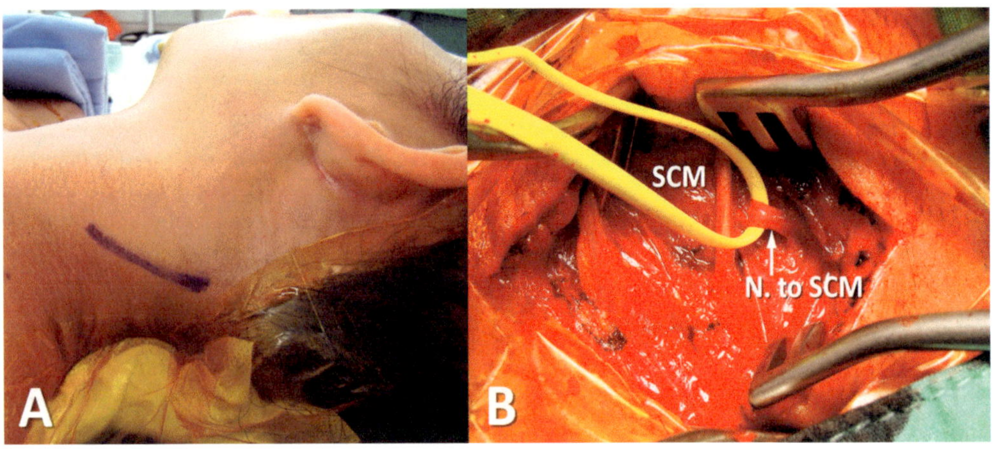

Fig. 12. Selective denervation of the left sternocleidomastoid (SCM). A, A small incision (blue line) along the posterior margin of the sternocleidomastoid. B, Operative exposure of nerve to the sternocleidomastoid (N. to SCM). It can be clearly found when the muscle is medially displaced.

Electrical stimulation of the correct nerve absolutely reveals contraction of the sternocleidomastoid without movement of the trapezius. On the other hand, isolated trapezius contraction indicates stimulation of the trapezius nerve which is inaccurate. If contraction occurs on both the muscles, that is a too proximal position. Besides, the additional nerve supply from the cervical plexus should be investigated and then sectioned. The potential complications are injury of nerve to the trapezius (Albanese et al., 2006; Braun & Richter, 1994, 2002; Taira, 2009) and numbness in the retro-auricular area caused by injury or excessive retraction of the great auricular nerve during the operation (Braun & Richter, 1994).

4.5 Anatomy of the levator scapulae and its nerve supply

The levator scapulae is the key muscle in emergence of laterocollis (Anderson et al., 2008; Taira et al., 2003), particularly when the lateral neck deviation is accompanied by elevation of the ipsilateral scapula. It extends from transverse processes of the 1st to 4th cervical vertebrae to insert at the medial aspect of the upper scapular border superior to the scapular spine (Roman, 1981) (Fig.13A). Contraction of the muscle brings about lateral inclination of the ipsilateral head and neck in the coronal plane together with upheaval of the shoulder on the same side (Clemente, 1985; Roman, 1981; Taira et al. 2003) (Fig.13B). Its major nerve supply originates from C3, C4, and C5 anterior rami. The twigs from C3-C4 nerve roots pass underneath the sternocleidomastoid and then enter the anteromedial aspect of the levator muscle. The dorsal scapular nerve arising from the C5 anterior ramus also participates in the innervation of the levator muscle through its inferomedial surface (Anderson et al., 2008; Clemente, 1985; Roman, 1981; Taira, 2009).

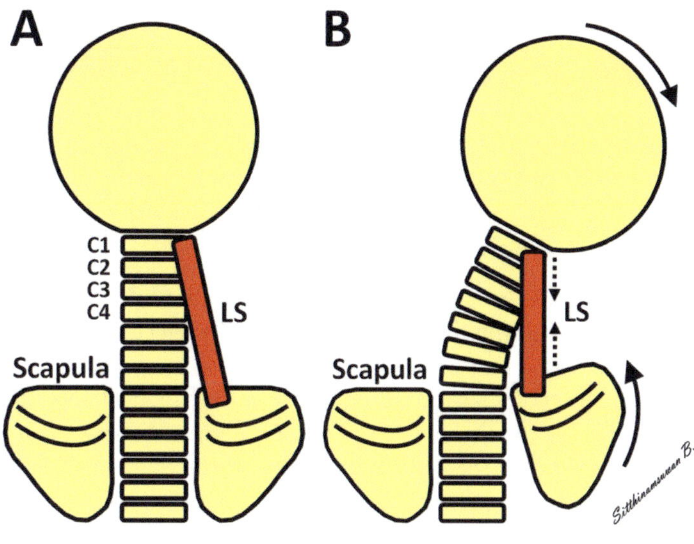

Fig. 13. Functional anatomy of the levator scapulae muscle. A, The muscle originates from the upper four cervical spines, then extends inferolaterally to the superior border of the scapula. B, Its main action consists of neck lateral deviation as well as shoulder elevation.

4.6 Levator scapulae muscle denervation

The operation is mainly indicated in laterocollic patients (Anderson et al., 2008) with marked shoulder elevation and minimal head rotation (Taira, 2009). The ascending shoulder points to the hyperactive levator muscle (Hernesniemi & Keränen, 1990; Taira & Hori, 2001; Taira, 2009). Importantly, noting palpable tense levator scapulae in the posterior cervical triangle is helpful in the diagnosis (Taira, 2009). The surgical incision is identical to that of the sternocleidomastoid denervation. The C3-C4 muscular branches can be encountered by using electrical nerve stimulator and then cutting on the anteromedial surface of the levator muscle (Fig.14). The further supply coming from the dorsal scapular nerve should be explored and eventually ablated. Care should be taken to preserve the adjacent phrenic nerve (Taira et al., 2003) and upper part of the brachial plexus.

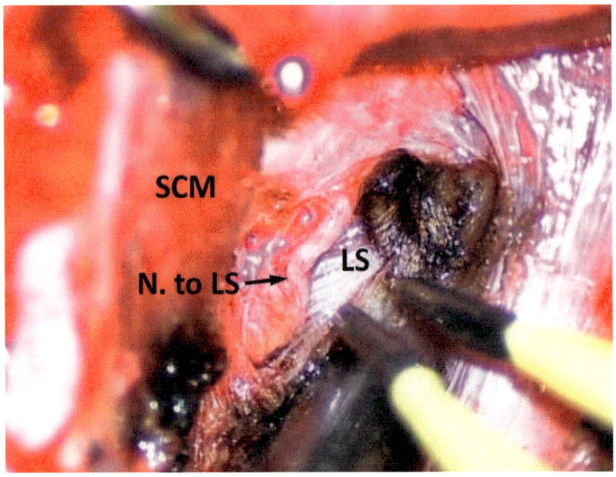

Fig. 14. Microsurgical exposure of the levator scapulae (LS) and its nerve supply (N. to LS) in the left posterior cervical triangle. The sternocleidomastoid (SCM) is retracted anteriorly. Nerve to the levator muscle can be identified on the anterior aspect of the innervated muscle.

4.7 Intraoperative electrical nerve stimulation

Aside from knowledge in the surgical anatomy, identification of accurate nerves by using intraoperative electrical nerve stimulator is very crucial in selective peripheral denervation for cervical dystonia. Intraoperative nerve stimulation has many benefits. It assists in exploration of nerves in the operative field (Brin & Benabou, 1999), in discrimination between motor and sensory nerves, and, importantly, defines muscle topography supplied by electrically stimulated nerve. Sensory nerve must be distinguished from motor nerve. The former has to be routinely preserved as much as possible to avoid neuropathic pain caused by injured or sectioned sensory nerve. Stimulation of motor nerve absolutely elicits contraction of the corresponding muscle (Ondo & Krauss, 2004) whereas there is nothing which occurs when sensory nerve is stimulated. Determination of innervation topography is valuable in selective nerve section. It can tell us which ones should be cut and left (Brin & Benabou, 1999; Sitthinamsuwan et al., 2010c). This strategy always results in the absence of adverse events caused by wrong nerve resection and unnecessary denervation (Sitthinamsuwan et al., 2010c). In utilization of the intraoperative electrical stimulator, short-acting muscle relaxants can be administered only for induction of general anesthesia and must be prohibited after that (Ondo & Krauss, 2004; Taira, 2009).

In posterior cervical muscle denervation, stimulation on each posterior cervical ramus gives rise to segmental contraction of the corresponding muscle. For instance, stimulation of the C2 posterior branch leads to vigorous contraction of the upper fibers of the splenius capitis, while movement of its lower portion is always elicited by electrical stimulation of the C5 or C6 posterior ramus. As discussed in denervation of the sternocleidomastoid, too proximal stimulation of the accessory nerve brings about concurrent contraction of both muscles innervated by the nerve. Isolated movement of either the sternocleidomastoid or trapezius indicates separated stimulation on the sternocleidomastoid or trapezius nerve, respectively. Furthermore, direct stimulation of nerve to the levator scapulae simply reveals contraction of the muscle. If movement of the diaphragm also appears, that means we are very close to the phrenic nerve. In the same manner, if the levator scapulae and rotator cuffs of the shoulder or pectoral muscles contract simultaneously during stimulation of the dorsal scapular nerve, this phenomenon indicates that the present location is too closely adjacent to the C5 spinal root or upper trunk of the brachial plexus.

4.8 Conclusion of the nerve supply

The nerves which contribute to the innervation of cervical dystonic muscles are summarized in Table 3 (Anderson et al., 2008; Aramrattana et al., 2005; Bertrand, 2004; Clemente, 1985; Dailiana et al., 2001; Frank et al., 1997; Kierner et al., 2000; Pu et al., 2008; Roman, 1981; Stacey et al., 1995; Taira, 2009; Zhao et al., 2006).

Cervical muscles	Nerve supply
Suboccipital muscles (rectus capitis posterior major and minor, obliguus superior capitis and obliguus inferior capitis)	Posterior rami of C1-C2 spinal nerves
Semispinalis capitis	Posterior rami of C1-C8 spinal nerves
Semispinalis cervicis	Posterior rami of C1-C8 spinal nerves
Splenius capitis	Posterior rami of C2-C6 spinal nerves
Longissimus cervicis	Posterior rami of C6-C8 spinal nerves
Levator scapulae	Anterior rami of C3-C4 spinal nerves Dorsal scapular nerve (from anterior ramus of C5 spinal nerve)
Trapezius	Accessory nerve Anterior rami of C2-C3 spinal nerves
Sternocleidomastoid	Accessory nerve Anterior rami of C2-C3 spinal nerves

Table 3. The muscles in the neck region associated with cervical dystonia and their nerve supply

4.9 Alternatives in selective peripheral denervation

In selective peripheral denervation, the procedure should be tailored according to the presenting dystonic forms (Sitthinamsuwan et al., 2010b). Surgical options for cervical dystonia are listed in Table 4 (Bertrand, 1993; Braun & Richter, 2002; Brin & Benabou, 1999; Chen et al., 2000; Huh et al., 2005, 2010; Münchau et al., 2001a; Taira et al., 2003). Selective peripheral denervation is not a good alternative for anterocollis because extensive bilateral denervation of both superficial and deep anterior cervical muscles can lead to significant disabling anterior neck muscle paresis and swallowing dysfunction. Furthermore, the operation is usually not effective in the treatment of anterocollis and complex cervical dystonia. Therefore, pallidal deep brain stimulation should be considered as the primary surgical therapy for such kinds of cervical dystonia.

Dystonic pattern	Common option in selective denervation
Torticollis	Selective C1-C6 denervation of the posterior cervical paraspinal muscles ipsilateral to the rotating head with contralateral sternocleidomastoid denervation
Retrocollis	Selective C1-C6 denervation of the bilateral posterior cervical paraspinal muscles; nevertheless, the unilateral C6 posterior ramus should be carefully preserved Selective denervation of the upper trapezius may be indicated either unilaterally or bilaterally in patients who have dystonia of this muscle
Laterocollis	Selective C1-C6 denervation of the posterior cervical muscles and levator scapula on the same side of the inclination Selective denervation of the ipsilateral sternocleidomastoid may be indicated in patients who have dystonia of this muscle
Torticollis + retrocollis	Bilateral posterior cervical muscle denervation (C1-C6 denervation on the ipsilateral side of the turning face with contralateral C1 - C4 or C5 denervation) plus contralateral sternocleidomastoid denervation If indicated, selective denervation of the upper trapezius should be done either unilaterally or bilaterally
Retrocollis + laterocollis	Bilateral posterior cervical muscle denervation (C1 - C6 denervation on the ipsilateral side of the tilting head with contralateral C1 - C4 or C5 denervation) plus ipsilateral levator scapulae denervation If indicated, the sternocleidomastoid ipsilateral to the tilting head should be denervated If indicated, selective denervation of the upper trapezius should be done either unilaterally or bilaterally
Anterocollis Complex cervical dystonia	Is not a good candidate for selective denervation Should be managed surgically by pallidal deep brain stimulation
Alternatives in C1-C6 denervation of the posterior cervical muscles	a. Extraspinal C1-C2 rhizotomy plus C3-C6 posterior ramisectomy (original Bertrand's denervation) b. Selective C1-C6 posterior ramisectomy c. Intradural C1-C2 anterior rhizotomy plus C3-C6 posterior ramisectomy (Taira's modified method)

Table 4. Alternatives in peripheral denervation for various patterns of cervical dystonia

4.10 Combined operative procedures

Our treatment of complex cervical dystonia and idiopathic generalized dystonia by using bilateral pallidal deep brain stimulation indicates that all of them dramatically respond to the operation. However, a few cases still had some residual cervical dystonia even though we attempted to adjust their implanted neurostimulators optimally. In such patients, we decided to add selective peripheral denervation to the muscles which have residual hypertonia. Postoperative improvement was encountered in all our cases who underwent the combined procedures. In summary, if the satisfactory outcome cannot be fulfilled by deep brain stimulation alone, selective peripheral denervation (or even selective muscle resection) is a good further surgical option in the treatment of refractory complex cervical dystonia. A demonstration of a case on whom we operated by using the combined procedures is presented in Fig.15.

5. Surgical outcome

By collecting surgical outcomes of selective denervation for cervical dystonia, the numerous studies revealed satisfactory results with minimal complications. Nonetheless, various methods in measure of outcome were utilized. Some of them were unvalidated and employed subjective methods whereas the remaining studies used widely accepted and validated measure tools, such as the TWSTRS or Tsui score. Overall therapeutic outcomes of selective peripheral denervation are displayed in Table 5 (Bertrand, 1993; Braun et al., 2002; Chen et al., 2000; Cohen-Gadol et al., 2003; Huh et al., 2005, 2010; Jang et al., 2005; Meyer, 2001; Münchau et al., 2001a; Nunta-aree et al., 2010a; Sitthinamsuwan et al., 2010b; Taira & Hori; 2003; Taira et al., 2003).

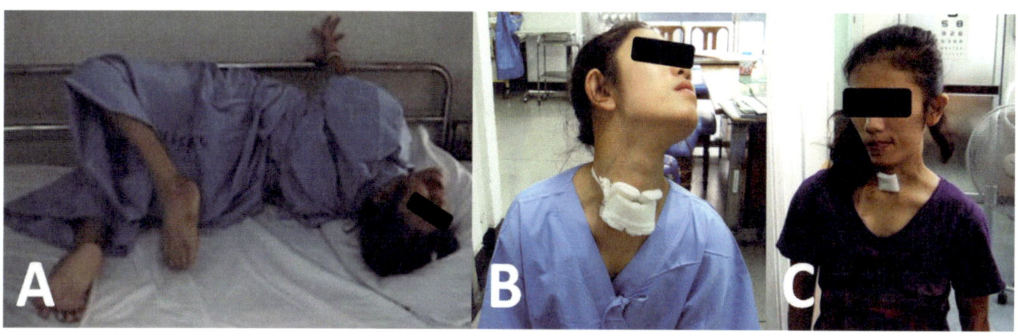

Fig. 15. A female patient with idiopathic generalized dystonia who underwent combined pallidal deep brain stimulation and selective peripheral denervation. A, Preoperative image reveals severe disabling generalized dystonia including mobile cervical dystonia. B, After the deep brain stimulation, her generalized and complex cervical dystonia was markedly improved. She could return to sitting and walking again. However, residual complex cervical dystonia (mobile left torticollis and retrocollis) was persistent even though we adjusted the implanted neurostimulator to achieve maximal benefit. Hence, we decided to denervate the remaining dystonic muscles. C, After multifocal selective denervation of the cervical muscles (left C1 - C6 and right C1 - C4 posterior ramisectomy, right sternocleidomastoid, and bilateral upper trapezius denervation), the residual dystonia was dramatically improved without complication.

Study	Outcome	Complication
Bertrand, 1993 n = 260 cases Age 29 - 61 years Follow-up period 64 cases: more than 10 years 167 cases: more than 5 years Outcome measure: unvalidated outcome scale	Excellent (no detectable abnormal movements): 40% Very good (slight deviation or slight residual movements): 48% Fair (appreciable amount of residual abnormal movements): 10% Poor (no improvement or worse): 1% Overall residual dystonia: 12%	No death Abscess: 1 patient Sensory loss in the distribution of the greater occipital nerve: unspecified number of cases Tic-like pain: 3 patients
Chen et al., 2000 The operation included selective peripheral denervation and myotomy n = 207 cases Mean age 39 years Follow-up 2 - 29 years Outcome measure: unvalidated outcome scale	Excellent (no detectable abnormal movements, normal movement of neck preserved): 70.5% Very good (slight deviation or slight residual movements): 7.4% Fair (appreciable amount of residual abnormal movements): 9.2% Poor (no improvement or worse): 2.9%	No death Sensory loss in distribution of the greater occipital nerve: most patients
Meyer, 2001 n = 30 cases Median age 55 years Median follow-up 26 months Outcome measure: - The severity score component of the TWSTRS - The scales for activities of daily living (ADL), whole person impairment, adverse life style effects and degree of incapacity	Overall improvement of the TWSTRS: 59% ADL score improvement: 90% Improvement of whole person impairment score: 59% Life style score improvement: 34% Improvement of incapacity score: 50%	Not mentioned
Münchau et al., 2001a n = 37 cases Mean age 50 years Mean follow-up 16.7 years Outcome measure: - The TWSTRS - Head tremor severity - Maximum degree of head rotation and head tilt - Self-assessed outcome - Psychological assessment	At 1-year follow-up Functional improvement: 68% of patients Mean total TWSTRS improvement: 30% Severity score reduction: 20% Disability score reduction: 40% Pain score reduction: 30% Head tremor severity did not change Self assessment outcome Comparable benefit of surgery and the past best response to botulinum toxin: 10% of patients Surgery was superior: 67% of patients Surgery was worse: 23% of patients Improvement in some psychological measures	No death Wound complication: 1 patient Progressive dystonia: 1 patient Transient imbalance: 3 patients Dysesthesia in the denervated posterior cervical segments: all patients Transient trapezius paresis: 1 patient Dysphagia: 7 patients Deterioration of dysphagia: 5 patients

Study	Outcome	Complication
Braun et al., 2002 n = 140 cases Mean age 39.7 years Mean follow-up 32.8 months Outcome measure: subjective assessment by the patients self-estimate questionaire	Satisfactory: 73% Complete relief: 13%, Significant improvement: 36% Moderate improvement: 24% Ineffective: 27% Minor relief: 14% No improvement: 14% Recurrent dystonia: 11%	No death Hematoma in the anterior neck: 3 patients Transient dysphagia: 4 patients Sensory deficit in the area of the greater occipital nerve: all patients Injury of trapezius branch of the accessory nerve: 2 patients
Taira & Hori, 2003 n = 82 cases Age: not mentioned Follow-up 3 months Outcome measure: Tsui score	Mean Tsui score improvement Group A (44 patients who underwent the modified Taira's procedure): 85% Group B (38 patients who underwent the traditional Bertrand procedure): 86.4 %	No death Sensory deficit in C2 dermatome Group A: 3 patients Group B: all (38) patients
Taira et al., 2003 n = 10 cases Mean age 34.8 years Mean follow-up 29.4 months Outcome measure: Tsui score	Mean Tsui score improvement: 88% Excellent: 40 % Good: 60 %	No death Transient C3 or C4 dysesthesia: 5 patients
Cohen-Gadol et al., 2003 n = 168 cases Mean age 53.4 years Mean follow-up 3.4 years in 130 cases Outcome measure: unvalidated outcome scale	At the 3-month follow-up Moderate to excellent improvement: 77% Pain improvement 81 % Long-term follow-up (mean 3.4 years) Moderate to excellent improvement: 70%	Death due to respiratory arrest: 1 patient Persistent C2 dysesthesia: 3 patients Slight shoulder weakness: 3 patients Wound infection: 1 patient
Jang et al., 2005 n = 5 cases Mean age 43.75 years Follow-up 3 months Outcome measure: - The TWSTRS - Cervical Dystonia Severity Scale (CDSS) - Visual Analogue Scale (VAS)	Mean total TWSTRS improvement: 76.5% CDSS improvement: 48.7% VAS improvement: 77.6%	No death or complication
Huh et al., 2005 n = 10 cases Mean age 52.4 years Mean follow-up 36 months Outcome measure: identical to that of the original Bertrand's study	Excellent :50% Good: 40% Fair: 10%	No death Wound infection: 2 patients Delirium: 1 patient Generalized weakness: 1 patient Transient neuralgia: unspecified number of cases

Study	Outcome	Complication
Huh et al., 2010 n = 24 cases Mean age 46.6 years Mean follow-up 29.5 months Outcome measure: - The TWSTRS - Subjective assessment by the patients	Mean total TWSTRS improvement In 16 patients who underwent selective peripheral denervation: 59% In 7 patients who underwent pallidal deep brain stimulation: 64.1% In 1 patient who underwent combined surgery: 92.5% The subjective result assessed by the patients Selective denervation group: excellent 25%, good 62.5%, and fair 12.5% Deep brain stimulation group (including a patient who underwent combined operation): excellent 25 %, good 62.5 %, and fair 12.5 %	No death Wound infection: 2 patients Occipital neuralgia: 3 patients Delirium: 1 patient Venous air embolism: 1 patient
Nunta-aree et al., 2010a n = 6 cases Age 24 - 62 years Mean follow-up 29.7 months Outcome measure: Tsui score	Mean Tsui score improvement: 70%	No death or complication
Sitthinamsuwan et al., 2010b Combined use of ablative neurosurgical operations for intractable spastic and dystonic cerebral palsy Single case report Age 27 years Follow-up period 12 months Outcome measure: - Unvalidated outcome scale for cervical dystonia (assessed by clinical observation and physical examination) - Modified Ashworth Scale (MAS) for spasticity	Disappearance of cervical dystonia following unilateral C1-C6 posterior ramisectomy Markedly improved neck control Improved swallowing Marked improvement of generalized spasticity Improved sitting balance and posture	No death or complication

Table 5. Therapeutic outcome of selective peripheral denervation in the treatment of cervical dystonia

6. Conclusion

Various surgical procedures should be considered in cervically dystonic individuals who do not respond to the conventional treatment. Among them, selective peripheral denervation usually yields a satisfactory result and has been one of the most popularly used operations for the disorder. It is mainly indicated in almost types of cervical dystonia, excluding anterocollis and complex patterns. The surgical planning and tailored resection of the nerve should be relied on the individual dystonic pattern. Good candidate selection, knowledge of the relevant anatomy, surgical skills in nerve exploration and precise identification are very significant in the operation through which they will lead to an excellent therapeutic outcome and avoidance of potential adverse effects.

7. References

Adams, C.B. (1984). Vascular Catastrophe Following the Dandy Mckenzie Operation for Spasmodic Torticollis. *Journal of Neurology Neurosurgery and Psychiatry*, Vol.47, No.9, (September 1984), pp. 990-994, ISSN 0022-3050

Albanese, A. (2005). Clinical Features of Dystonia and European Guideline for Diagnosis and Treatment. In: *Proceedings of the Medtronic Forum for Neuroscience and Neuro-Technology 2005*, van Hilten, B. & Nuttin, B., (Ed.), pp. 289-321, Springer, ISBN 978-354-032-745-5, Germany

Albanese, A.; Barnes, M.P.; Bhatia, K.P.; Fernandez-Alvarez, E.; Filippini, G.; Gasser, T.; Krauss, J.K.; Newton, A.; Rektor, I.; Savoiardo, M. & Valls-Solè J. (2006). A Systematic Review on the Diagnosis and Treatment of Primary (Idiopathic) Dystonia and Dystonia Plus Syndromes: Report of an EFNS/MDS-ES Task Force. *European Journal of Neurology*, Vol.13, No.5, (May 2006), pp. 433-444, ISSN 1351-1501

Albright, A.L.; Barry, M.J.; Shafton, D.H. & Ferson, S.S. (2001). Intrathecal Baclofen for Generalized Dystonia. *Developmental Medicine and Child Neurology*, Vol.43, No.10, (October 2001), pp. 652-657, ISSN 1469-8749

Anderson, W.S.; Lawson, H.C.; Belzberg, A.J. & Lenz, F.A. (2008). Selective Denervation of the Levator Scapulae Muscle: An Amendment to the Bertrand Procedure for the Treatment of Spasmodic Torticollis. *Journal of Neurosurgery*, Vol.108, No.4, (April 2008), pp. 757-763, ISSN 0022-3085

Aramrattana, A.; Sittitrai, P. & Harnsiriwattanagit, K. (2005). Surgical Anatomy of the Spinal Accessory Nerve in the Posterior Triangle of the Neck. *Asian Journal of Surgery*, Vol.28, No.3, (2005), pp. 171-173, ISSN 1015-9584

Benedetti, A.; Carbonin, C. & Colombo, F. (1977). Extended Posterior Cervical Rhizotomy for Severe Spastic Syndromes with Dyskinesias. *Applied Neurophysiology*, Vol.40, No.1, (1977-1978), pp. 41-47, ISSN 0302-2773

Bertelli, J.A.; Ghizoni, M.F. & Michels, A. (2000). Brachial Plexus Dorsal Rhizotomy in the Treatment of Upper-limb Spasticity. *Journal of Neurosurgery*, Vol.93, No.1, (July 2000), pp. 26-32, ISSN 0022-3085

Bertelli, J.A.; Ghizoni, M.F.; Frasson, T.R. & Borges, K.S. (2003). Brachial Plexus Dorsal Rhizotomy in Hemiplegic Cerebral Palsy. *Hand Clinics*. Vol.19, No.4, (November 2003), pp. 687-699, ISSN 1158-1969

Bertrand, C.; Molina-Negro, P.; Bouvier, G. & Gorczyca, W. (1987). Observations and Analysis of Results in 131 Cases of Spasmodic Torticollis After Selective Denervation. *Applied Neurophysiology*, Vol.50, No.1-6, (1987), pp. 319-323, ISSN 0302-2773

Bertrand, C.M. (1988). Operative Management of Spasmodic Torticollis and Adult-Onset Dystonia with Emphasis on Selective Denervation, In: *Operative Neurosurgical*

Techniques 2nd Edition, Schmidek, H.H., & Sweet, W.H., (Ed.), 1261-1269, Grune & Stratton, Orlando, United States of America

Bertrand, C.M. (1993). Selective Peripheral Denervation for Spasmodic Torticollis. Surgical Technique, Results, and Observation in 260 Cases. *Surgical Neurology*, Vol.40, No.2, (August 1993), pp. 96-103, ISSN 1879-3339

Bertrand, C.M. (2004). Surgery of Involuntary Movements, Particularly Stereotactic Surgery: Reminiscences. *Neurosurgery*, Vol.55, No.3, (September 2004), pp. 698-703, ISSN 1524-4040

Bittar, R.G.; Yianni, J.; Wang, S.; Liu, X.; Nandi, D.; Joint, C.; Scott, R.; Bain, P.G.; Gregory, R.; Stein, J.F. & Aziz, T.Z. (2005). Deep Brain Stimulation for Generalised Dystonia and Spasmodic Torticollis. *Journal of Clinical Neuroscience*, Vol.12, No.1, (January 2005), pp. 12-16, ISSN 0697-5868

Brashear, A. (2004). Treatment of Cervical Dystonia with Botulinum Toxin Injection. *Operative Techniques in Otolaryngology - Head and Neck Surgery*, Vol.15, No.2, (June 2004), pp. 122-127, ISSN 1043-1810

Braun, V. & Richter, H.P. (1994). Selective Peripheral Denervation for the Treatment of Spasmodic Torticollis. *Neurosurgery*, Vol.35, No.1, (July 1994), pp. 58-62, ISSN 1524-4040

Braun, V.; Richter, H.P. & Schröder, J.M. (1995). Selective Peripheral Denervation for Spasmodic Torticollis: Is the Outcome Predictable? *Journal of Neurology*, Vol.242, No.8, (August 1995), pp. 504-507, ISSN 1432-1459

Braun, V. & Richter, H.P. (2002). Selective Peripheral Denervation for Spasmodic Torticollis: 13-Year Experience with 155 Patients. *Journal of Neurosurgery*, Vol.97, No.2 Supplement, (September 2002), pp. 207-212, ISSN 0022-3085

Brennan, P.A.; Smith, G. & Ilankovan, V. (2002). Trapezius Muscle Innervation by a Cervical Nerve - A Rare Anatomical Variant. *The British Journal of Oral and Maxillofacial Surgery*, Vol.40, No.3, (June 2002), pp. 263-264, ISSN 1532-1940

Brin, M.F. & Benabou, R. (1999). Cervical Dystonia (Torticollis). *Current Treatment Options in Neurology*, Vol.1, No.1, (March 1999), pp. 33-43, ISSN 1092-8480

Bronte-Stewart, H. (2003). Surgical Therapy for Dystonia. *Current Neurology and Neuroscience Reports*, Vol.3, No.4, (July 2003), pp. 296-305, ISSN 1528-4042

Brown, H.; Burns, S. & Keiser, W. (1988). The Spinal Accessory Nerve Plexus, The Trapezius Muscles, and Shoulder Stabilization After Radical Neck Cancer Surgery. *Annals of Surgery*, Vol.208, No.5, (November 1988), pp. 654-661, ISSN 1528-1140

Cacciola, F.; Farah, J.O.; Eldridge, P.R.; Byrne, P. & Varma, T.K. (2010). Bilateral Deep Brain Stimulation for Cervical Dystonia: Long-term Outcome in a Series of 10 Patients. *Neurosurgery*, Vol.67, No.4, (October 2010), pp. 957-963, ISSN 1524-4040

Caliot, P.; Cabanié, P.; Bousquet, V. & Midy, D. (1984). A Contribution to the Study of the Innervation of the Sternocleidomastoid Muscle. *Anatomia Clinica*, Vol.6, No.1, (1984), pp. 21-28, ISSN 0343-6098

Caliot, P.; Bousquet, V.; Midy, D. & Cabanié, P. (1989). A Contribution to the Study of the Accessory Nerve: Surgical Implications. *Surgical and Radiologic Anatomy*, Vol.11, No.1, (1989), pp. 11-15, ISSN 1279-8517

Cano, S.J.; Hobart, J.C.; Fitzpatrick, R.; Bhatia, K.; Thompson, A.J. & Warner, T.T. (2004). Patient-Based Outcomes of Cervical Dystonia: A Review of Rating Scales. *Movement Disorders*, Vol.19, No.9, (September 2004), pp. 1054-1059. ISSN 1531-8257

Ceballos-Baumann, A.O. (2001). Evidence-Based Medicine in Botulinum Toxin Therapy for Cervical Dystonia. *Journal of Neurology*, Vol.248, No. Supplement 1, (April 2001), pp. 14-20, ISSN 1432-1459

Chawda, S.J.; Münchau, A.; Johnson, D.; Bhatia, K.; Quinn, N.P.; Stevens, J.; Lees, A.J. & Palmer, J.D. (2000). Pattern of Premature Degenerative Changes of the Cervical Spine in Patients with Spasmodic Torticollis and the Impact on the Outcome of Selective Peripheral Denervation. *Journal of Neurology Neurosurgery and Psychiatry*, Vol.68, No.4, (April 2000), pp. 465-471, ISSN 0022-3050

Chen, X.; Ma, A.; Liang, J.; Ji, S. & Pei, S. (2000). Selective Denervation and Resection of Cervical Muscles in the Treatment of Spasmodic Torticollis: Long-term Follow-up Results in 207 cases. *Stereotactic and Functional Neurosurgery*, Vol.75, No.2-3, (2000), pp. 92-95, ISSN 1423-0372

Clemente, C.D. (1985). *Gray's Anatomy 30th Edition*. Lea & Febiger, ISBN 978-0-812-10644-2, Philadelphia, United States of America

Comella, C.L.; Stebbins, G.T.; Goetz, C.G.; Chmura, T.A.; Bressman, S.B. & Lang, A.E. (1997). Teaching Tape for the Motor Section of the Toronto Western Spasmodic Torticollis Scale. *Movement Disorders*, Vol.12, No.4, (July 1997), pp. 570-575, ISSN 1531-8257

Comella, C.L.; Leurgans, S.; Wuu, J.; Stebbins, G.T.; Chmura, T. & Dystonia Study Group. (2003). Rating Scales for Dystonia: A Multicenter Assessment. *Movement Disorders*, Vol.18, No.3, (March 2004), pp. 303-312, ISSN 1531-8257

Dailiana, Z.H.; Mehdian, H. & Gilbert, A. (2001). Surgical Anatomy of Spinal Accessory Nerve: Is Trapezius Functional Deficit Inevitable After Division of the Nerve? *The Journal of Hand Surgery*, Vol.26, No.2, (April 2001), pp. 137-141, ISSN 1532-2211

Dashtipour, K.; Barahimi, M. & Karkar, S. (2007). Cervical Dystonia. *Journal of Pharmacy Practice*, Vol.20, No. 4, (December 2007), pp. 449-457, ISSN 0897-1900

Dent, T.H.S. (March 2002). Selective Denervation for Spasmodic Torticollis, In: *Succinct and Timely Evaluated Evidence Review (STEER)*, 01.04.2011, Available from http://www.wihrd.soton.ac.uk/projx/signpost/steers/STEER_2002(10).pdf

Dressler, D. (2000). Electromyographic Evaluation of Cervical Dystonia for Planning of Botulinum Toxin Therapy. *European Journal of Neurology*, Vol.7, No.6, (November 2000), pp. 713-718, ISSN 1468-1331

Dykstra, D.D.; Mendez, A.; Chappuis, D.; Baxter, T.; DesLauriers, L. & Stuckey, M. (2002). Treatment of Cervical Dystonia and Focal Hand Dystonia by High Cervical Continuously Infused Intrathecal Baclofen: A Report of 2 Cases. *Archives of Physical Medicine and Rehabilitation*, Vol.86, No.4, (April 2005), pp. 830-833, ISSN 0003-9993

Fahn, S. (1985). Lack of Benefit from Cervical Cord Stimulation for Dystonia. *New England Journal of Medicine*, Vol.313, No.19, (November 1985), pp. 1229, ISSN 1533-4406

Feeley, J. (December 2003). Surgical Intervention for Dystonia, In: *Dystonia Medical Research Foundation Booklet*, 01.04.2011, Available from http://www.dystonia-foundation.org/filebin/pdf/surgweb.pdf

Forouzanfar, T.; Kemler, M.A.; Weber, W.E.; Kessels, A.G. & van Kleef, M. (2004). Spinal Cord Stimulation in Complex Regional Pain Syndrome: Cervical and Lumbar Devices are Comparably Effective. *British Journal of Anaesthesiology*, Vol.92, No.3, (March 2004), pp. 348-353, ISSN 1471-6771

Fraioli, B.; Nucci, F. & Baldassarre, L. (1977). Bilateral Cervical Posterior Rhizotomy: Effects on Dystonia and Athetosis, on Respiration and Other Autonomic Functions. *Applied Neurophysiology*, Vol.40, No.1, (1977-1978), pp. 26-40, ISSN 0302-2773

Frank, D.K.; Wenk, E.; Stern, J.C.; Gottlieb, R.D. & Moscatello, A.L. (1997). A Cadaveric Study of the Motor Nerves to the Levator Scapulae Muscle. *Otolaryngology and Head and Neck Surgery*, Vol.117, No.6, (December 1997), pp. 671–680, ISSN 1097-6817

Hagenah, J.M.; Vieregge, A. & Vieregge, P. (2001). Radiculopathy and Myelopathy in Patients with Primary Cervical Dystonia. *European Neurology*, Vol.45, No.4, (2001), pp. 236-240, ISSN 0014-3022

Heimburger, R.F.; Slominski, A. & Griswold, P. (1973). Cervical Posterior Rhizotomy for Reducing Spasticity in Cerebral Palsy. *Journal of Neurosurgery*, Vol.39, No.1, (July 1973), pp. 30-34, ISSN 0022-3085

Hernesniemi, J. & Keränen, T. (1990). Long-term Outcome After Surgery for Spasmodic Torticollis. *Acta Neurochirurgica*, Vol.103, No.3-4, (1990), pp. 128-130, ISSN 0001-6268

Hsin, Y.L.; Harnod, T.; Kuo, T.B.J.; Su, C.F. & Lin, S.Z. (2004). Selective Cervical Dorsal Rhizotomy to Relieve Upper-limb Spasticity After Stroke or Spinal Cord Injury - Report of Five Cases. *Tzu Chi Medical Journal*, Vol.16, No.6, (2004), pp. 371-375, ISSN 1016-3190

Huh, R.; Ahn, J.Y.; Chung, Y.S.; Chang, J.H.; Chang, J.W. & Chung, S.S. (2005). Effectiveness of Selective Peripheral Denervation for the Treatment of Spasmodic Torticollis. *Journal of Korean Neurosurgical Society*, Vol.38, No.5, (November 2005), pp. 344-349, ISSN 1225-8245

Huh, R.; Han, I.B.; Chung, M. & Chung, S. (2010). Comparison of Treatment Results Between Selective Peripheral Denervation and Deep Brain Stimulation in Patients with Cervical Dystonia. *Stereotactic and Functional Neurosurgery*, Vol.88, No.4, (May 2010), pp. 234-238, ISSN 1423-0372

Hung, S.W.; Hamani, C.; Lozano, A.M.; Poon, Y.Y.; Piboolnurak, P.; Miyasaki, J.M.; Lang, A.E.; Dostrovsky, J.O.; Hutchison, W.D. & Moro, E. (2007). Long-term Outcome of Bilateral Pallidal Deep Brain Stimulation for Primary Cervical Dystonia. *Neurology*, Vol.68, No.6, (February 2007), pp. 457-459, ISSN 0028-3878

Imer, M.; Ozeren, B.; Karadereler, S.; Yapici, Z.; Omay, B.; Hanağasi, H. & Eraksoy, M. (2005). Destructive Stereotactic Surgery for Treatment of Dystonia. *Surgical Neurology*, Vol.64, No. Supplement 2, (2005), pp. S89-94, ISSN 1879-3339

Jameson, R.; Rech, C. & Garreau de Loubresse, C. (2010). Cervical Myelopathy in Athetoid and Dystonic Cerebral Palsy: Retrospective Study and Literature Review. *European Spine Journal*, Vol.19, No.5, (May 2010), pp. 706-712, ISSN 0940-6719

Kahle, W. & Frotscher, M. (2003). *Color Atlas and Textbook of Human Anatomy: Nervous System and Sensory Organs 5th Edition*. Thieme, ISBN 978-1-58890-064-7, Stuttgart, Germany

Kayalioglu, G. (2009). The Spinal Nerves, In: *The Spinal Cord*, Watson, C.; Paxinds, G. & Kayalioglu, G., (Ed.), pp. 37-56, Elsevier, ISBN 078-0-12-374247-6, China

Kierner, A.C.; Zelenka, I.; Heller, S. & Burian, M. (2000). Surgical Anatomy of the Spinal Accessory Nerve and the Trapezius Branches of the Cervical Plexus. *Archives of Surgery*, Vol.135, No.12, (December 2000), pp. 1428-1431, ISSN 1538-3644

Konrad, C.; Vollmer-Haase, J.; Anneken, K. & Knecht, S. (2004). Orthopedic and Neurological Complications of Cervical Dystonia--Review of the Literature. *Acta Neurolica Scandinavica*, Vol.109, No.6, (June 2004), pp. 369-373, ISSN 0001-6314

Krauss, J.K.; Toups, E.G.; Jankovic, J. & Grossman, R.G. (1997). Symptomatic and Functional Outcome of Surgical Treatment of Cervical Dystonia. *Journal of Neurology Neurosurgery and Psychiatry*, Vol.63, No.5, (November 1997), pp. 642-648, ISSN 0022-3050

Krauss, J.K.; Pohle, T.; Weber, S.; Ozdoba, C. & Burgunder, J.M. (1999). Bilateral Stimulation of Globus Pallidus Internus for Treatment of Cervical Dystonia. *Lancet*, Vol.354, No.9181, (September 1999), pp. 837-838, ISSN 0140-6736

Krauss, J.K.; Loher, T.J.; Pohle, T.; Weber, S.; Taub, E., Bärlocher, C.B. & Burgunder, J.M. (2002). Pallidal Deep Brain Stimulation in Patients with Cervical Dystonia and Severe Cervical Dyskinesias with Cervical Myelopathy. *Journal of Neurology Neurosurgery and Psychiatry*, Vol.72, No.2, (February 2002), pp. 249-256, ISSN 0022-3050

Krauss, J.K.; Yianni, J.; Loher, T.J. & Aziz, T.Z. (2004). Deep Brain Stimulation for Dystonia. *Journal of Clinical Neurophysiology*, Vol.21, No.1, (January-February 2004), pp. 18-30, ISSN 1537-1603

Krauss, J.K. (2007). Deep Brain Stimulation for Treatment of Cervical Dystonia. (2007). *Acta Neurochirurgica Supplement*, Vol.97, No. Pt 2, (2007), pp. 201-205, ISSN 0065-1419

Krauss, J.K. (2010). Surgical Treatment of Dystonia. *European Journal of Neurology*, Vol.17, No. Supplement 1, (July 2010), pp. 97-101, ISSN 1351-1501

Kunnumpurath, S.; Srinivasagopalan, R. & Vadivelu, N. (2009). Spinal Cord Stimulation: Principles of Past, Present and Future Practice: A Review. *Journal of Clinical Monitoring and Computing*, Vol.23, No.5, (October 2009), pp. 333-339, ISSN 1573-2614

Laitinen, L.V.; Nilsson, S. & Fugl-Meyer, A.R. (1983). Selective Posterior Rhizotomy for Treatment of Spasticity. *Journal of Neurosurgery*, Vol.58, No.6, (June 1983), pp. 895-899, ISSN 0022-3085

Latarjet, A. (1948). *Testut's Traité d'Anatomie Humaine 9th Edition*. G. Doin & Cie, Paris, France

Moore, A.P & Blumhardt, L.D. (1991). A Double Blind Trial of Botulinum Toxin "A" in Torticollis, with One Year Follow Up. *Journal of Neurology Neurosurgery and Psychiatry*, Vol.54, No.9, (September 1991), pp. 813-816, ISSN 0022-3050

Münchau, A.; Palmer, J.D.; Dressler, D.; O'Sullivan, J.D.; Tsang, K.L.; Jahanshahi, M.; Quinn, N.P.; Lees, A.J. & Bhatia, K.P. (2001a). Prospective Study of Selective Peripheral Denervation for Botulinum-Toxin Resistant Patients with Cervical Dystonia. *Brain: A Journal of Neurology*, Vol.124, No.Pt 4, (April 2001), pp. 769-783, ISSN 1460-2156

Münchau, A.; Good, C.D.; McGowan, S.; Quinn, N.P.; Palmer, J.D. & Bhatia, K.P. (2001b). Prospective Study of Swallowing Function in Patients with Cervical Dystonia Undergoing Selective Peripheral Denervation. *Journal of Neurology Neurosurgery and Psychiatry*, Vol.71, No.1, (July 2001), pp. 67-72, ISSN 0022-3050

Nunta-aree, S. & Sitthinamsuwan, B. (2009). Efficacy of Movement Disorder Surgery. In: *Contemporary Medicine 2nd Edition*, Rattanachaiyanont, M. & Tantawichien, T., (Ed), pp. 853-856, P.A. Living Publishing, ISBN 978-974-11-1145-9, Bangkok, Thailand

Nunta-Aree, S.; Sitthinamsuwan, B. & Itthimathin, P. (2010a). Overview and Outcomes of Movement Disorder Surgery. *Neurological Surgery*, Vol.1, No.1, (January-March 2010), pp. 21-26, ISSN 1906-7984

Nunta-aree, S.; Sitthinamsuwan, B.; Nitising, A.; Boonyapisit, K. & Pisarnpong, A. (2010b). Movement Disorder Surgery. In: *Medical Update 2010*, Rattanachaiyanont, M.; Wanachiwanawin, D.; Wisutsareevong, W.; Chinswangwatanakul, V. & Pithukpakorn, M., (Ed), pp. 433-440, P.A. Living Publishing, ISBN 978-974-11-1329-3, Bangkok, Thailand

Ondo, W.G. & Krauss, J.K. (2004). Surgical Therapies for Dystonia. In: *Dystonia: Etiology, Clinical Features, and Treatment*, Brin, M.F.; Comella, C. & Jankovic, J., (Ed.), pp. 125-148, Lippincott Williams & Wilkins, ISBN 0-7817-4114-9, Philadelphia, USA

Ostergaard, L.; Fuglsang-Frederiksen, A.; Sjö, O.; Werdelin, L. & Winkel H. (1996). Quantitative EMG in Cervical Dystonia. *Electromyography and Clinical Neurophysiology*. Vol.36, No.3, (May 1996), pp. 179-185, ISSN 0301-150X

Parkin, S.; Aziz, T.; Gregory, R. & Bain, P. (2001). Bilateral Internal Globus Pallidus Stimulation for the Treatment of Spasmodic Torticollis. *Movement Disorders*, Vol.16, No.3, (May 2001), pp. 489-493, ISSN 1531-8257

Pu, Y.M.; Tang, E.Y. & Yang, X.D. (2008). Trapezius Muscle Innervation from the Spinal Accessory Nerve and Branches of the Cervical Plexus. *International Journal of Oral and Maxillofacial Surgery*, Vol.37, No.6, (June 2008), pp. 567-572, ISSN 1399-0020

Roman, G.J. (1981). *Cunningham's Textbook of Anatomy 12th Edition*. Oxford University Press, ISBN 978-0-192-69031-9, India

Schim, J.D. (2006). Cervical Dystonia Associated with Headache. *Johns Hopkins Advanced Studies in Medicine*, Vol.6, No.9C, (October 2006), pp. S901-903, ISSN 1558-0334

Shiozaki, K.; Abe, S.; Agematsu, H.; Mitarashi, S.; Sakiyama, K.; Hashimoto, M. & Ide, Y. (2007). Anatomical Study of Accessory Nerve Innervation Relating to Functional Neck Dissection. *Journal of Oral and Maxillofacial Surgery*, Vol.65, No.1, (January 2007), pp. 22-29, ISSN 1531-5053

Sitthinamsuwan, B. & Nunta-aree, S. (2010). Functional Peripheral Nerve Surgery. *Siriraj Medical Journal*, Vol.62, No.2, (March-April 2010), pp. 106-111, ISSN 2228-8082

Sitthinamsuwan, B.; Nunta-Aree, S. & Itthimathin, P. (2010a). Neurosurgery for Spasticity. In: *20th Year Anniversary Scientific Congress of Sirindhorn National Medical Rehabilitation Center (SNMRC)*, Solanda, S., (Ed), pp. 113-130, Funny Publishing, ISBN 978-974-422-593-1,Bangkok, Thailand

Sitthinamsuwan, B.; Chanvanitkulchai, K.; Nunta-aree, S.; Kumthornthip, W.; Pisarnpong, A. & Ploypetch, T. (2010b). Combined Ablative Neurosurgical Procedures in a Patient with Mixed Spastic and Dystonic Cerebral Palsy. *Stereotactic and Functional Neurosurgery*, Vol.3, (May 2010), pp. 187-192, ISSN 1524-4040

Sitthinamsuwan, B.; Parnnang, C.; Nunta-Aree, S.; Chankaew, E. & Papatthanaporn, A. (2010c). An Innovation of Intraoperative Electrical Nerve Stimulator. *Neurological Surgery*, Vol.1, No.3, (July-September 2010), pp. 65-82, ISSN 1906-7984

Sorensen, B.F. & Hamby, W.B. (1965). Spasmodic Torticollis. Result in 71 Surgically Treated Patients. *The Journal of The American Medical Association*. Vol.194, No.7, (1965), pp. 706-708, ISSN 1538-3598

Spitz, M.; Goncalves, L.; Silveira, L. & Barbosa E. (2006). Myelopathy as a Complication of Cervical Dystonia. *Movement Disorders*, Vol.21, No.5, (May 2006), pp. 726-727, ISSN 0885-3185

Stacey, R.J.; O'Leary, S.T. & Hamlyn, P.J. (1995). The Innervation of the Trapezius Muscle: A Cervical Motor Supply. *Journal of Cranio-maxillo-facial Surgery*, Vol.23, No.4, (August 1995), pp. 250-251, ISSN 1878-4119

Sun, K.; Lu, Y.; Hu, G.; Luo, C.; Hou, L.; Chen, J.; Wu, X. & Mei, Q. (2009). Microvascular Decompression of the Accessory Nerve for Treatment of Spasmodic Torticollis: Early Results in 12 Cases. *Acta Neurochirurgica*, Vol.151, No.10, (October 2009), pp. 1251-1257, ISSN 0942-0940

Sung, D.H.; Choi, J.Y.; Kim, D.H.; Kim, E.S.; Son, Y.I.; Cho, Y.S.; Lee, S.J.; Lee, K.H. & Kim, B.T. (2007). Localization of Dystonic Muscles with 18F-FDG PET/CT in Idiopathic Cervical Dystonia. *Journal of Nuclear Medicine*, Vol.48, No.11, (November 2007), pp. 1790-1795, ISSN 1535-5667

Taira, T, & Hori, T. (2001). Peripheral Neurotomy for Torticollis: A New Approach. *Stereotactic and Functional Neurosurgery*, Vol.77, No.1-4, (2001), pp. 40-43, ISSN 1423-0372

Taira, T.; Kobayashi, T.; Takahashi, K. & Hori, T. (2002). A New Denervation Procedure for Idiopathic Cervical Dystonia. *Journal of Neurosurgery*, Vol.97, No.2 Supplement, (September 2002), pp. 201-206, ISSN 0022-3085

Taira, T. & Hori, T. (2003). A Novel Denervation Procedure for Idiopathic Cervical Dystonia. *Stereotactic and Functional Neurosurgery*, Vol.80, No.1-4, (2003), pp. 92-95, ISSN 1423-0372

Taira, T.; Kobayashi, T. & Hori, T. (2003). Selective Peripheral Denervation of the Levator Scapulae Muscle for Laterocollic Cervical Dystonia. *Journal of Clinical Neuroscience*, Vol.10, No.4, (July 2003), pp. 449-452, ISSN 1532-2653

Taira, T.; Ochiai, T.; Koto, S. & Hori, T. (2006). Multimodal Neurosurgical Strategies for the Management of Dystonias. *Acta Neurochirurgica Supplement*, Vol.99, (2006), pp. 29-31, ISSN 0065-1419

Taira, T & Hori, T. (2007). Intrathecal Baclofen in the Treatment of Post-Stroke Central Pain, Dystonia, and Persistent Vegetative State. *Acta Neurochirurgica Supplement*, Vol.97, No.Pt 1, (2007), pp. 227-229, ISSN 0065-1419

Taira T. Peripheral Procedures for Cervical Dystonia. (2009). In: *Textbook of Stereotactic and Functional Neurosurgery 2nd Edition*, Lozano, A.M.; Gildenberg, P.L. & Tasker, R.R., (Ed), pp. 1885-1909, Springer, ISBN 978-3-540-69959-0, Retrieved from http://www.springer.com/medicine/surgery/book/978-3-540-69959-0

Tonomura, Y.; Kataoka, H.; Sugie, K.; Hirabayashi, H.; Nakase, H. & Ueno, S. (2007). Atlantoaxial Rotatory Subluxation Associated with Cervical Dystonia. *Spine*, Vol.32, No.19, (September 2007), pp. E561-E564, ISSN 0362-2436

Tsui, J.K.; Eisen, A.; Stoessl, A.J.; Calne, S. & Calne, D.B. (1986). Double-Blind Study of Botulinum Toxin in Spasmodic Torticollis. *Lancet*, Vol.2, No.8501, (August 1986), pp. 245-247, ISSN 1474-547X

Tubbs, R.S.; Loukas, M.; Slappey, J.B.; Shoja, M.M.; Oakes, W.J. & Salter, E.G. (2007). Clinical Anatomy of the C1 Dorsal Root, Ganglion, and Ramus: A Review and Anatomical Study. *Clinical Anatomy*, Vol.20, No.6, (August 2007), pp. 624-627, ISSN 1098-2353

Vercueil, L. (2003). Fifty Years of Brain Surgery for Dystonia: Revisiting The Irving S. Cooper's legacy, and Looking Forward. *Acta Neurologica Belgica,* Vol.103, No.3, (September 2003), pp. 125-8, ISSN 0300-9009

Vogel, T.D.; Pendleton, C.; Quinoñes-Hinojosa, A. & Cohen-Gadol, A.A. (2010). Surgery for Cervical Dystonia: the Emergence of Denervation and Myotomy Techniques and the Contributions of Early Surgeons at The Johns Hopkins Hospital. *Journal of Neurosurgery Spine,* Vol.12, No.3, (March 2010), pp. 280-285, ISSN 1547-5654

Volkmann, J. & Benecke, R. (2002). Deep Brain Stimulation for Dystonia: Patient Selection and Evaluation. *Movement Disorders,* Vol.17, No. Supplement 3, (2002), pp. S112-5, ISSN 1531-8257

Waterston, J.A.; Swash, M., & Watkins, E.S. (1989). Idiopathic Dystonia and Cervical Spondylotic Myelopathy. *Journal of Neurology Neurosurgery and Psychiatry,* Vol.52, No.12, (December 1989), pp. 1424-1426, ISSN 0022-3050

Xinkang, C. (1981). Selective Resection and Denervation of Cervical Muscles in the Treatment of Spasmodic Torticollis: results in 60 cases. *Neurosurgery,* Vol.8, No.6, (June 1981), pp. 680-688, ISSN 1524-4040

Yianni, J.; Bain, P.G.; Gregory, R.P.; Nandi, D.; Joint, C.; Scott, R.B.; Stein, J.F. & Aziz, T.Z. (2003). Post-operative Progress of Dystonia Patients Following Globus Pallidus Internus Deep Brain Stimulation. *European Journal of Neurology,* Vol.10, No.3, (May 2003), pp. 239–247, ISSN 1468-1331

Zhao, W.; Sun, J.; Zheng, J.W.; Li, J.; He, Y. & Zhang, Z.Y. (2006). Innervation of the Trapezius Muscle: Is Cervical Contribution Important to Its Function? *Otolaryngology and Head and Neck Surgery,* Vol.135, No.5, (November 2006), pp. 758–764, ISSN 1097-6817

13

Dystonia and Muscle Spindles: The Link in Idiopathic Focal Dystonias

Richard Grünewald
Department of Neurology,
Sheffield Teaching Hospitals NHS Foundation Trust,
Royal Hallamshire Hospital, Sheffield
UK

1. Introduction

Idiopathic focal dystonia (IFD) is the commonest type of dystonia, characterised by more or less fixed abnormalities of posture, involuntary movements and muscular spasm. Published estimates of prevalence vary [1-4]. The condition appears to run in families [5]. As certain groups, such as musicians, seem to be at much higher risk [6, 7], it would seem that one or more common genes with low penetrance may be responsible, but such genes interact with physical factors, overuse being one. Damage to several different brain areas, including the basal ganglia, has been associated with secondary dystonia [8]. This, and the lack of demonstrable neurodegeneration, has contributed to the idea that the pathophysiology of IFD relates to subtle abnormalities of the circuits between cerebral cortex and basal ganglia [9], perhaps involving defective sensory processing, abnormal central nervous system excitability or loss of inhibition of motor control. Some authors have hypothesized a deficiency in a specific class of brain interneurons [10].

Experiments based on research that has been undertaken at the University of Sheffield over the last 14 years [11-14] have demonstrated that there is a predisposing proprioceptive sensory abnormality in subjects with dystonia. Fatigue-induced distortion of the proprioceptive feedback subserved by muscle spindles appears to characterise the condition. The primary abnormality in IFD is likely to be a physical property of muscle spindles, specialised stretch receptors present in skeletal muscle, which are responsible for signalling to the brain proprioceptive information about body position, velocity, muscle load, fatigue and muscular effort. Our experiments do not suggest a primary abnormality of sensory processing in the neural networks of the brain. Instead the experiments imply that the abnormality is in the genetically determined, elastic property of muscle spindles that produces distortion of feedback when the muscle spindles are over-stretched. It is plausible that this endophenotype interacts with other predispositions, such as other genes which predispose to generalised dystonia (for example DYT1), the effects of drugs such as those which block dopamine receptors in the brain, or disorders of the basal ganglia, such as idiopathic parkinson's disease, to produce the dystonic phenotype. The evidence, its interpretation and the resulting hypothetical pathophyisological basis for IFD are discussed below.

2. Clinical features and what they tell us about dystonia

IFD (e.g. torticollis, blepharospasm, writer's cramp and other dystonias affecting localised areas of the body) involves abnormality of posture or positioning of part of the body. A hypothesis to account for the underlying mechanisms of IFD must account for the clinical features of the condition:

1. The commonest form, neck dystonia, is "task-independent", but many dystonias may be apparent only with particular learned movements (so-called task-specfic dystonia). For example, a patient may develop dystonic posturing of the hand whilst typing but not whilst playing the piano, despite the same muscles being involved (although there may be a tendency for the dystonia gradually to evolve and interfere with more tasks). This implies that the condition involves corruption of sensorimotor programming specific to particular learned activities, rather than an abnormality of the motor control of specific muscle groups.
2. After treatment of neck dystonia with botulinum toxin, patients may return to the clinic with weakness of head rotation in one direction as an effect of the treatment. Despite the imbalance in the strength of the muscles of the neck, the postural abnormal posture at rest may persist, though it may be easier for the patient to correct voluntarily. Another feature of idiopathic focal dystonia that has to be accounted for in models of the disorder, is the phenomenon of the '*geste antagonistique*', the relief of the abnormal posture, typically in patients with cervical dystonia, by touching, or approximating, the affected part with the patient's own hand. The *geste antagonistique* does not involve physical force to oppose muscle spasm. These observations imply that dystonia involves a problem with proprioceptive feedback, and the pathophysiology is likely to involve the way the brain senses body posture, i.e. to involve proprioception.
3. Contrary to some assertions in the literature, IFD does not necessarily involve co-contraction of agonist and antagonist muscles (though this is usual when the patient tries to achieve function with the affected body part). With hand dystonias, especially in early stages, a single muscle, such as the extensor of the index finger, may be over-active during the dystonic movement. Hand and arm dystonia is often highly task-specific initially, though there is a tendency for the dystonia gradually to evolve to affect other skilled movements, at least to some extent. These features imply a role of abnormal motor learning in the pathophysiology of IFD.

We can conclude that the essential clinical features imply that IFD is a disorder of the way posture and learned movement is programmed by the central nervous system, rather than spasm, inadequate inhibition or overactivity of a muscle or group of muscles.

3. A disorder of the basal ganglia?

A common concept is that dystonia is primarily a disorder of the basal ganglia and its connections. This is based partly on the observation that pathology in the basal ganglia, such as vascular insult, neurodegenerative disorders and kernicterus, can sometimes lead to types of dystonia. This type of dystonia differs from IFD in that it is constant, "task-independent", and affects large contiguous areas of the body. In contrast, no structural or biochemical abnormality has been demonstrated in association with IFD, and the subjects with the condition generally retain high skill levels in the dystonic limb when undertaking tasks which do not trigger the dystonia (for example, musicians with IFD can often write without difficulty or play another musical instrument without dystonia). There is therefore little reason to postulate that structural abnormalities of the basal ganglia are the prime cause of IFD. However, the observation of improvement of IFD after neurosurgical implantation and stimulation of electrodes in the corpus striatum suggest that basal ganglia may have an important role in the generation of dystonia.

Physiological abnormalities of the brain and spinal cord have been documented in subjects with IFD. Interpretation of such abnormalities is problematic - some may represent adaptive changes in response to the presence of dystonic muscle contractions rather than being related to processes that predispose to, and antedate, the development of dystonia. Physiological abnormalities that are found bilaterally in subjects with unilateral dystonia and in areas of the nervous system that serve parts of the body remote from the site of dystonia are less likely to be adaptive and more likely to reflect predisposing factors. Such predisposing abnormalities include reduced short latency intracortical inhibition [15]. Increased excitability of the motor cortex during voluntary muscle contraction [16], and excessive excitability of primary motor cortex upon magnetic stimulation [17] are not invariably found in dystonic subjects. Abnormalities in the 'silent period' of electromyographic activity following transcranial magnetic stimulation (TMS) and of long interval intracortical inhibition assessed by paired suprathreshold transcranial magnetic stimulation pulses have been documented, but are restricted to the symptomatic hand [18,19] as are inhibitory effects in TMS threshold on peripheral nerve stimulation [20]. In the spinal cord there is also abnormal excitability, demonstrable by reduced reciprocal inhibition of forearm H reflexes [21-23]. The importance of such abnormalities in the pathophysiology of IFD is undermined by the demonstration of similar abnormalities in psychogenic dystonia [24]. Such phenomena remain difficult to interpret and translate into a coherent theory of IFD pathophysiology.

Subtle sensory abnormalities have also been demonstrated in IFD and in asymptomatic relatives, including reduced tactile spatial discrimination [25]. The sensory pathways involved in such perception are complex and such observations, whilst of undoubted importance, do not in themselves clarify the understanding of the pathophysiology of the condition.

4. Muscle spindles, proprioception and basal ganglia in movement control

It has been known since the 1970's that stretch receptors within skeletal muscle, the muscle spindles, subserve proprioceptive sensation [26], and since it is apparent that IFD involves a prioprioceptive problem it makes sense to examine muscle spindle responses in IFD. A review of the role of muscle spindles in dystonia has been published [27].

The function of muscle spindles is complex [28]. In a situation of maintained posture, muscle spindle stretch reflects muscle load, and signals to the brain how to vary drive to the skeletal muscle to maintain the posture. If the muscle is contracted voluntarily, this shortens the muscle spindle stretch receptor, 'unloading' it. The resulting loss of proprioceptive information would be catastrophic for maintenance of posture. To circumvent this, each muscle spindle has its own muscle and nerve supply (fig 3). When a muscle contracts voluntarily, the intrafusal muscle of the muscle spindle simultaneously contracts (so-called alpha gamma co-activation) to maintain muscle spindle stretch, thus maintaining sensitivity to changes in applied load.

In order to undertake willed movement the brain has to appreciate body position, posture, centre of gravity and velocity so as to maintain balance during movement. This relies mainly on proprioceptive information with some contribution from visual or vestibular feedback. To determine hand position relative to the body, activity from muscle spindles of the forearm and hand must be interpreted in the context of in the context of proprioceptive proprioceptive information from muscle spindles situated more proximally, in the upper arm, shoulder and neck. All this information has to be integrated with that from the legs and trunk, interpreted in the context of the afferent volleys to the intrafusal fibres, for the body to maintain posture and balance during a hand movement. Muscle spindles also encode information about muscle fatigue [29, 30].

It is likely that a major function of the basal ganglia is to interpret muscle spindle feedback to facilitate maintenance of posture and balance in the face of superimposed willed movements. This is consistent with the observation that most neurones of the globus pallidus interna are sensitive to passive movement [31]. In broad conceptual terms, extrapyramidal systems may dominate control of posture and balance, are inhibited focally during superimposed voluntary movement, and re-established when the movement is completed.

5. What is the evidence that muscle spindles are involved in dystonia?

Muscle or muscle tendon vibration at a rate of 50-100 cycles a second produces a tendency for that muscle to contract (known as the 'tonic vibration reflex' [29]). It also produces a sensation of movement of the vibrated limb that is not dependent on physical movement of the limb, known as the vibration-induced illusion of movement. This is likely to be caused by stimulation of the muscle spindle afferents near the vibrator [32]. This phenomenon enables quantitative study of muscle spindle function in human subjects.

Our experimental protocol involved a subject sitting with elbows resting on a table and with one arm resting relaxed in a splint to stop it moving. The splint maintained the elbow joint at approximately a right angle. The subject was blindfolded to remove visual feedback of arm position and the biceps tendon was vibrated at 50 to 100 cycles a second. This produced a feeling of slow extension of the arm around the elbow joint, the 'vibration induced illusion of movement', despite the arm being fixed in a splint. This sensation results from the brain interpreting the vibration-induced muscle spindle afferent volleys from the biceps muscle as the biceps being stretched. Since the arm is relaxed, the brain infers that the muscle spindle afferent discharge from the biceps implies that the arm is extending at the elbow (if the arm were actively maintaining a posture the vibration induced muscle spindle afferent activity would be interpreted as an increased load on the muscle, the basis of the tonic vibration reflex).

We quantified this illusion by asking the experimental subject to match the movement felt in the vibrated arm using the opposite arm which was free to move. Movement of the 'tracking' arm in 45 seconds was recorded using a digital camera. These simple experiments demonstrated that in subjects with IFD, the vibration-induced illusion of movement is reliably *subnormal* [12], figure 1. This abnormal perception occurs all over the body, in parts unaffected by IFD as well as parts that are [11]. It is found in patients who have received treatment with botulinum toxin and those who have not, implying that it is not a phenomenon associated with treatment or spread of botulinum toxin. It thus appears to represent a factor that predisposes to IFD [14]. Initially we interpreted this as an abnormality of interpretation of the sensory information from the muscle spindles somewhere in the central nervous sensory pathways to the cerebral cortex. However, a second series of experiments made us revise this view.

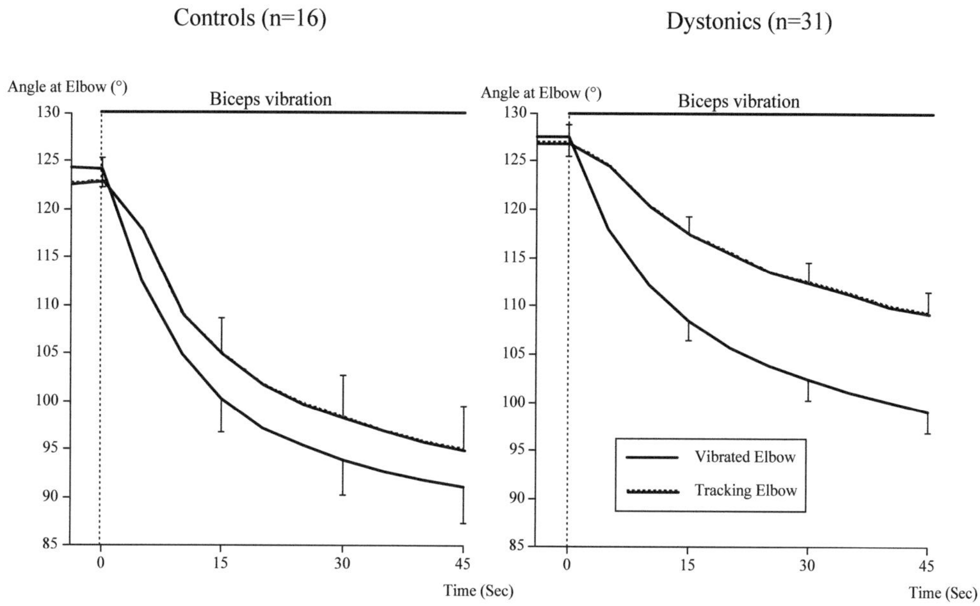

Fig. 1. The tonic vibration reflex differs in dystonic subjects and controls. Mean angular displacement of the elbow vibrated arm and tracking arm in the groups of healthy control subjects and dystonic subjects on stimulation of the biceps brachii tendon. The tonic vibration reflex is similar in both groups, but the tracking movements are smaller in the dystonic patients.

6. The vibration-induced illusion of movement and fatigue

Subjects with and without IFD were required repeatedly to lift a dumbbell with the arm we were going to vibrate until they could lift it no longer, and then immediately slip the arm back into the splint [13]. We then immediately retested the vibration-induced illusion of movement, vibrating the fatigued biceps tendon.

Immediately after fatigue the vibration-induced illusion of movement in the subjects with IFD *increased* so that it was now similar to normal subjects. This was temporary - the effect only lasted as long as the biceps remained fatigued. In contrast, the healthy control subjects *showed no change* in the vibration-induced illusion of movement with muscle fatigue (figure 2).

It is difficult to imagine how the manoeuvre of lifting a dumbbell a dozen or so times could have any effect on the way in which the central nervous system processes sensory information. It is easier to imagine a direct effect on peripheral muscle. Lifting a dumbbell until the muscle fails physically stretches the muscle spindles to their physiological limit. We were attracted by the idea that we were likely to be looking at an effect of lifting the dumbbell on the elastic properties of the muscle spindles themselves. Muscle spindles thixotropic properties are critical to their function as stretch receptors [32]. A simple explanation is that the muscle spindles in dystonic subjects are stiffer than those in normal subjects, but become more elastic after they are over-stretched, rather like an elastic band when warmed by stretching.

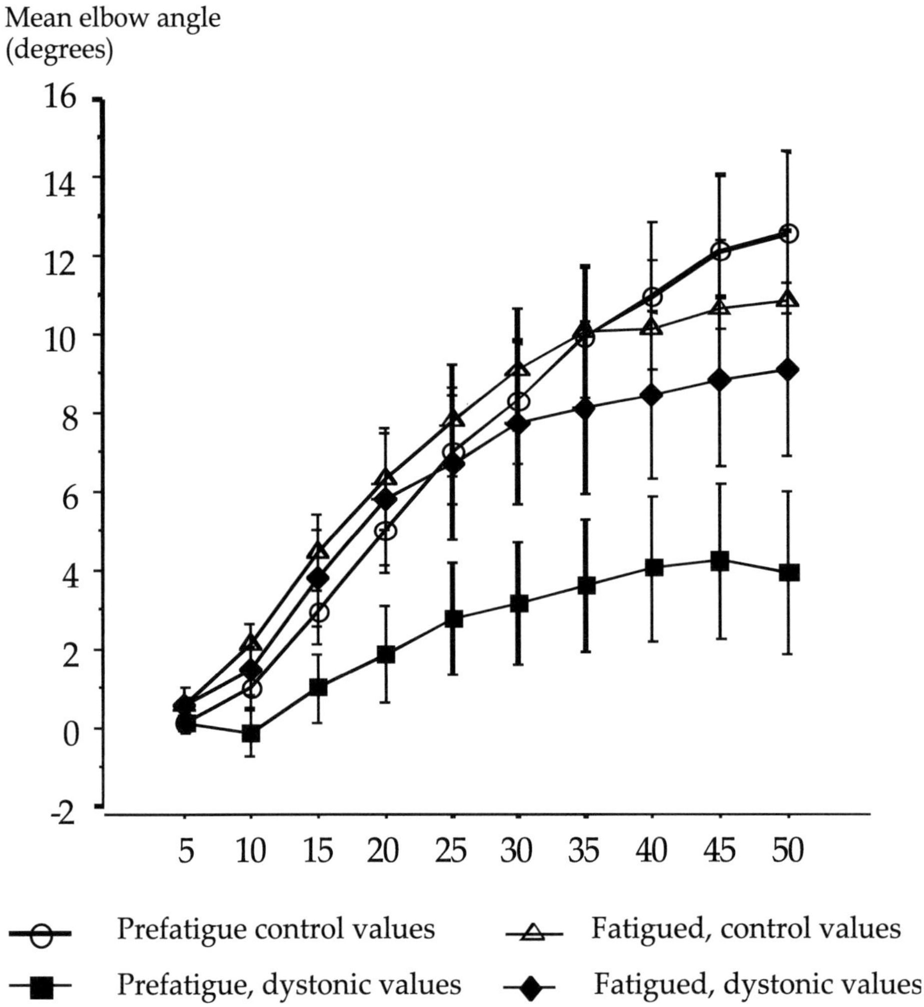

Fig. 2. Assessment of the vibration-induced illusion of movement in dystonic and healthy control subjects. Extension of the tracking arm in response to 50Hz vibration of opposite biceps tendon over 50s in ten dystonic and 10 healthy control subjects. Dystonic subjects (black squares) show significantly less extension of the tracking arm than healthy subjects (white circles), implying subnormal vibration-induced illusion of movement. When the vibrated arm is fatigued after lifting a dumbbell (black diamonds), the vibration-induced illusion of movement improves to become indistinguishable from control subjects. In contrast, fatigue does not affect the vibration-induced illusion of movement in control subjects (white diamonds).

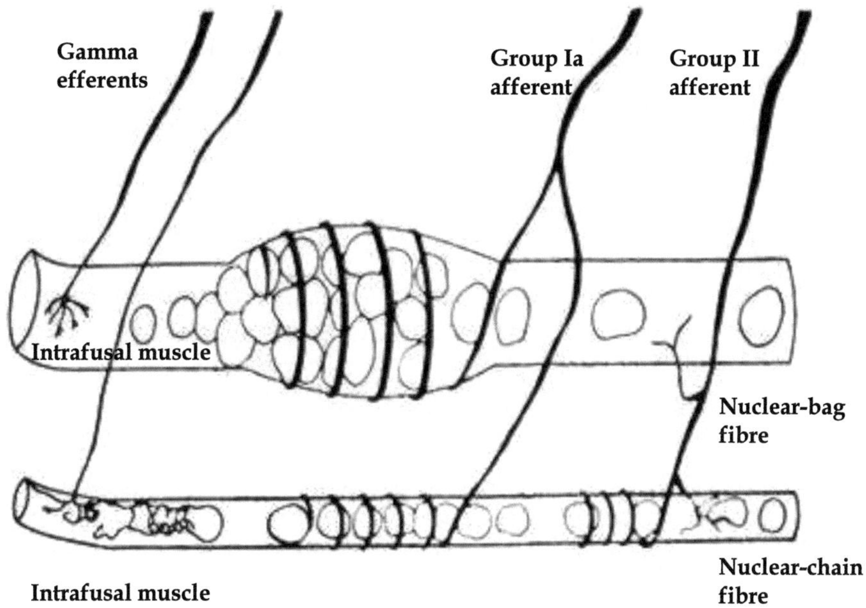

Fig. 3. Diagram of a muscle spindle (after Matthews, 1972). Muscle spindle afferents provide information on position, load, fatigue and effort that are integrated by the nervous system to ensure the maintenance of posture and balance during a willed movement. Interpretation of this afferent activity has to be undertaken in the context of gamma efferent discharge, which contracts intrafusal muscle fibres of the spindle and increases the afferent discharge frequency. This is necessary in order to maintain the sensitivity of the spindles to applied load when the surrounding skeletal muscle contracts.

The idea that a peripheral muscular abnormality such as the mechanical properties of muscles spindles predispose to the development of IFD, and represents a significant change in the way we think about dystonia, hitherto considered a disorder of higher central nervous system functioning. The observation that limb cooling improves IFD is also consistent with the suggestion that it is a disorder generated in the periphery [33].

An implication of this experiment is that IFD develops when the brain attempts to use information from muscle spindles that changes disproportionately that changes disproportionately as muscles fatigue. Writer's cramp, musician's cramp, and other occupational dystonias such as those which effect sports players, occur in muscle groups which are used repeatedly when practising a particular skill so that the subject will be learning the movement sequence whilst the muscle is fatigued. In contrast to normal subjects, the relationship between body position and muscle spindle afferent information in dystonic subjects differs in the fatigued state from the unfatigued state (figure 4). This provides insight into why dystonic subjects may develop involuntary muscle spasm with learned movements [35].

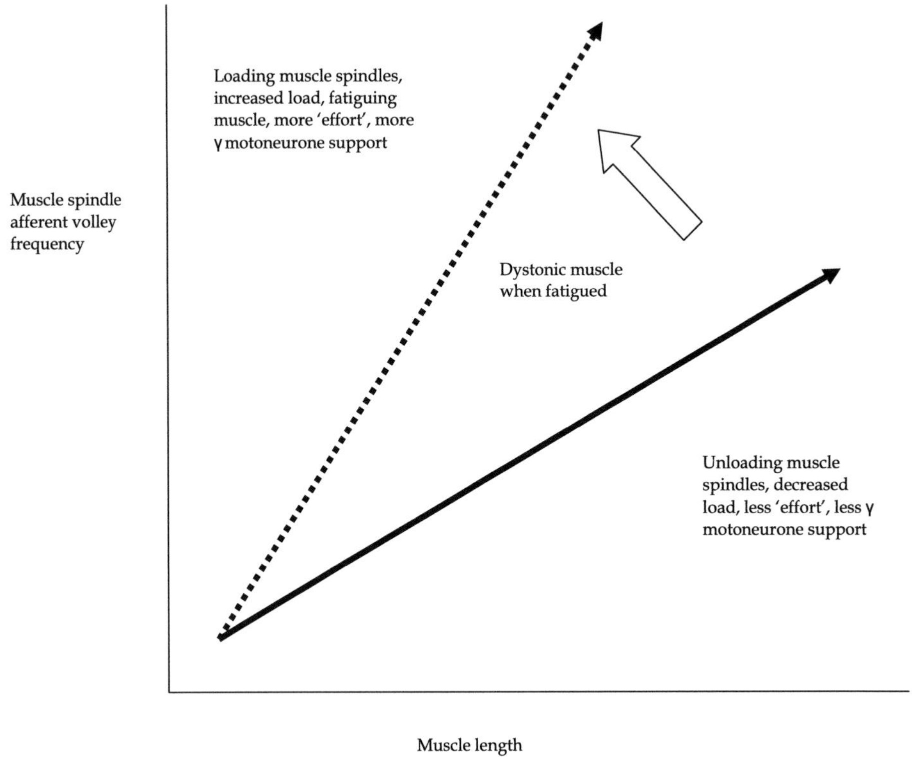

Fig. 4. Factors which influence muscle spindle afferent activity. In healthy subjects the nervous system can interpret changes in muscle spindle afferent activity in terms of load and position. In dystonic subjects the relationship between muscle spindle stretch and afferent discharge becomes steeper after fatigue. In such circumstances the increase in muscle spindle afferent activity is interpreted as weakening of the surrounding muscle. This corrupts the motor program for overlearned movements of the limb, causing muscles to be driven excessively (i.e. dystonic spasm).

7. Role of muscle spindles in motor learning and the evolution of symptoms

Writing is a motor skill which is commonly affected in IFD. The skill of writing is sophisticated. We can write using a variety of materials on surfaces of variable texture, and our signature will usually remain recognisable throughout. Writing can be undertaken without visual feedback and scaled as required. The movements of the hand whilst writing have to be able to adapt to different resistance to the movement of the pen and the size of the letters required. This implies that the motor subroutines of writing involve proprioceptive feedback. If affected by writer's cramp, the grip of the pen becomes abnormal soon after writing starts and the effort required to control writing increases. Pain in the hand or arm results as muscles contract to control the hand as writing posture becomes distorted.

The patterns of movements required to write seem likely to be stored in motor memory as a pattern of proprioceptive feedback (possibly in frontostriatal circuits) from arm and hand during the neuronal acitivity driving the muscles involved in writing. In order to control the pen, the brain must continuously compare proprioceptive feedback with efferent volleys in order to adapt to resistance to movement of the pen and the fatigue of the muscles involved in writing. The relationships between the effort to drive muscles and the feedback from muscle spindles is continuously over-learned as motor skills are repeated or practiced.

In dystonic subjects, afferent muscle spindle activity increases disproportionately as writing occurs whilst muscles fatigue. Increased muscle spindle afferent discharge is interpreted by the brain as meaning either increased load or weakening muscle, i.e. an increase in effort or drive to the muscle is required (figure 4). Since increased muscle spindle afferent activity for a particular muscle position implies to the brain that the muscle is disproportionately fatiguing, the motor 'subroutine' for that movement adapts to one appropriate for an excessively weakened or fatigued muscle. This results in the corrupted motor subroutine for that movement over-driving the affected muscle group when the motor subroutine is activated. The dystonic subject sees this as spasm or over-activity of particular muscles involved in the learned movement.

Thus, the abnormalities of the vibration induce illusion of movement suggest a mechanism whereby motor subroutines become corrupted when movements are over-learned in the fatigued state. This provides an explanation for why IFD symptoms tend to affect skilled and heavily practiced movements. It also may explain why sometimes dystonic symptoms evolve with time [35,36]. For example dystonia dystonia may affect writing, then perhaps involve typing or holding a cup. When learning a manual motor skill, abnormally enhanced fatigue resulting from attempts to counter the dystonic muscle spasm places extra stress on the other muscles of the hand involved in the movement. Other muscles, therefore, fatigue more rapidly when the motor subroutines for writing are activated (which is felt as the 'cramp' of writer's cramp). As writing continues, other muscles of the hand fatigue faster than normal, and as with continued motor learning in this state the motor subroutines of other muscles become corrupted and dystonia evolves. This may explain why injuries, myasthenia and spinal scoliosis may occasionally precipitate IFD. The phenomenon may also explain the tendency of the geste antagonistique to disappear with time. As a greater proportion of neck muscles provide corrupted proprioceptive information to the basal ganglia as the dystonia evolve, the contribution of 'correct' proprioceptive input obtained by touching the affected part with the hand may become relatively less influential.

8. Why is cervical dystonia the commonest IFD?

Although this is a plausible explanation for the development of writer's cramp or occupational dystonias where motor activity is practiced in the fatigued state, it provides no explanation for the most common dystonia, that of the neck (torticollis).

Assuming that the same principal of fatigue-induced distortion of muscle spindle feedback leads to abnormal of motor programming in cervical dystonia, a plausible explanation of the development of torticollis is that a twisted posture and poorly supported neck during sleep might result in asymmetric patterns of fatigue, and corruption of the motor program to position the head straight.

9. What is the physical substrate of abnormal muscle spindle function in IFD?

A plausible explanation is that in individuals with a predisposition to IFD the muscle spindles have abnormal elastic, or more precisely 'thixotropic', properties (see reference 31 for a review of the topic). In order to reflect optimally how the surrounding muscle is moving, the elastic properties of muscle spindles must match the surrounding muscle. The simplest explanation of the abnormal vibration-induced illusion of movement in dystonic subjects is that the muscle spindles are too stiff, and are therefore relatively insensitive to any change in muscle load.

For the most part the elastic properties of the muscle spindles are not critical to motor control, as the neural networks learn the relationship between movement and the feedback from muscle spindles with practice as motor skills develop. Indeed the learning of the relationship between proprioceptive feedback and movement occurs as we practice movement from birth onwards. Subjects with IFD are therefore not generally clumsy before the onset of dystonia. In IFD it is not only that the muscle spindles too stiff, but rather that their elastic properties change as they are stretched, as demonstrated by the change in perception of the vibration-induced illusion of movement with muscle fatigue, which poses problems for motor learning. It is the inconstancy of elastic properties of the dystonic muscle spindle that leads to the corruption of the motor subroutine.

10. Inheritance of the trait and the endophenotype

We examined the vibration-induced illusion of movement in both patients with IFD, members of their family and in unrelated healthy subjects [14]. First degree relatives of those with dystonia had a higher rate of abnormal vibration-induced illusion of movement than control subjects. This implied that the vibration induced illusion of movement was a true endophenotype.

Thus, abnormal thixotropy of the muscle spindles is likely to be determined genetically. It may be, for example, that the elastic properties of the muscle spindles are determined by genetically determined structural properties of the muscle spindles.

Our experiments revealed that many people who inherit the abnormal vibration-induced illusion of movement do not develop dystonia. Of the other genes which are involved in dystonia, the best defined, DYT1, has low penetrance, with only about one third of those with the gene abnormality developing the disorder. It is likely that this gene interacts with others to producing dystonia, and it is plausible that patients with DYT1 only develop symptoms if they happen also to inherit abnormal vibration-induced illusion of movement as well. Whilst consistent with our own observations, we have not systematically studied asymptomatic families with DYT1 to confirm this observation. How genes other than those which are involved in the vibration induced illusion of movement influence the pathophysiology of dystonia is unclear. Some genes involved in the dystonic phenotype may act peripherally, at the level of the muscle spindle, whereas others may act centrally to influence, say, flexibility of motor learning.

11. What about tremor?

Many people with dystonia have an associated tremor, and tremor may be commoner in first degree family members [37,38]. For this reason we looked at whether other people with tremor had abnormal vibration-induced illusion of movement [39]. About half of people with apparently 'essential' tremor and no family history of dystonia showed the same abnormality of the vibration-induced illusion of movement as those with IFD.

The maintenance of posture is an active process involving feedback from muscle spindles to the brain. If the muscle spindle thixotropic properties are abnormal this may be expected distort the phase of their feedback response to perturbation of the posture. If phase of the feedback is so delayed as to reinforce rather than damp the perturbation, tremor may result. We have suggested that the increased prevalence of tremor with age might be related to age-related changes in elastic properties of muscle spindles. That essential tremor is suppressed by limb cooling supports the notion that peripheral factors are involved in its generation [40].

12. Why do only some subjects with the endophenotype develop symptoms?

The relationship between afferent feedback and efferent drive changes as limbs grow and muscle strength changes, so some flexibility in motor learning is essential. On the other hand, to develop exquisitely refined skills, such as those of a musician or athlete, such learning must result in precise, reliable and stable motor subroutines. The nervous system therefore has to provide both for plasticity and consistency. It may be that abnormal plasticity demonstrated in dystonic subjects by the abnormalities of cortical and spinal neural inhibition facilitate corruption of established motor programmes by distorted muscle spindle feedback, but represent no more than an extreme of a continuum of normal motor plasticity of the nervous system.

I propose that the development of IFD requires both an abnormality of muscle spindle thixotropy and an abnormality of neural inhibition or plasticity of the cortical and spinal pathways involved in motor learning to produce the phenotype [41,42]. If the former only is present, the endophenotype may be asymptomatic or result in tremor only, but if there are abnormalities of cortical plasticity the motor subroutines are more readily corrupted by overlearning of motor subroutines in the fatigued state using distorted muscle spindle feedback.

13. Conclusions

The hypothesis within this paper is based on the premise that there is an underlying proprioceptive disorder in subjects predisposed to IFD caused by abnormal thoixotropic properties of the muscle spindles. Testable predictions which follow from this hypothesis include:

1. that a gene contributing to the phenotype will code for a structural muscle spindle protein,
2. that adequate head support in sleep might prevent cervical dystonia in predisposed individuals or reduce its progression,
3. that abnormalities of sensorimotor integration in IFD will be interpretable mainly in terms of abnormal proprioception, and
4. that despite symptomatic improvement, deep brain stimulation treatment of dystonia will have little effect on the abnormal vibration-induced illusion of movement of patients with IFD.

The interaction between this endophenotype and the other genes identified as associated with dystonia is intriguing as are the insights that these processes provide into the functioning of the motor systems in health and disease. The substantial literature on abnormal sensorimotor integration in dystonia is difficult to interpret in this context, as physiological abnormalities such as reduced tactile discrimination are complex perceptions involving many different sensory modalities, but these observations should trigger a re-interpretation of some of the experimental evidence which has accumulated concerning this intriguing disorder.

14. Acknowledgements

I should like to thank the research workers involved in this work over the years, including Prof Harvey Sagar, Dr Yuki Yonada, Dr Susan Rome and Dr Nausika Frima, for their invaluable contributions and enthusiasm for the work.

15. References

[1] A prevalence study of primary dystonia in eight European countries. Journal of Neurology 2000; , 247: 787-792

[2] J. Müller, MD, S. Kiechl, MD, G. K. Wenning, MD, K. Seppi, MD, J. Willeit, MD, A. Gasperi, MD, J. Wissel, MD, T. Gasser, MD and W. Poewe, The prevalence of primary dystonia in the general community. Neurology 2002; 59 (6): 941-943.

[3] C. Marras, MD, S. K. Van den Eeden, PhD, R. D. Fross, MD, K. S. Benedict-Albers, MPH, J. Klingman, MD, A. D. Leimpeter, MS, L. M. Nelson, PhD, N. Risch, PhD, A. J. Karter, PhD, A. L. Bernstein, MD and C. M. Tanner, MD, PhD. Minimum incidence of primary cervical dystonia in a multiethnic health care population. Neurology 2007; 69 (7): 676-680.

[4] Khanh-Dung Le, Beate Nilsen and Espen Dietrichs. Prevalence of primary focal and segmental dystonia in Oslo. Neurology 2003; 61 (9): 1294-1296.

[5] Leube B, Kessler KR, Goecke T, Auburger G, Benecke R. Frequency of familial inheritance among 488 index patients with idiopathic focal dystonia and clinical variability in a large family. Mov Disord. 1997;12(6):1000-6.

[6] Nutt JG, Muenter MD, Melton LJ, Aronson A, Kurland LT Epidemiology of dystonia in Rochester, Minnesota. Adv Neurol 1988; 50:361–365.

[7] Altenmüller E. Focal dystonia: advances in brain imaging and understanding of fine motor control in musicians. Hand Clin 2003; 19:523–538.

[8] Loher TJ, Krauss JK. Dystonia associated with pontomesencephalic lesions. Mov Disord. 2009; 24(2):157-67.

[9] Jerrold L. Vitek, Pathophysiology of Dystonia: A Neuronal Model. Movement Disorders 2002; 17 (supl.3): S49–S62.

[10] Hallett M. Neurophysiology of dystonia: The role of inhibition. Neurobiology of Disease 2011; 42 (2): 177-184.

[11] RA Grunewald, Y Yoneda, JM Shipman and HJ Sagar Idiopathic focal dystonia: a disorder of muscle spindle afferent processing? Brain 1997; 120 (12): 2179-2185.

[12] S. Rome and R. A. Grünewald. Abnormal perception of vibration-induced illusion of movement in dystonia. Neurology 1999; 53: 1794-1800.

[13] N Frima, S M Rome, R A Grünewald. The effect of fatigue on abnormal vibration-induced illusion of movement in idiopathic focal dystonia. Journal of Neurology Neurosurgery and Psychiatry 2003;74:1154-1156.
[14] Nafsika Frima, Jamal Nasir, and Richard A. Grunewald. Abnormal Vibration-Induced Illusion of Movement in idiopathic Focal dystonia: An Endophenotypic Marker? Movement Disorders 2007; 23 (3); 373-377..
[15] Ridding MC, Sheean G, Rothwell JC, InzelbergR, Kujirai T. Changes in the balance between motor cortical excitation and inhibition in focal, task specific dystonia. JNNP 1995; 59(5): 493-498.
[16] F. Gilio, A. Curra, M. Inghilleri, C. Lorenzano, A. Suppa, M. Manfredi and A. Berardelli. Abnormalities of motor cortex excitability preceding movement in patients with dystonia. Brain 2003; 126:1745-1754.
[17] Ikoma K, Samii A, Mercuri B, Wassermann EM, Hallett M. Abnormal cortical motor excitability in dystonia. Neurology 1996; 46(5): 1371-1376..
[18] Chen, R., et al.,. Impaired inhibition in writer's cramp during voluntary muscle activation. Neurology 1997; 49: 1054–1059.
[19] Kimberley, T.J., et al.,. Establishing the definition and inter-rater reliability of cortical silent period calculation in subjects with focal hand dystonia and healthy controls. Neurosci. Lett. 2009; 464: 84–87.
[20] Abbruzzese, G., et al.,. Abnormalities of sensorimotor integration in focal dystonia: a transcranial magnetic stimulation study. Brain 2001; 124: 537–545.
[21] Nakashima K, Rothewell J C, Day B L, Thompson P D, Shannon K, Marsden C D. Reciprocal inhibition between forearm muscles in patients with writer's cramp and other occupational cramps, symptomatic hemidystonia and hemiparesis due to stroke' Brain 1989; 112 (3): 681-697.
[22] Panizza ME, Hallett M, Nilsson J. Reciprocal inhibition in patients with hand cramps. Neurology 1989; 39(1): 85-89.
[23] Panizza M E, HallettM, Nilsson J. reciprocal inhibition in patients with hand cramps. Neurology 1989; 39(1): 85-89..
[24] Espay, A.J., et al.,. Cortical and spinal abnormalities in psychogenic dystonia. Ann.Neurol. 2006; 59: 825–834.
[25] Walsh R, O'Dwyer JP, Sheikh IH, O'Riordan S, Lynch T, Hutchinson M Sporadic adult onset dystonia: sensory abnormalities as an endophenotype in unaffected relatives. J Neurol Neurosurg Psychiatry 2007; 78:980-983.
[26] GM Goodwin, DI McCloskey, PB Matthews. The contribution of muscle afferents to kinaesthesia shown by vibration-induced illusions of movement and by the effects of paralysing joint afferents. Brain 1972; 95(4):705-48.
[27] On muscle spindles, dystonia and botulinum toxin, R. L. Rosales and D. Dressler: European Journal of Neurology 2010, 17 (Suppl. 1): 71–80.
[28] Matthews PBC: Mammalian Muscle Receptors and Their Central Actions. Baltimore, Williams and Wilkins, 1972.
[29] Guy M. Goodwin 1, D. Ian McCloskey 1, and Peter B. C. Matthews. Proprioceptive Illusions Induced by Muscle Vibration: Contribution by Muscle Spindles to Perception? Science 1972; 175(4028): 1382 - 1384.
[30] A. Biro, L. Griffin and E. Cafarelli. Reflex gain of muscle spindle pathways during fatigue. Exp Brain Res 2006; 177 (2): 157-166.()

[31] Chang, E F, Turner R S, Osterm, J L, Davis VR, Starr PA. Neuronal responses to passive movement in the globus pallidus internus in primary dystonia. J Neuorphysiol 2007; 98(6): 3696-707..

[32] Matthews, P. B. C. (). The reflex excitation of the soleus muscle of the decerebrate cat caused by vibration applied to its tendon. J. Physiol. 1966; 184; 450-472.

[33] Proske W, Morgan D L, Gregory JE. Thixotrophy in skeletal muscle and in muscle spindles: a review. Progress in Neurobiology 1993;41:705-721..

[34] Pohl C, Happe J, Klockgether T. Cooling improves the writing performance of patients with writer's cramp. Move Disord. 2002; 17(6): 1341-4.

[35] Grünewald RA. Progression of dystonia: learning from distorted feedback? J Neurol Neurosurg Psychiatry. 2007 78(9): 914.

[36] M D Rosset-Llobet J, Candia V, Fabregas S, et al. Secondary motor disturbances in 101 patients with musician's dystonia. J Neurol Neurosurg Psychiatry 2007; 78:949-953.

[37] Ferraz HB, De Andrade LA, Silva SM, Borges V, Rocha MS. Postural tremor and dystonia. Clinical aspects and physiopathological considerations. Arq Neuropsiquiatr. 1994 Dec;52(4):466-70

[38] Jankovic J, Leder S, Warner DR, Schwartz K. Cervical dystonia: clinical findings and associated movement disorders. Neurology 1991;41:1088-1091.

[39] N Frima and R Grunewald Abnormal vibration-induced illusion of movement in essential tremor: evidence for abnormal muscle spindle afferent function. J Neurol Neurosurg Psychiatry. 2005; 76(1): 55–57.

[40] Cooper C, Evidente VG, Hentz JG, Adler CH, Caviness JN, Gwinn-Hardy K. The effect of temperature on hand function in patients with tremor. Journal of Hand Therapy 2000;13(4):276-8.

[41] Tamura Y, Ueki YH, Lin P, Vorback S, Mima T, Kakigi R, Hallett M. Disordered plasticity in the primary somatosensory cortex in focal hand dystonia. Brain 2009; 132(3):749-55.

[42] Quartarone A, Morgante F, Sant'Angelo A, Rizzo V, Bagnato S, Terranova C, Siebner H, Berardelli A, Girlanda P. Abnromal plasticity of sensorimotor circuits extends beyond the affected body part in focal dystonia. JNNP 2008; 79:985-990

14

Dystonia Pathophysiology: A Critical Review

Pierre Burbaud
Department of Clinical Neurophysiology, Centre Hospitalier de Bordeaux, Institut des Maladies Neurodégénératives (CNRS UMR5293), Université Victor Segalen, Bordeaux, France

1. Introduction

During the past years, dramatic progress have been achieved in our knowledge of the pathophysiology of dystonia on the basis of imaging and electrophysiological data collected in human patients. Converging arguments now support the role of combined corticostriatal and cerebellar dysfunctions in the genesis of this movement disorder (1). Several excellent reviews have been recently proposed on this topic (2-8). Moreover, animals models of dystonia can help us to investigate the pathogenesis since they provide the opportunity to dissect more precisely the abnormal neuronal networks leading to primary dystonia and its genetic background (9-12).

However, many points remain to be clarified. Here, we discuss some of the findings previously reviewed but will detail more specifically less recognized aspects of the pathophysiology of dystonia, such as the link between phenomenology and physiology and the lessons that we can get from animal models.

2. Phenomenological considerations

Dystonia is defined as a syndrom of sustained muscular contractions leading to repetitive movements and abnormal postures. However, a rapid overview of the litterature reveals that this term is broadly used in very different contexts and can be associated with various pathological conditions. Thus, there is a need for clarification, not only for highlightening the concept of dystonia, but above all because of the pathophysiological and therapeutical consequences. In dystonia, abnormal posture is linked to repetitive muscular spasms triggered or worsened by voluntary movement (13). The overspreading of muscular activity to muscles usually not involved in the movement corresponds to a loss of inhibition during movement execution (3, 14). However, dystonia can be observed in different conditions such as spasticity, primary dystonia, secondary dystonia, levodopa-induced dystonia and off-dystonia in parkinsonian patients, among others.

Initially, several types of dystonia have been proposed depending on the age of onset, topography of clinical signs, and primary or secondary origin of dystonia (13). Focal dystonia is the most frequent form with a categorization depending on localization in the facial musculature (blepharospasm, oromandibular dystonia), cervical region (spasmodic torticolis), limb (occupational dystonia e.g. writer'scramp or musician's cramp) or the larynx (laryngeal dystonia). Segmental dystonia involves two or more contiguous regions e.g. the cervical region and one limb, and corresponds to the diffusion of the dystonic process to close anatomic regions. This point suggests a spreading of abnormal motor command in a somatotopic manner. Although multifocal dystonia encompasses non-adjacent body part, it is less frequent in clinical practice. Hemidystonia is limited to one hemibody and frequently associated with lesions of the controlateral hemisphere. However, as for most of secondary dystonia, it is characterized by permanent tonic postures very different from the clinical pattern seen in primary dystonia. General dystonia have a broader distribution than focal dystonia but also frequently encompasses adjacent parts of the body e.g lower limb and trunks and/or upper limbs. Dystonia is primary when no lesions of the central nervous system or metabolic abnormalities are found (15) whereas it is associated with other neurological troubles in dystonia-plus syndroms (2). In secondary dystonia, lesions generally concern the basal ganglia and more particularly the putamen although lesions in other regions have been reported (16).

It is critical to be precise as to which type of dystonia we are dealing with. The fixed focal dystonia frequently observed in untreated Parkinson's disease (off-dystonia) or in various neurological disorders encompassing dystonia and parkinsonism is likely to correspond to a form of focal akineto-rigid syndrome There are clinical and experimental arguments supporting this view. For instance, off-dystonia in Parkinsonian patients is observed in a state of low dopaminergic plasma levels either before treatment (off-state) or as a end-of-dose effect. A fixed focal dystonia, generally in the lower limb, is frequently noticed in MPTP-treated monkey at the onset of intoxication and before the development of a full akinetic-rigid syndrome in a situation where dopaminergic neurons are only partially destroyed (17). In dopa-sensitive dystonia (DRD), tonic postures are frequently encountered, sometimes in association with a parkinsonian syndrome ; the use of dopaminergic treatment is effective because there is a decrease in the production and consequently the availability of dopamine at the nigro-striatal synapsis. In secondary dystonia where most of the lesions involve the putamen, a fixed dystonia with a somatotopic organisation is most frequently observed. In this case, lesions seriously disrupt the organisation of motor patterns at the striatal level, the support of procedural memory. This point explains the inability of patients to control accurately the spatio-temporal pattern of agonist and antagonist muscles necessary to achieve a smooth and goal-directed movement.

Primary dystonia is clearly an hyperkinetic movement provoked or accentuated by voluntary movement. Fixed posture at rest are observed only in the most evoluated forms of the disease such as long-lasting DYT1 dystonia or spasmodic torticollis. A critical feature of mobile dystonia is that each patient exhibits his own abnormal motor pattern, repetitive in time and space. For instance, a patient with cervical dystonia will have a specific pattern of neck posture, a patient with generalized dystonia the same kind of back-arching movements and lower limb movements. Similar remarks could be made for levodopa-induced dyskinesia (LID) and/or dystonia: each patient exhibits his own pattern of LID. In addition, we must point out the fact that by many aspects, LID are more dystonic in nature than choreic: they frequently associate repetitive myoclonic jerks and mobile abnormal postures but are rarely eratic as the choreic movements observed in Huntington's disease. One interpretation of the phenomenon could be that in primary dystonia the disorganization of networks controlling movement occurs in patch within the striatum (18, 19).

3. Lessons form primate models of dystonia: The physiological approach

Primate models of dystonia are informative, first because of the tight phylogenetic link between monkeys and humans, but also because they provide the possibility to obtain phenotypes of dystonia in the monkey using a more invasive physiological approach than in humans.

It was found initially that brain regions involved in the regulation of muscular tone, such as the red nucleus or dorsomedial mesencephalic tegmentum, provoked the appearance of a spasmodic torticollis (20). The head was turning to the side of the tegmental lesion. Moreover, electrical stimulations or pharmacological inactivation of the interstitial nucleus of Cajal (NIC) induced neck dystonia, a result which can be explained by the role of NIC in the control of head posture (21). The cervical dystonia observed in this condition is characterized by lateral flexion of the head to the shoulder opposite to the site of the lesion and intermittent co-contraction of neck muscles resulting in spasmodic head movements. Muscimol (22) or histamine (23) injections within the red nucleus also induced a cervical dystonia as well as pharmacological manipulations of vestibular nucleii (24).

In monkeys, as in humans, systematic treatments acting on the dopaminergic system induce dystonia. These models could provide some lights on two aspects of the pathophysiology of primary dystonia : 1) the putative role of dopaminergic receptors, 2) the implication of the direct and indirect striato-pallidal pathways. Acute dystonia was first reported in the primate after haloperidol injections (25) with a response to anti-cholinergic drugs (26, 27) and reserpine (28). On the other hand, clozapine (a second generation antipsychotic agent) compared to classical neuroleptics (first generation antipsychotic agents) did not provoke acute dystonia possibly due to its particular post-synaptic receptor affinity to D1 receptors (29). Conversely, injections of D1 agonists induced less frequently acute dystonia than D2 receptor antagonists (30, 31). Thus, it seems that acute dystonia, frequently hypertonic in its clinical expression, is mainly trigerred by the blockade of D2 receptors. Tardive dystonia can be induced by a chronic treatment with neuroleptics (32-35). As for acute dystonia, drugs that prevent dopamine storage (reserpine), synthesis (α-methyl-p-tyrosine) or block dopamine receptors decrease tardive dyskinesias (36). However, there is some pharmacologic evidences for a peculiar implication of D1 dopaminergic receptors in orofacial dystonia (37). The substitution of a D2 antagonist by a D1 antagonist decreases the clinical expression of dystonia (38). Thus, in tardive dystonia which is frequently mobile, the overactivity of the direct pathways could play a preponderant role.

When Bicuculline (Bic), a potent antagonist of $GABA_A$ receptors, is injected directly within the GPi or SNr, it induces at high volumes (10µl) a severe parkinsonian syndrome similar to that observed in MPTP-treated monkeys. However, when lower volumes (2µl) are used, abnormal focal postures in the lower limbs close to off-dystonia are observed (39). Severe hypertonic postures in controlateral limbs are noticed after GPi injections whereas SNr injections generally induce more axial symptoms, particularly in the neck. Thus, this type of dystonia characterized by hypertonia and bradykinesia corresponds to a form of focal akinetic-rigid syndrome, the somatotopy of which depending on the targeted basal ganglia. In MPTP monkeys, chronic treatment with levodopa or apomorphine induces dyskinesia (40-42). Metabolic studies relying on 2-Desoxyglucose (2-DG) show an increase of GABAergic inhibition of the subthalamic nucleus, suggesting a diminished subthalamopallidal activity (40-42). This data would suggest an increased activity within the thalamo-cortical network although thalamotomy did not improve dystonia in MPTP-treated monkeys (43, 44). During peak-dose dystonia, an increase in the expression of D1 dopaminergic receptors was observed and interpreted as an overactivity of the direct striato-pallidal pathway. On the other hand, D1 agonists induce less dyskinesias than D2 agonists (45, 46).

Bic injection into the STN blocks GABAergic inputs, increases activity and leads to a tonic dystonia (42). Conversely, the injection of muscimol, a GABAergic agonist, within the basal ganglia output structures, namely the internal pallidum (GPi), and pars reticulata of the substantia nigra (SNr) induces a mobile dyskinesias encompassing mixed choreic and dystonic features mimicking the hyperkinetic movements observed in idiopathic dystonias (39). The mechanism could be related to an inhibition of neuronal activity in these regions (47).

A line of evidence also suggest that manipulations of the striatum might induce dystonia. Bicuculline injections within the putamen in the cat provoked neck dystonic movements directed towards the controlateral side, associated with an increased activity within the striatum and concomitent inhibition in the substantia nigra pars reticulata (SNr) (48). Injection of the same drug within the putamen also induced contralateral dyskinesia in the monkey (49). The blockade of striatal $GABA_A$-receptors in the striatum increases GPI neuronal activity and induces EEG spikes in the primary motor cortex (50). Direct electric stimulation of the putamen in the monkey using various duration of stimulation trains induces movement disorders the nature of which depending on the duration of the stimulation train (51). With short duration (100ms), myoclonic jerks of the contralateral hemibody are observed whereas dystonic and stereotyped movements are noticed with longer duration trains (>500ms). These data suggest that the difference between myoclonus and dystonia relies on the duration of the abnormal neuronal activity generated within the putamen.

An increased activity in the direct striato-pallidal pathway is likely to induce changes in the motor thalamus. Lesion studies in humans indicate that dystonia is mainly observed after lesions of the caudal motor thalamus (Vc, VIM) but not of the rostral pallidal segment (Vop) (52, 53). In monkey, the motor thalamus is a complex structure encompassing several regions (54). Its rostral part, corresponding to the ventrolateral pars oralis (VLo) and ventral anterior (VA) nucleii, receives inputs from basal ganglia output structures and send projections to the supplementary motor area (55). The caudal part corresponding to the ventroposterolateral, pars oralis (VPLo) and ventrolateral, pars caudalis (VLc) nucleii mainly receive cerebellar inputs. The projections are directed to the primary motor cortex (54). Several lines of evidence suggest that the thalamus plays a role in the synchronization of cortical activity in time and space (56). Thus, its dysfunction could potentially inducea loss of selectivity in the implementation of cortical modules during motor planning. Injection of bicuculline within the rostral part (VLo and VA) provoked a mobile contralateral dystonia whereas a myoclonic dystonia was observed after injections into the caudal region (VPLo, VLc) (57, 58). These bicuculline injections increased the discharge frequency of thalamic neurons and decreased the threshold of current necessary to evoke motor responses after intrathalamic microstimulation (58). Moreover, a bursty pattern correlating with myoclonic jerks was observed for most neurons in the caudal region. These results suggest that the tonic and myoclonic components frequently associated in dystonic patients could be the result of a dysfunction in both the rostral (pallidal) and caudal (cerebellar) parts of the motor thalamus. These notions are also in congruity with the view that an hyperexcitability of thalamo-cortical pathway induces dystonia as proposed by Berardelli et al. (59). Interestingly, a greater number of thalamic neurons responded to passive joint manipulations after bicuculline injection (58). The data obtained in an acute experimental situation reveal the drastic and immediate modifications of somesthesic receptive fields that thalamic neurons may exhibit, highlighting the role of the motor thalamus in sensori-motor processing.

Taken as a whole, the results of pharmacological studies in monkeys suggest that in primary dystonia there would be an overactivity in the direct striato-palidal pathway, potentially associated with a decreased activity in the indirect striato-palidal pathway leading to a disrupted activation of the thalamo-cortical projections.

So far, the only phenotypic model of primary dystonia in the primate was that obtained in monkeys trained to perform repetitive movements (60-62). The animals performed the same movement of grasping 2 hours a day 5 days a week for 12 to 25 weeks and experienced difficulties removing their hands from the handpiece after 5-8 weeks of training, associated with a reduction in the number of trials correctly performed (60). The animals also exhibited difficulties in hand motor control during feeding, a loss of digital dexterity, evoking dystonia. In parallel, a disorganization of hand somatotopy was observed in area 3b of the primary somaesthetic cortex (S1). Receptive fields of recorded neurons became larger, encompassing more than one digit and segregation between glabrous and hairy skin was altered. Moreover, it was found that hand-face border in S1 normally sharp became patchy and spread over 1 mm of cortex (60). Thus focal dystonia induced by repetitive behaviors generates aberrant sensory representations which interfere with motor control (63). Abnormal motor control strengthens sensory abnormalities and the positive feed-back loop reinforces the dystonic condition.

4. Lessons from rodent models of dystonia: The genetic approach

Models of dystonia in the rodent provide valuable tools for exploring the contribution of genetic factors in the pathophysiology of dystonia. They can be divided into those that mimic the dystonic phenotype and those that duplicate the genetic abnormalities (2). In genotypic models, the mutations that produce dystonia in humans have been introduced into mice. Several models have been developed (11). Mouse models of DYT1 include both transgenic mice expressing human mutant torsin A (hMT) (64, 65), and heterozygous knock-in mice in which the GAG mutation has been introduced in the mouse torsin A gene (Dyt1) (66, 67). These mice do not have obvious dystonic features (65, 66) but exhibit some learning motor deficit (64). In striatal explant slices from transgenic hMT mice, cholinergic interneurons manifest an abnormal physiology: they respond to dopamine receptor (D2) activation with an increase in spiking, rather than an inhibition as observed in normal mice (68). Genotypic mouse models have also been generated for DYT5, DYT11 and DYT12 (2).

The role of dopaminergic dysfunction in dystonia is supported by several studies in the rodent (1). In a transgenic model of dopa-responsive dystonia, a depletion of tyrosine hydroxylase was found in the striatum (69). There was a marked posterior to anterior gradient with a predominant loss of striosome tyrosine hydroxylase expression in the remaining tyrosine hydroxylase staining areas at an early stage of the postnatal development. A DYT1 mouse model had a decreased amphetamine-induced dopamine release and evidence for an increased dopamine turnover was found (70).

In phenotypic models, mutations that produce dystonic movements occur naturally (12). The dt/dt rat has an autosomal, recessive condition with dystonic posturing appearing 10 days after birth encompassing twisting movements of the neck, padding motions of the limbs and postural instability of increasing severity (71). Purkinje cell soma are smaller (10) and the defective protein, caytaxin, is a lipophilic binding protein that is expressed at high levels in cerebellar neurons during development (11, 72). This protein might be involved in signalling pathways that use calcium and phosphatidyl-inositol, and in regulating the synthesis of glutamate. Cerebellectomy eliminates the motor syndrome and rescues animals from juvenile lethality. In the df/dt mouse model, neuronal degeneration results from loss of a cytolinker protein (dystonin), which is expressed in the central and peripheral nervous systems and resembles the proposed function of torsinA (73). The tottering mice carry a homozygous mutation in a P/Q-type calcium channel expressed abundantly within Purkinje cells (10). The animals exhibit episodic dyskinetic attacks reminiscent of the attacks experienced by patients with paroxysmal non-kinesigenic dyskinesia (2). At the most advanced stages of attacks, tottering mice assume prolonged twisting postures involving the whole body and a mild ataxia. Lethargic mice also exhibit paroxysmal dyskinesia triggered by procedures that promote motor activity (12). In these animals, cytochrome oxydase histochemistry revealed increased activity in the red nucleus. Surgical removal of the cerebellum worsens ataxia but improved dyskinesias.

Thus, lesions of the cerebellum in rodents models of dystonia abolish the motor disorder suggesting that the cerebellum is necessary for the expression of dystonia (12). Morevover, it was shown in the dt rat that abnormal signaling in cerebellar cortex can lead to abnormal cerebellar output (11, 74). Moreover, microinjections of low doses of kainic acid into the cerebellar vermis of the mice elicited reliable and reproductible dystonic postures of the trunk and limbs (75). Peripheral administration of 3-nitropropionic acid to rodents, as in the primate, induced a dystonic phenotype associated to striatal lesions (76). In comparison with controls, hMT1 mice show increased glucose utilization (GU) in the inferior olive (IO) medial nucleus (IOM), IO dorsal accessory nucleus and substantia nigra compacta, and decreased GU in the medial globus pallidus (MGP) and lateral globus pallidus (77). They also showed increased CO activity in the IOM and Purkinje cell layer of cerebellar cortex, and decreased CO activity in the caudal caudate-putamen, substantia nigra reticulata and MGP. These findings suggest that the DYT1 carrier state increases energy demand in the olivocerebellar network and the IO may be a pivotal node for abnormal basal ganglia-cerebellar interactions in dystonia (77).

The dtSZ/dtSZ hamster, which manifests as an autosomal recessive condition with episodes of generalized dystonia induced by stress is a robust model of paroxysmal non-kinesigenic dyskinesias (78, 79). Attacks can last for hours and appear to be age-dependent (10). A line of evidence suggests a GABA-mediated neurotransmission defect and drugs that target these molecules are able to relieve the dystonic symptoms (80). The dtSZ hamster also exhibit highly irregular pattern of electrical activity within the striatum and globus pallidus (81).

The interaction between the basal ganglia and cerebellum in the expression of dystonic movement has been studies in two rodent models of dystonia (82). One of the model involved tottering mice, the other one was obtained by local application of kainic acid into the cerebellar cortex. Subthreshold lesions of the striatum exaggerated dystonic attacks in both models. In tottering mice, microdyalisis of the striatum revealed that dystonic attacks were associated with a significant reduction in extracellular dopamine. This interesting result demonstrates the functional interactions between cerebellar and basal ganglia circuits in dystonia.

However, some forms of focal dystonia could be related to different mechanisms. Blepharospasm corresponds to involuntary spasms of bilateral eyelid closure. The increased spontaneous blink rate may result from the increased excitability of the trigeminal system which is dependent on the basal ganglia (83, 84). It seems that reduction in dopamine induces a reduction in nucleus raphe magnus activity via the subtantia nigra pars reticulata and superior colliculus (85, 86). Schicatano and collegues created a two component model of benign blepharospasm based on the combination of a permissive condition (dopamine depletion) and a precipitating event (corneal irritation and dry eye caused by partial lesion of the zygomatic branch of the facial nerve). They considered that spasms of eye lid closure was an exaggeration of the normally compensatory process evoked by eye irritation (87). In this situation, there was a dysfunctional sensorimotor integration in which the central nervous system either misinterpret sensory signals or misrepresents the desired movement.

Taken as a whole most of these rodent models reveal that dysfunctional cerebellar output is sufficient for the expression of generalized dystonia. However, it is important to be aware that the organization and physiology of the central nervous system is quite different between rodents and primates. For instance, the main basal ganglia output structure is represented by the subtantia nigra pars reticulata (SNr) in the rodent, a region involved in the control of the axial musculature, whereas it is the internal pallidum (GPi) in the primate, a region associated with the development of sophisticated hand dexterity. It is likely that the respective roles of the basal ganglia and cerebellum in motor control are different between rodents and primates.

5. Loss of inhibitory control

Electrophysiological studies are easier to perform in humans than in animals but must be based on non invasive techniques that limits exploration to a specific brain region. Two main techniques have been used : 1) Transcranial magnetic stimulation (TMS) of the cerebral cortex, 2) neuronal recordings in the basal ganglia during surgery.

Concerning the TMS, an excellent review has been recently proposed (Hallett, 2011) and here we we will only focus on specific segments. A line of evidence suggests that inhibition processes are defective during movement execution in dystonia. The loss of selectivity and overflow of muscular activity to muscles not usually involved in the on-going movement is clearly increased by voluntary action (3, 14, 88, 89). TMS allowed to show a decrease in both intra-cortical inhibition and silent period (3, 4). The coupling of a peripheral stimulation delivered prior to TMS shocks (PAS) at different intervals between the two stimuli also revealed an abnormal inhibition in dystonia (3, 8, 90, 91). As mentionned by Hallett (3), the results obtained with TMS are valuable, but they remain at a phenomenological level and focused the primary cortex whereas there have been only few data reporting stimulation of the premotor cortex (92) or cerebellum (93).

While dystonia is mainly a motor problem, mild sensory abnormalities have been reported in patients with hand dystonia both in the spatial (94-97) and temporal (98-100) domains. Kinesthesia is also impaired (101-103) and abnormal somatotopy was demonstrated by somatosensory evoked potential mapping based on EEG (94), MEG (94, 104, 105) and fMRI (106-108). As for motor control, a loss of lateral inhibition in sensory processing in space and time was reported (109-111). Moreover, the existence of bilateral abnormalities in the dystonic and non dystonic sides, suggests that this phenomenon is an endophenotypic trait (104) leading to changes in sensorimotor integration (3, 105).

Single unit recording of pallidal or thalamic nucleii have been performed in dystonic patients candidate to deep brain stimulation (DBS). They revealed interesting but contradictory data. A trend for low firing rate with a bursty pattern and oscillations was reported in the internal pallidum (112-116) and subthalamic nucleus (117). However, the role of anaesthesia was debated because some authors found no difference between dystonic and PD patients (118, 119). The current pathophysiological model of dystonia was also questioned by data showing that pallidal DBS was able to inihibit a subpopulation of motor thalamic neurons (120) and the abscence of difference between GPe and GPi firing rate (119). However, clear correlation between abnormal neuronal activitiy and EMG activity was reported in the basal ganglia and thalamus of patients with dystonia (116, 121-123). Moreover, single unit recording performed in cerebellar relays of the thalamus revealed abnormal firing pattern and increased response to peripheral inputs in dystonic patients (123-125). The technique of local field potentials (LFPs) allows to study local populations of neurons within a given brain region. Low oscillatory activity was recorded in the GPi of dystonic patients (126). This activity was found to be correlated with dystonic EMG (112, 114, 127) and single unit neuronal activity (112, 128). The conclusion was that the frequency of synchronization in the basal ganglia is a critical problem in dystonia, as in other movement disorders (129).

Thus, electrophysiological data revealed an impaired surround inhibition in several régions including the cerebral cortex, thalamus and basal ganglia with a trend for low and bursty firing rate in the GPi in line with the current models of dystonia (18, 19, 59). It is noteworthy that an abnormal pattern in the thalamus was observed in relays receiving cerebellar inputs (124).

6. Neuronal networks (imaging data)

Most of structural MRIs studies failed to show robust evidence of neural degeneration in patients with primary dystonia (130) although subtle grey and white matter micro-structural alterations were reported (131). Contradictory results have been found with voxel-based morphometry. Some studies noticed increased volumes in the sensorimotor cortex (132), putamen (133), globus pallidus (134) and cerebellum (135), but other decreased volumes in the putamen (136) sensorimotor cortex (137), cerebellum and thalamus (136, 137). These results must be interpreted in a phenomenological perspective since dfferent types of dystonia may yield different results.

Diffusion-weighted imaging (DWI) is sensitive to the random motion of water molecules and provide an estimate of the micro-structural integrity of the brain parenchyma and the directionality of molecular diffusion. The last parameter, also called anisotropy, is measured using indices such as fractional anisotropy (FA). Changes in FA are interpreted as "micro-structural" changes in axonal amounts, axonal integrity, myelination, and has also been used to trace specific fiber tracts and to quantify abnormalities along them (4). DTI tractography is interesting in primary dystonia because this neurodevelopment disorder might disrupt cortico-striatal and/or cerebello-thalamic pathways. Indeed, abnormalities have been reported in the cortex (138-140), basal ganglia (141, 142), internal capsule (143), or thalamocortical pathways (144).

Initial PET studies with $^{[O15]}$H2O revealed an overactivity in the cerebral cortex (particularly the rostral supplementary motor area i.e. pre-SMA), basal ganglia, cerebellum, and thalamus. The role of the caudal supplementary motor area (SMAp) and primary sensory-motor cortex was debated. Metabolism was deceased during execution of a learned movement (145-147) but increased when primary dystonia occurs at rest or in secondary dystonia (148). These abnormalities were also found in non-symptomatic patients carrying the DYT1 gene (149). In line with electrophysiological studies, abnormal sensory processing was reported in focal hand dystonia (150), blepharospasm (151), and cervical dystonia (152). Similar results were also obtained in non-manifesting DYT1 carriers (153, 154). The loss of inhibition in motor control was supported by the finding that an impaired GABA was observed in the striatum of dystonic patients (155).

The involvement of the dopaminergic system in primary dystonia was also demontrated with imaging techniques. Indeed, reduced D2 receptor availability in the striatum was reported in DYT1 (156-160) as well as in DYT6 patients (158). This data is compatible with dysfunction or loss of D2-bearing neurons, increased synaptic dopamine levels, or both. These changes, which may be present to different degrees in the DYT1 and DYT6 genotypes, are likely to represent susceptibility factors for the development of clinical manifestations. Moreover, abnormalities in motor sequence learning associated with increased cerebellar activation during task performance was observed in non-manifesting carriers of the DYT1 and DYT6 mutation but did not correlate with striatal D2 receptor binding (161). In a recent study, sequence learning deficits and concomitant increases in cerebellar activation were found to be specific features of the DYT1 genotype versus DYT6 carriers (162).

Disruption in information processing within the cortico-striato-pallido-thalamo-cortical and cerebello-thalamo-cortical pathways at rest was analyzed using sophisticated statistical tools (5). FDG-PET studies revealed abnormal functional connectivity with a specific pattern characterized by relative increase of metabolic activity in the posterior putamen/globus pallidus, cerebellum and SMA in DYT1 patients. In DYT6 patients, slight different results were obtained since opposite patterns of tracer uptake in the putamen were observed (154, 163, 164). In blepharospasm, there was a predominent role of the thalamus and midbrain/brainstem rather than basal ganglia and cortex. Thus, it appears clearly that different types of dystonia may be associated with different metabolic patterns (5).

Among a larger number of fMRI studies, the most commonly affected regions included various portions of the cerebral cortex, basal ganglia, and cerebellum (4, 5). Most studies reported either normal or increased basal ganglia activation during motor or sensory tasks. In the cortex, activation level was variably altered, depending on the task, the type of dystonia, and whether patients expressed dystonia during task performance or not. The primary sensory cortex was activated frequently (165-167) but not always (107, 166, 168).

Dystonic movements were commonly associated with overactivation in the sensorimotor cortex (166, 167, 169, 170), whereas activation levels may be normal (171) or decreased (168) during non-dystonic movements. However, reduced sensorimotor activation also may occur during dystonic movements (165, 166). The abnormal fMRI signals for representation of digits in the primary sensory cortex (107, 108) or other body parts in the basal ganglia (171) have been interpreted as a loss of neuronal selectivity. It is noteworthy that although fMRI presumably monitors neuronal activation, results only partially correlate with PET studies of blood flow.

Thus, imaging studies point to the role of combined corticostriatal and cerebellar pathways in the pathophysiology of dystonia. Anatomical disruption of the cerebellar outflow was found in non manifesting carriers and manifesting mutation carriers, and a second downstream disruption in thalamo-cortical projections appeared clinically protective in non-manifestationg carriers (5).

7. Plasticity in dystonia: A central mechanism

Dystonia seems to be a motor circuit disorder rather than an abnormality of a specific brain region (7). There are lines of evidences showing that dytonia is associated with abnormal plasticity (6, 172-174). On a phenomenological point of view, primary dystonia, appears in the young age when procedural motor learning and plasticity are optimal (6, 172-174). Even in secondary dystonia, the delayed appearence of symptoms after brain lesion suggests some form of plasticity (175) as well as the delayed therapeutic effect of pallidal stimulation in primary dystonia (176, 177). Long term potentiation (LTP) and long term depression (LTD) are the most widely recognized physiological models of plasticity. In humans, the physiological basis of LTP and LTD is limited to TMS and transcranial direct current stimulation (TDCS) of the cerebral cortex (7). Two main techiques have been used to study plasticity at the cortical level: repetitive TMS (rTMS) with variable frequencies inducing either LTP or LTD (172, 178) and paired-associative stimulation (PAS) combining electrical stimulation of a peripheral nerve and cortical TMS (172, 179, 180). It was shown that the sensorimotor cortex (SM) exhibited an exaggerated responsiveness to rTMS responding protocols (90, 181-184). Associative plasticity (LTP, LTD, PAS) is enhanced with a loss of spatial specificity explained by a failure of surround inhibition (3, 7). Morever, somatosensory evoked response in SM was more enhanced by PAS in dystonic patients than in normal controls (182) revealing an increased susceptibility to peripheral events. Another way to test cortical plasiticity is to use theta burst stimulation (TBS) which relies on short trains of pulses (5Hz) with an high intra-burst frequency (50Hz). TBS after-effect was enhanced in dystonic patients but not in their symptomatic relatives (185). Moreover, in dystonic patients, cortical responses to 1Hz rTMS is unaffected by pre-conditionning with anodal TDCS contrarily to normal controls (179, 181). In dystonia, there would be an increased tendency to form associations between sensory inputs and motor inputs which may lead to de-differentiation of motor representations in accordance with the theory of synaptic homeostatis (7, 186, 187).

The question remains to whether the loss of surround inhibition and synaptic homeostasis is a trait of the whole sensorimotor system or the result of dysfuntionning of specific regions such as the striatum and the cerebellum. The processing of sensory inputs is for instance altered either in the basal ganglia (187), the thalamus (124) and cerebral cortex (3).

Moreover, pharmacological manipulations of the thalamus induce immediate changes in the receptive fields of thalamic neurons (58) probably mimicking the effect of plasticity occuring in dystonic patients. Thus, abnormal plasticity seems to be an endophenotypic trait of dystonia (6, 7, 179).

Several lines of evidence suggest that dystonic symptoms are generated by an abnormal functionning of the putamen, a basal ganglia region involved in motor control (188). The striatofugal medium spiny cells (MSC) receive strong cortical glutamatergic inputs and represent the main projection neurons of the striatum. They are modulated by a complex interneuronal network in which local cholinergic interneurons (Ach-I), GABAergic interneurons and mesencephalic dopaminergic inputs play critical roles. In the current accepted model of dystonia, there is an imbalance between the direct and indirect striato-pallidal output pathways (189). Use-dependent long lasting changes in synaptic efficacy at cortico-striatal synpases has been proposed as a model of motor learning and memory (7). As in humans, LTP and LTD can be obtained by high frequency stimulation of cortico-striatal afferents. Moreover, LTP can be reversed by low frequency afferent stimulation (synaptic depotentiation). These phenomena are modulated by striatal interneurons. A series of elegant experiments performed in a rodent genetic model of DYT1 dystonia recently revealed the close interaction between cholinergic and dopaminergic transmission (68, 190, 191). In trangenic mice expression of the mutant form of the torsinA, increased long-term potentiation (LTP) but decreased long-term depression (LTD) and depotentiation (SD). Hence, these phenomena were reversed by lowering endogenous Ach level or by antagonizing muscarinic M1 receptors (191). On the other hand, no difference was found in electrophysiological and morphological characteristics of MSC and Ach-I between mutant and non-mutant mice (190, 191). These results may provide an explanation for the efficacy of anticholinergic drugs in dystonia. Thus, long-term modifications of synaptic strength at the cortico-striatal synapse exhibit a highly dynamic organization ensuring the maintenance of a synaptic homeostasis within basal ganglia circuitry (7).

As we saw previously, strong evidences have recently emerged suggesting that the cerebellum also actively contributes to the pathophysiology of dystonia. Indeed, dystonia can be associated with cerebellar dysfunction in different forms of genetic ataxia and the neuronal network involved in primary dystonia consistently encompasses the cerebellum (4, 5). Conversely, the cerebellum has the ability to inhibit cortical activity, control sensori-motor integration and play a part in maladaptative neural plasticity (4). The fundamental mechanism may be the ability of the cerebellum to control cortico-striatal long-term depression, a mechanism thought to underlie neural plasticity. As previously noticed, the paradox is that most of genetic rodent model of dystonia associated with cerebellar dysfunctionning do not exhibit a clear phenotype of dystonia (2).

8. Conclusion and perspectives

Primary dystonia is a developement disorder with a strong genetic basis but the phenotype is likely to be triggered by risk factors such as environment insults, increased sensory inputs or physiological stress (2). Several lines of evidence suggest that dystonia corresponds to a disruption in the homeostatic regulation of neural plasticity within the sensorimotor circuitry (1, 3). However, the term dystonia encompasses a broad spectrum of disease and it is important to take up its pathophysiology on the basis of clear phenomenological considerations. In addition, different pathophysiological mechanisms may underlie similar phenotypes whereas different genotypes (e.g. DT6 and DYT1) may share similar functional abnormalities (1).

Imaging data support the hypotheses of the respective roles of basal ganglia and cerebellum by showing that dystonia disrupts the whole motor circuits involved in motor learning (5). Disruption in surround inhibition and aberrant plasticity are critical features of dystonia but we do not know whether this phenomenon occurs in a critical region (striatum, cerebellum) or is a feature of the whole sensorimotor network. How and where cerebellar circuits interact with basal ganglia circuits still remains a partially unsolved question. The thalamus which receive inputs from both systems in anatomically close nucleii could potentially play a critical rôle in the intégration of pallidal and cerbellar inputs. Indeed, disruption in sensory information and increased activity were reported in this region either in dystonic patients and in a primate model of the disease.

We began to have an idea of the disrupted networks within the striatum based on experimental models of dystonia showing that plasticity is impaired by an abnormal functionning of acetylcholine interneurones and their paradoxical response to D2 dopaminergic stimulation (7). The net result is a disequilibrium between LTP and LTD, the bases of plasticity at the cortico-striatal synapsis. The impairment of surround inhibition could also be related to decreased GABA transmission within the striatum as suggested by data obtained in human patients (3, 155) but also by the loss of parvalbumin-reactive GABArgic interneurones in a hamster model of paroxysmal dystonia (192). The cellular mechanisms leading to a dysfunctionning of the cerebellum remains less clear but some observations in rodent models suggest a possible dysfunctionning of Purkinje cells potentially related to some forms of channelopathy (11). Thus, animal models are promising although none of them can perfectly mimic the complexity of the clinical features observed in humans (1, 12). A problem in the genotypic rodent models is that they do not induce a phenotypic of dystonia. As stated above, it is possible that this discrepancy is due to the different organization of the subcortico-cortical networks between rodents and primates. However, the rodent models may be particularly challenging to make the gap between genes and the functional brain abnormalitites associated with primary dystonia (2). They can also be useful to develop experimental therapeutics. In primates, most models have focused on basal ganglia dysfunction. However, the elegant model proposed by Mink several years ago on this basis (18, 189) still lacks a direct experimental demonstration in the monkey. It will be probably necessary in the near future to develop more sophisticated models of dystonia in the sub-human primate to test directly some pathophysiological hypotheses concerning the disruption of information processing within the striato-pallidal and/or cerebello-cortical pathways.

Finally, a great challenge will be to understand how the ubiquitous cellular mechanisms disrupted by genetic mutations might explain the focal phenotypic expression of dystonia. As recently pointed by Pisani and collegues, dystonia would represent a high priority for medical reseach in the field of movement disorders for several reasons (193). First, this pathological model is unique because it represents a window to study the role of plasticity in the development of the central nervous system. Second, it provides the opportunity to explore the subtle interactions between the basal ganglia and cerebellum networks in motor control. Third, there is a fascinating challenge to undestand how the genetic defects will be translated into phenotypic effects. Finally, the development of new therapeutics may necessitate novel strategies based on original technologies. There is no doubt that a large collaboration of scientists with different expertises will be necessary to achieve this goal.

9. References

[1] Vidailhet M, Grabli D, Roze E. Pathophysiology of dystonia. Curr Opin Neurol 2009;22:406-413.

[2] Breakefield XO, Blood AJ, Li Y, Hallett M, Hanson PI, Standaert DG. The pathophysiological basis of dystonias. Nat Rev Neurosci 2008;9:222-234.

[3] Hallett M. Neurophysiology of dystonia: The role of inhibition. Neurobiol Dis 2011;42:177-184.

[4] Neychev VK, Gross RE, Lehericy S, Hess EJ, Jinnah HA. The functional neuroanatomy of dystonia. Neurobiol Dis 2011;42:185-201.

[5] Niethammer M, Carbon M, Argyelan M, Eidelberg D. Hereditary dystonia as a neurodevelopmental circuit disorder: Evidence from neuroimaging. Neurobiol Dis 2011;42:202-209.

[6] Peterson DA, Sejnowski TJ, Poizner H. Convergent evidence for abnormal striatal synaptic plasticity in dystonia. Neurobiol Dis 2010;37:558-573.

[7] Quartarone A, Pisani A. Abnormal plasticity in dystonia: Disruption of synaptic homeostasis. Neurobiol Dis 2011;42:162-170.

[8] Quartarone A, Rizzo V, Morgante F. Clinical features of dystonia: a pathophysiological revisitation. Curr Opin Neurol 2008;21:484-490.

[9] Guehl D, Cuny E, Ghorayeb I, Michelet T, Bioulac B, Burbaud P. Primate models of dystonia. Prog Neurobiol 2009;87:118-131.

[10] Jinnah HA, Hess EJ, Ledoux MS, Sharma N, Baxter MG, Delong MR. Rodent models for dystonia research: characteristics, evaluation, and utility. Mov Disord 2005;20:283-292.

[11] LeDoux MS. Animal models of dystonia: Lessons from a mutant rat. Neurobiol Dis 2011;42:152-161.

[12] Raike RS, Jinnah HA, Hess EJ. Animal models of generalized dystonia. NeuroRx 2005;2:504-512.

[13] Fahn S. Concept and classification of dystonia. Adv Neurol 1988;50:1-8.

[14] Hallett M. Dystonia: abnormal movements result from loss of inhibition. Adv Neurol 2004;94:1-9.

[15] Calne DB, Lang AE. Secondary dystonia. Adv Neurol 1988;50:9-33.

[16] Bhatia KP, Bhatt MH, Marsden CD. The causalgia-dystonia syndrome. Brain 1993;116 (Pt 4):843-851.

[17] Perlmutter JS, Tempel LW, Black KJ, Parkinson D, Todd RD. MPTP induces dystonia and parkinsonism. Clues to the pathophysiology of dystonia. Neurology 1997;49:1432-1438.

[18] Mink JW. The Basal Ganglia and involuntary movements: impaired inhibition of competing motor patterns. Arch Neurol 2003;60:1365-1368.

[19] Mink JW. Abnormal circuit function in dystonia. Neurology 2006;66:959.

[20] Malouin F, Bedard PJ. Frontal torticollis (head tilt) induced by electrolytic lesion and kainic acid injection in monkeys and cats. Exp Neurol 1982;78:551-560.

[21] Klier EM, Wang H, Constantin AG, Crawford JD. Midbrain control of three-dimensional head orientation. Science 2002;295:1314-1316.

[22] Schmied A, Amalric M, Dormont JF, Farin D. GABAergic mechanisms in the cat red nucleus: effects of intracerebral microinjections of muscimol or bicuculline on a conditioned motor task. Exp Brain Res 1990;81:523-532.
[23] van't Groenewout JL, Stone MR, Vo VN, Truong DD, Matsumoto RR. Evidence for the involvement of histamine in the antidystonic effects of diphenhydramine. Exp Neurol 1995;134:253-260.
[24] Burke RE, Fahn S. An evaluation of sustained postural abnormalities in rats induced by intracerebro-ventricular injection of chlorpromazine methiodide or somatostatin as models of dystonia. Adv Neurol 1988;50:335-342.
[25] Casey DE, Gerlach J, Christensson E. Dopamine, acetylcholine, and GABA effects in acute dystonia in primates. Psychopharmacology (Berl) 1980;70:83-87.
[26] Heintz R, Casey DE. Pargyline reduces/prevents neuroleptic-induced acute dystonia in monkeys. Psychopharmacology (Berl) 1987;93:207-213.
[27] Povlsen UJ, Noring U, Laursen AL, Korsgaard S, Gerlach J. Effects of serotonergic and anticholinergic drugs in haloperidol-induced dystonia in Cebus monkeys. Clin Neuropharmacol 1986;9:84-90.
[28] Jenner P, Clow A, Reavill C, Theodorou A, Marsden CD. Stereoselective actions of substituted benzamide drugs on cerebral dopamine mechanisms. J Pharm Pharmacol 1980;32:39-44.
[29] Casey DE. Extrapyramidal syndromes in nonhuman primates: typical and atypical neuroleptics. Psychopharmacol Bull 1991;27:47-50.
[30] Casey DE. Dopamine D1 (SCH 23390) and D2 (haloperidol) antagonists in drug-naive monkeys. Psychopharmacology (Berl) 1992;107:18-22.
[31] Lublin H, Gerlach J, Morkeberg F. Long-term treatment with low doses of the D1 antagonist NNC 756 and the D2 antagonist raclopride in monkeys previously exposed to dopamine antagonists. Psychopharmacology (Berl) 1994;114:495-504.
[32] Barany S, Haggstrom JE, Gunne LM. Application of a primate model for tardive dyskinesia. Acta Pharmacol Toxicol (Copenh) 1983;52:86-89.
[33] Kistrup K, Gerlach J. Selective D1 and D2 receptor manipulation in Cebus monkeys: relevance for dystonia and dyskinesia in humans. Pharmacol Toxicol 1987;61:157-161.
[34] Klintenberg R, Gunne L, Andren PE. Tardive dyskinesia model in the common marmoset. Mov Disord 2002;17:360-365.
[35] Marsden CD, Jenner P. The pathophysiology of extrapyramidal side-effects of neuroleptic drugs. Psychol Med 1980;10:55-72.
[36] Gerlach J, Bjorndal N, Christensson E. Methylphenidate, apomorphine, THIP, and diazepam in monkeys: dopamine-GABA behavior related to psychoses and tardive dyskinesia. Psychopharmacology (Berl) 1984;82:131-134.
[37] Peacock L, Lublin H, Gerlach J. The effects of dopamine D1 and D2 receptor agonists and antagonists in monkeys withdrawn from long-term neuroleptic treatment. Eur J Pharmacol 1990;186:49-59.
[38] Peacock L, Jensen G, Nicholson K, Gerlach J. Extrapyramidal side effects during chronic combined dopamine D1 and D2 antagonist treatment in Cebus apella monkeys. Eur Arch Psychiatry Clin Neurosci 1999;249:221-226.
[39] Burbaud P, Bonnet B, Guehl D, Lagueny A, Bioulac B. Movement disorders induced by gamma-aminobutyric agonist and antagonist injections into the internal globus pallidus and substantia nigra pars reticulata of the monkey. Brain Res 1998;780:102-107.

[40] Boyce S, Clarke CE, Luquin R, et al. Induction of chorea and dystonia in parkinsonian primates. Mov Disord 1990;5:3-7.
[41] Crossman AR, Sambrook MA. Experimental torticollis in the monkey produced by unilateral 6-hydroxy-dopamine brain lesions. Brain Res 1978;149:498-502.
[42] Mitchell IJ, Luquin R, Boyce S, et al. Neural mechanisms of dystonia: evidence from a 2-deoxyglucose uptake study in a primate model of dopamine agonist-induced dystonia. Mov Disord 1990;5:49-54.
[43] Page RD. The use of thalamotomy in the treatment of levodopa-induced dyskinesia. Acta Neurochir (Wien) 1992;114:77-117.
[44] Page RD, Sambrook MA, Crossman AR. Thalamotomy for the alleviation of levodopa-induced dyskinesia: experimental studies in the 1-methyl-4-phenyl-1,2,3,6-tetrahydropyridine-treated parkinsonian monkey. Neuroscience 1993;55:147-165.
[45] Pearce RK, Jackson M, Britton DR, Shiosaki K, Jenner P, Marsden CD. Actions of the D1 agonists A-77636 and A-86929 on locomotion and dyskinesia in MPTP-treated L-dopa-primed common marmosets. Psychopharmacology (Berl) 1999;142:51-60.
[46] Pearce RK, Jackson M, Smith L, Jenner P, Marsden CD. Chronic L-DOPA administration induces dyskinesias in the 1-methyl-4- phenyl-1,2,3,6-tetrahydropyridine-treated common marmoset (Callithrix Jacchus). Mov Disord 1995;10:731-740.
[47] Galvan A, Villalba RM, West SM, et al. GABAergic modulation of the activity of globus pallidus neurons in primates: in vivo analysis of the functions of GABA receptors and GABA transporters. J Neurophysiol 2005;94:990-1000.
[48] Yamada H, Fujimoto K, Yoshida M. Neuronal mechanism underlying dystonia induced by bicuculline injection into the putamen of the cat. Brain Res 1995;677:333-336.
[49] Worbe Y, Baup N, Grabli D, et al. Behavioral and movement disorders induced by local inhibitory dysfunction in primate striatum. Cereb Cortex 2009;19:1844-1856.
[50] Darbin O, Wichmann T. Effects of striatal GABA A-receptor blockade on striatal and cortical activity in monkeys. J Neurophysiol 2008;99:1294-1305.
[51] Worbe Y, Epinat J, Feger J, Tremblay L. Discontinuous Long-Train Stimulation in the Anterior Striatum in Monkeys Induces Abnormal Behavioral States. Cereb Cortex 2011.
[52] Lehericy S, Grand S, Pollak P, et al. Clinical characteristics and topography of lesions in movement disorders due to thalamic lesions. Neurology 2001;57:1055-1066.
[53] Lehericy S, Vidailhet M, Dormont D, et al. Striatopallidal and thalamic dystonia. A magnetic resonance imaging anatomoclinical study. Arch Neurol 1996;53:241-250.
[54] Hoover JE, Strick PL. The organization of cerebellar and basal ganglia outputs to primary motor cortex as revealed by retrograde transneuronal transport of herpes simplex virus type 1. J Neurosci 1999;19:1446-1463.
[55] Matelli M, Luppino G. Thalamic input to mesial and superior area 6 in the macaque monkey. J Comp Neurol 1996;372:59-87.
[56] Steriade M. Impact of network activities on neuronal properties in corticothalamic systems. J Neurophysiol 2001;86:1-39.
[57] Guehl D, Burbaud P, Boraud T, Bioulac B. Bicuculline injections into the rostral and caudal motor thalamus of the monkey induce different types of dystonia. Eur J Neurosci 2000;12:1033-1037.

[58] Macia F, Escola L, Guehl D, Michelet T, Bioulac B, Burbaud P. Neuronal activity in the monkey motor thalamus during bicuculline-induced dystonia. Eur J Neurosci 2002;15:1353-1362.
[59] Berardelli A, Rothwell JC, Hallett M, Thompson PD, Manfredi M, Marsden CD. The pathophysiology of primary dystonia. Brain 1998;121 (Pt 7):1195-1212.
[60] Byl NN. What can we learn from animal models of focal hand dystonia? Rev Neurol (Paris) 2003;159:857-873.
[61] Byl NN, Merzenich MM, Cheung S, Bedenbaugh P, Nagarajan SS, Jenkins WM. A primate model for studying focal dystonia and repetitive strain injury: effects on the primary somatosensory cortex. Phys Ther 1997;77:269-284.
[62] Topp KS, Byl NN. Movement dysfunction following repetitive hand opening and closing: anatomical analysis in Owl monkeys. Mov Disord 1999;14:295-306.
[63] Blake DT, Strata F, Churchland AK, Merzenich MM. Neural correlates of instrumental learning in primary auditory cortex. Proc Natl Acad Sci U S A 2002;99:10114-10119.
[64] Sharma N, Baxter MG, Petravicz J, et al. Impaired motor learning in mice expressing torsinA with the DYT1 dystonia mutation. J Neurosci 2005;25:5351-5355.
[65] Shashidharan P, Sandu D, Potla U, et al. Transgenic mouse model of early-onset DYT1 dystonia. Hum Mol Genet 2005;14:125-133.
[66] Dang MT, Yokoi F, McNaught KS, et al. Generation and characterization of Dyt1 DeltaGAG knock-in mouse as a model for early-onset dystonia. Exp Neurol 2005;196:452-463.
[67] Goodchild RE, Kim CE, Dauer WT. Loss of the dystonia-associated protein torsinA selectively disrupts the neuronal nuclear envelope. Neuron 2005;48:923-932.
[68] Pisani A, Martella G, Tscherter A, et al. Altered responses to dopaminergic D2 receptor activation and N-type calcium currents in striatal cholinergic interneurons in a mouse model of DYT1 dystonia. Neurobiol Dis 2006;24:318-325.
[69] Sato K, Sumi-Ichinose C, Kaji R, et al. Differential involvement of striosome and matrix dopamine systems in a transgenic model of dopa-responsive dystonia. Proc Natl Acad Sci U S A 2008;105:12551-12556.
[70] Balcioglu A, Kim MO, Sharma N, Cha JH, Breakefield XO, Standaert DG. Dopamine release is impaired in a mouse model of DYT1 dystonia. J Neurochem 2007;102:783-788.
[71] Lorden JF, McKeon TW, Baker HJ, Cox N, Walkley SU. Characterization of the rat mutant dystonic (dt): a new animal model of dystonia musculorum deformans. J Neurosci 1984;4:1925-1932.
[72] Xiao J, Ledoux MS. Caytaxin deficiency causes generalized dystonia in rats. Brain Res Mol Brain Res 2005;141:181-192.
[73] Young KG, De Repentigny Y, Kothary R. Re: "A possible cellular mechanism of neuronal loss in the dorsal root ganglia of dystonia musculorum (dt) mice". J Neuropathol Exp Neurol 2007;66:248-249; author reply 249.
[74] Campbell RM, Peterson AC. An intrinsic neuronal defect operates in dystonia musculorum: a study of dt/dt<==>+/+ chimeras. Neuron 1992;9:693-703.
[75] Pizoli CE, Jinnah HA, Billingsley ML, Hess EJ. Abnormal cerebellar signaling induces dystonia in mice. J Neurosci 2002;22:7825-7833.
[76] Fernagut PO, Diguet E, Stefanova N, et al. Subacute systemic 3-nitropropionic acid intoxication induces a distinct motor disorder in adult C57Bl/6 mice: behavioural and histopathological characterisation. Neuroscience 2002;114:1005-1017.

[77] Xiao J, Zhao Y, Bastian RW, et al. The c.-237_236GA>TT THAP1 sequence variant does not increase risk for primary dystonia. Mov Disord 2011;26:549-552.

[78] Richter A, Loscher W. Pathology of idiopathic dystonia: findings from genetic animal models. Prog Neurobiol 1998;54:633-677.

[79] Richter A, Loscher W. Animal models of paroxysmal dystonia. Adv Neurol 2002;89:443-451.

[80] Sander SE, Richter A. Effects of intrastriatal injections of glutamate receptor antagonists on the severity of paroxysmal dystonia in the dtsz mutant. Eur J Pharmacol 2007;563:102-108.

[81] Kohling R, Koch UR, Hamann M, Richter A. Increased excitability in cortico-striatal synaptic pathway in a model of paroxysmal dystonia. Neurobiol Dis 2004;16:236-245.

[82] Neychev VK, Fan X, Mitev VI, Hess EJ, Jinnah HA. The basal ganglia and cerebellum interact in the expression of dystonic movement. Brain 2008;131:2499-2509.

[83] Evinger C. Animal models of focal dystonia. NeuroRx 2005;2:513-524.

[84] Evinger C, Bao JB, Powers AS, et al. Dry eye, blinking, and blepharospasm. Mov Disord 2002;17 Suppl 2:S75-78.

[85] Basso MA, Evinger C. An explanation for reflex blink hyperexcitability in Parkinson's disease. II. Nucleus raphe magnus. J Neurosci 1996;16:7318-7330.

[86] Basso MA, Powers AS, Evinger C. An explanation for reflex blink hyperexcitability in Parkinson's disease. I. Superior colliculus. J Neurosci 1996;16:7308-7317.

[87] Schicatano EJ, Basso MA, Evinger C. Animal model explains the origins of the cranial dystonia benign essential blepharospasm. J Neurophysiol 1997;77:2842-2846.

[88] Obeso JA, Rothwell JC, Lang AE, Marsden CD. Myoclonic dystonia. Neurology 1983;33:825-830.

[89] Sohn YH, Voller B, Dimyan M, et al. Cortical control of voluntary blinking: a transcranial magnetic stimulation study. Clin Neurophysiol 2004;115:341-347.

[90] Quartarone A, Morgante F, Sant'angelo A, et al. Abnormal plasticity of sensorimotor circuits extends beyond the affected body part in focal dystonia. J Neurol Neurosurg Psychiatry 2008;79:985-990.

[91] Quartarone A, Rizzo V, Terranova C, et al. Abnormal sensorimotor plasticity in organic but not in psychogenic dystonia. Brain 2009;132:2871-2877.

[92] Koch G, Schneider S, Baumer T, et al. Altered dorsal premotor-motor interhemispheric pathway activity in focal arm dystonia. Mov Disord 2008;23:660-668.

[93] Ugawa Y. [Electromyographic analysis of cortical myoclonus and focal dystonia]. Rinsho Shinkeigaku 1995;35:1387-1389.

[94] Bara-Jimenez W, Catalan MJ, Hallett M, Gerloff C. Abnormal somatosensory homunculus in dystonia of the hand. Ann Neurol 1998;44:828-831.

[95] Sanger TD, Pascual-Leone A, Tarsy D, Schlaug G. Nonlinear sensory cortex response to simultaneous tactile stimuli in writer's cramp. Mov Disord 2002;17:105-111.

[96] Sanger TD, Tarsy D, Pascual-Leone A. Abnormalities of spatial and temporal sensory discrimination in writer's cramp. Mov Disord 2001;16:94-99.

[97] Serrien DJ, Burgunder JM, Wiesendanger M. Disturbed sensorimotor processing during control of precision grip in patients with writer's cramp. Mov Disord 2000;15:965-972.

[98] Bara-Jimenez W, Shelton P, Sanger TD, Hallett M. Sensory discrimination capabilities in patients with focal hand dystonia. Ann Neurol 2000;47:377-380.

[99] Fiorio M, Tinazzi M, Bertolasi L, Aglioti SM. Temporal processing of visuotactile and tactile stimuli in writer's cramp. Ann Neurol 2003;53:630-635.
[100] Tinazzi M, Fiaschi A, Frasson E, Fiorio M, Cortese F, Aglioti SM. Deficits of temporal discrimination in dystonia are independent from the spatial distance between the loci of tactile stimulation. Mov Disord 2002;17:333-338.
[101] Frima N, Nasir J, Grunewald RA. Abnormal vibration-induced illusion of movement in idiopathic focal dystonia: an endophenotypic marker? Mov Disord 2008;23:373-377.
[102] Grunewald RA, Yoneda Y, Shipman JM, Sagar HJ. Idiopathic focal dystonia: a disorder of muscle spindle afferent processing? Brain 1997;120 (Pt 12):2179-2185.
[103] Putzki N, Stude P, Konczak J, Graf K, Diener HC, Maschke M. Kinesthesia is impaired in focal dystonia. Mov Disord 2006;21:754-760.
[104] Meunier S, Garnero L, Ducorps A, et al. Human brain mapping in dystonia reveals both endophenotypic traits and adaptive reorganization. Ann Neurol 2001;50:521-527.
[105] Meunier S, Hallett M. Endophenotyping: a window to the pathophysiology of dystonia. Neurology 2005;65:792-793.
[106] Butterworth S, Francis S, Kelly E, McGlone F, Bowtell R, Sawle GV. Abnormal cortical sensory activation in dystonia: an fMRI study. Mov Disord 2003;18:673-682.
[107] Nelson AJ, Blake DT, Chen R. Digit-specific aberrations in the primary somatosensory cortex in Writer's cramp. Ann Neurol 2009;66:146-154.
[108] Peller M, Zeuner KE, Munchau A, et al. The basal ganglia are hyperactive during the discrimination of tactile stimuli in writer's cramp. Brain 2006;129:2697-2708.
[109] Frasson E, Priori A, Bertolasi L, Mauguiere F, Fiaschi A, Tinazzi M. Somatosensory disinhibition in dystonia. Mov Disord 2001;16:674-682.
[110] Tamura Y, Matsuhashi M, Lin P, et al. Impaired intracortical inhibition in the primary somatosensory cortex in focal hand dystonia. Mov Disord 2008;23:558-565.
[111] Tinazzi M, Priori A, Bertolasi L, Frasson E, Mauguiere F, Fiaschi A. Abnormal central integration of a dual somatosensory input in dystonia. Evidence for sensory overflow. Brain 2000;123 (Pt 1):42-50.
[112] Chen CC, Kuhn AA, Trottenberg T, Kupsch A, Schneider GH, Brown P. Neuronal activity in globus pallidus interna can be synchronized to local field potential activity over 3-12 Hz in patients with dystonia. Exp Neurol 2006;202:480-486.
[113] Liu X, Yianni J, Wang S, Bain PG, Stein JF, Aziz TZ. Different mechanisms may generate sustained hypertonic and rhythmic bursting muscle activity in idiopathic dystonia. Exp Neurol 2006;198:204-213.
[114] Sharott A, Grosse P, Kuhn AA, et al. Is the synchronization between pallidal and muscle activity in primary dystonia due to peripheral afferance or a motor drive? Brain 2008;131:473-484.
[115] Starr PA, Rau GM, Davis V, et al. Spontaneous pallidal neuronal activity in human dystonia: comparison with Parkinson's disease and normal macaque. J Neurophysiol 2005;93:3165-3176.
[116] Tang JK, Moro E, Mahant N, et al. Neuronal firing rates and patterns in the globus pallidus internus of patients with cervical dystonia differ from those with Parkinson's disease. J Neurophysiol 2007;98:720-729.
[117] Schrock LE, Ostrem JL, Turner RS, Shimamoto SA, Starr PA. The subthalamic nucleus in primary dystonia: single-unit discharge characteristics. J Neurophysiol 2009;102:3740-3752.

[118] Hashimoto T. Neuronal activity in the globus pallidus in primary dystonia and off-period dystonia. J Neurol 2000;247 Suppl 5:V49-52.
[119] Merello M, Cerquetti D, Cammarota A, et al. Neuronal globus pallidus activity in patients with generalised dystonia. Mov Disord 2004;19:548-554.
[120] Pralong E, Debatisse D, Maeder M, Vingerhoets F, Ghika J, Villemure JG. Effect of deep brain stimulation of GPI on neuronal activity of the thalamic nucleus ventralis oralis in a dystonic patient. Neurophysiol Clin 2003;33:169-173.
[121] Foncke EM, Bour LJ, van der Meer JN, Koelman JH, Tijssen MA. Abnormal low frequency drive in myoclonus-dystonia patients correlates with presence of dystonia. Mov Disord 2007;22:1299-1307.
[122] Tang JK, Mahant N, Cunic D, et al. Changes in cortical and pallidal oscillatory activity during the execution of a sensory trick in patients with cervical dystonia. Exp Neurol 2007;204:845-848.
[123] Zhuang P, Li Y, Hallett M. Neuronal activity in the basal ganglia and thalamus in patients with dystonia. Clin Neurophysiol 2004;115:2542-2557.
[124] Lenz FA, Suarez JI, Metman LV, et al. Pallidal activity during dystonia: somatosensory reorganisation and changes with severity. J Neurol Neurosurg Psychiatry 1998;65:767-770.
[125] Zirh TA, Reich SG, Perry V, Lenz FA. Thalamic single neuron and electromyographic activities in patients with dystonia. Adv Neurol 1998;78:27-32.
[126] Silberstein P, Kuhn AA, Kupsch A, et al. Patterning of globus pallidus local field potentials differs between Parkinson's disease and dystonia. Brain 2003;126:2597-2608.
[127] Chen CC, Kuhn AA, Hoffmann KT, et al. Oscillatory pallidal local field potential activity correlates with involuntary EMG in dystonia. Neurology 2006;66:418-420.
[128] Foncke EM, Bour LJ, Speelman JD, Koelman JH, Tijssen MA. Local field potentials and oscillatory activity of the internal globus pallidus in myoclonus-dystonia. Mov Disord 2007;22:369-376.
[129] Eusebio A, Brown P. Oscillatory activity in the basal ganglia. Parkinsonism Relat Disord 2007;13 Suppl 3:S434-436.
[130] Rutledge JN, Hilal SK, Silver AJ, Defendini R, Fahn S. Magnetic resonance imaging of dystonic states. Adv Neurol 1988;50:265-275.
[131] Black KJ, Ongur D, Perlmutter JS. Putamen volume in idiopathic focal dystonia. Neurology 1998;51:819-824.
[132] Garraux G, Bauer A, Hanakawa T, Wu T, Kansaku K, Hallett M. Changes in brain anatomy in focal hand dystonia. Ann Neurol 2004;55:736-739.
[133] Etgen T, Muhlau M, Gaser C, Sander D. Bilateral grey-matter increase in the putamen in primary blepharospasm. J Neurol Neurosurg Psychiatry 2006;77:1017-1020.
[134] Egger K, Mueller J, Schocke M, et al. Voxel based morphometry reveals specific gray matter changes in primary dystonia. Mov Disord 2007;22:1538-1542.
[135] Obermann M, Yaldizli O, De Greiff A, et al. Morphometric changes of sensorimotor structures in focal dystonia. Mov Disord 2007;22:1117-1123.
[136] Draganski B, Thun-Hohenstein C, Bogdahn U, Winkler J, May A. "Motor circuit" gray matter changes in idiopathic cervical dystonia. Neurology 2003;61:1228-1231.
[137] Delmaire C, Vidailhet M, Elbaz A, et al. Structural abnormalities in the cerebellum and sensorimotor circuit in writer's cramp. Neurology 2007;69:376-380.
[138] Bonilha L, de Vries PM, Vincent DJ, et al. Structural white matter abnormalities in patients with idiopathic dystonia. Mov Disord 2007;22:1110-1116.

[139] Carbon M, Kingsley PB, Su S, et al. Microstructural white matter changes in carriers of the DYT1 gene mutation. Ann Neurol 2004;56:283-286.
[140] Carbon M, Kingsley PB, Tang C, Bressman S, Eidelberg D. Microstructural white matter changes in primary torsion dystonia. Mov Disord 2008;23:234-239.
[141] Colosimo C, Pantano P, Calistri V, Totaro P, Fabbrini G, Berardelli A. Diffusion tensor imaging in primary cervical dystonia. J Neurol Neurosurg Psychiatry 2005;76:1591-1593.
[142] Fabbrini G, Pantano P, Totaro P, et al. Diffusion tensor imaging in patients with primary cervical dystonia and in patients with blepharospasm. Eur J Neurol 2008;15:185-189.
[143] Delmaire C, Vidailhet M, Wassermann D, et al. Diffusion abnormalities in the primary sensorimotor pathways in writer's cramp. Arch Neurol 2009;66:502-508.
[144] Argyelan M, Carbon M, Niethammer M, et al. Cerebellothalamocortical connectivity regulates penetrance in dystonia. J Neurosci 2009;29:9740-9747.
[145] Ceballos-Baumann AO, Passingham RE, Warner T, Playford ED, Marsden CD, Brooks DJ. Overactive prefrontal and underactive motor cortical areas in idiopathic dystonia. Ann Neurol 1995;37:363-372.
[146] Eidelberg D, Moeller JR, Ishikawa T, et al. The metabolic topography of idiopathic torsion dystonia. Brain 1995;118 (Pt 6):1473-1484.
[147] Playford ED, Passingham RE, Marsden CD, Brooks DJ. Increased activation of frontal areas during arm movement in idiopathic torsion dystonia. Mov Disord 1998;13:309-318.
[148] Ceballos-Baumann AO, Brooks DJ. Activation positron emission tomography scanning in dystonia. Adv Neurol 1998;78:135-152.
[149] Eidelberg D. Functional brain networks in movement disorders. Curr Opin Neurol 1998;11:319-326.
[150] Tempel LW, Perlmutter JS. Abnormal vibration-induced cerebral blood flow responses in idiopathic dystonia. Brain 1990;113 (Pt 3):691-707.
[151] Feiwell RJ, Black KJ, McGee-Minnich LA, Snyder AZ, MacLeod AM, Perlmutter JS. Diminished regional cerebral blood flow response to vibration in patients with blepharospasm. Neurology 1999;52:291-297.
[152] Naumann M, Magyar-Lehmann S, Reiners K, Erbguth F, Leenders KL. Sensory tricks in cervical dystonia: perceptual dysbalance of parietal cortex modulates frontal motor programming. Ann Neurol 2000;47:322-328.
[153] Carbon M, Ghilardi MF, Argyelan M, Dhawan V, Bressman SB, Eidelberg D. Increased cerebellar activation during sequence learning in DYT1 carriers: an equiperformance study. Brain 2008;131:146-154.
[154] Carbon M, Su S, Dhawan V, Raymond D, Bressman S, Eidelberg D. Regional metabolism in primary torsion dystonia: effects of penetrance and genotype. Neurology 2004;62:1384-1390.
[155] Levy LM, Hallett M. Impaired brain GABA in focal dystonia. Ann Neurol 2002;51:93-101.
[156] Asanuma K, Ma Y, Okulski J, et al. Decreased striatal D2 receptor binding in non-manifesting carriers of the DYT1 dystonia mutation. Neurology 2005;64:347-349.
[157] Beukers RJ, Booij J, Weisscher N, Zijlstra F, van Amelsvoort TA, Tijssen MA. Reduced striatal D2 receptor binding in myoclonus-dystonia. Eur J Nucl Med Mol Imaging 2009;36:269-274.

[158] Carbon M, Argyelan M, Eidelberg D. Functional imaging in hereditary dystonia. Eur J Neurol 2010;17 Suppl 1:58-64.
[159] Karimi M, Moerlein SM, Videen TO, et al. Decreased striatal dopamine receptor binding in primary focal dystonia: A D2 or D3 defect? Mov Disord 2010.
[160] Kishore A, Nygaard TG, de la Fuente-Fernandez R, et al. Striatal D2 receptors in symptomatic and asymptomatic carriers of dopa-responsive dystonia measured with [11C]-raclopride and positron-emission tomography. Neurology 1998;50:1028-1032.
[161] Carbon M, Niethammer M, Peng S, et al. Abnormal striatal and thalamic dopamine neurotransmission: Genotype-related features of dystonia. Neurology 2009;72:2097-2103.
[162] Carbon M, Argyelan M, Ghilardi MF, et al. Impaired sequence learning in dystonia mutation carriers: a genotypic effect. Brain 2011;134:1416-1427.
[163] Carbon M, Eidelberg D. Abnormal structure-function relationships in hereditary dystonia. Neuroscience 2009;164:220-229.
[164] Carbon M, Trost M, Ghilardi MF, Eidelberg D. Abnormal brain networks in primary torsion dystonia. Adv Neurol 2004;94:155-161.
[165] Dresel C, Haslinger B, Castrop F, Wohlschlaeger AM, Ceballos-Baumann AO. Silent event-related fMRI reveals deficient motor and enhanced somatosensory activation in orofacial dystonia. Brain 2006;129:36-46.
[166] Haslinger B, Erhard P, Dresel C, Castrop F, Roettinger M, Ceballos-Baumann AO. "Silent event-related" fMRI reveals reduced sensorimotor activation in laryngeal dystonia. Neurology 2005;65:1562-1569.
[167] Simonyan K, Ludlow CL. Abnormal activation of the primary somatosensory cortex in spasmodic dysphonia: an FMRI study. Cereb Cortex 2010;20:2749-2759.
[168] Oga T, Honda M, Toma K, et al. Abnormal cortical mechanisms of voluntary muscle relaxation in patients with writer's cramp: an fMRI study. Brain 2002;125:895-903.
[169] Hu XY, Wang L, Liu H, Zhang SZ. Functional magnetic resonance imaging study of writer's cramp. Chin Med J (Engl) 2006;119:1263-1271.
[170] Pujol J, Roset-Llobet J, Rosines-Cubells D, et al. Brain cortical activation during guitar-induced hand dystonia studied by functional MRI. Neuroimage 2000;12:257-267.
[171] Delmaire C, Krainik A, Tezenas du Montcel S, et al. Disorganized somatotopy in the putamen of patients with focal hand dystonia. Neurology 2005;64:1391-1396.
[172] Quartarone A, Bagnato S, Rizzo V, et al. Abnormal associative plasticity of the human motor cortex in writer's cramp. Brain 2003;126:2586-2596.
[173] Quartarone A, Sant'Angelo A, Battaglia F, et al. Enhanced long-term potentiation-like plasticity of the trigeminal blink reflex circuit in blepharospasm. J Neurosci 2006;26:716-721.
[174] Rothwell JC, Huang YZ. Systems-level studies of movement disorders in dystonia and Parkinson's disease. Curr Opin Neurobiol 2003;13:691-695.
[175] Scott BL, Jankovic J. Delayed-onset progressive movement disorders after static brain lesions. Neurology 1996;46:68-74.
[176] Vidailhet M, Vercueil L, Houeto JL, et al. Bilateral deep-brain stimulation of the globus pallidus in primary generalized dystonia. N Engl J Med 2005;352:459-467.
[177] Vidailhet M, Vercueil L, Houeto JL, et al. Bilateral, pallidal, deep-brain stimulation in primary generalised dystonia: a prospective 3 year follow-up study. Lancet Neurol 2007;6:223-229.

[178] Quartarone A, Classen J, Morgante F, Rosenkranz K, Hallett M. Consensus paper: use of transcranial magnetic stimulation to probe motor cortex plasticity in dystonia and levodopa-induced dyskinesia. Brain Stimul 2009;2:108-117.

[179] Quartarone A, Rizzo V, Bagnato S, et al. Homeostatic-like plasticity of the primary motor hand area is impaired in focal hand dystonia. Brain 2005;128:1943-1950.

[180] Stefan K, Kunesch E, Cohen LG, Benecke R, Classen J. Induction of plasticity in the human motor cortex by paired associative stimulation. Brain 2000;123 Pt 3:572-584.

[181] Quartarone A, Siebner HR, Rothwell JC. Task-specific hand dystonia: can too much plasticity be bad for you? Trends Neurosci 2006;29:192-199.

[182] Tamura Y, Ueki Y, Lin P, et al. Disordered plasticity in the primary somatosensory cortex in focal hand dystonia. Brain 2009;132:749-755.

[183] Weise D, Schramm A, Beck M, Reiners K, Classen J. Loss of topographic specificity of LTD-like plasticity is a trait marker in focal dystonia. Neurobiol Dis 2011;42:171-176.

[184] Weise D, Schramm A, Stefan K, et al. The two sides of associative plasticity in writer's cramp. Brain 2006;129:2709-2721.

[185] Edwards MJ, Huang YZ, Mir P, Rothwell JC, Bhatia KP. Abnormalities in motor cortical plasticity differentiate manifesting and nonmanifesting DYT1 carriers. Mov Disord 2006;21:2181-2186.

[186] Magarinos-Ascone CM, Figueiras-Mendez R, Riva-Meana C, Cordoba-Fernandez A. Subthalamic neuron activity related to tremor and movement in Parkinson's disease. Eur J Neurosci 2000;12:2597-2607.

[187] Magarinos-Ascone CM, Regidor I, Gomez-Galan M, Cabanes-Martinez L, Figueiras-Mendez R. Deep brain stimulation in the globus pallidus to treat dystonia: electrophysiological characteristics and 2 years' follow-up in 10 patients. Neuroscience 2008;152:558-571.

[188] Bhatia KP, Marsden CD. The behavioural and motor consequences of focal lesions of the basal ganglia in man. Brain 1994;117 (Pt 4):859-876.

[189] Mink JW. The basal ganglia: focused selection and inhibition of competing motor programs. Prog Neurobiol 1996;50:381-425.

[190] Bonsi P, Martella G, Cuomo D, et al. Loss of muscarinic autoreceptor function impairs long-term depression but not long-term potentiation in the striatum. J Neurosci 2008;28:6258-6263.

[191] Martella G, Tassone A, Sciamanna G, et al. Impairment of bidirectional synaptic plasticity in the striatum of a mouse model of DYT1 dystonia: role of endogenous acetylcholine. Brain 2009;132:2336-2349.

[192] Gernert M, Hamann M, Bennay M, Loscher W, Richter A. Deficit of striatal parvalbumin-reactive GABAergic interneurons and decreased basal ganglia output in a genetic rodent model of idiopathic paroxysmal dystonia. J Neurosci 2000;20:7052-7058.

[193] Pisani A. Towards a new era for dystonia, a high priority for biomedical research. Neurobiol Dis 2011;42:125-126.